RELATE
Nottinghamshire Marriage Guidance
96 Mansfield Road
Nottingham NG1 3HD

THE NEW GUIDE TO SEXUAL FULFILMENT

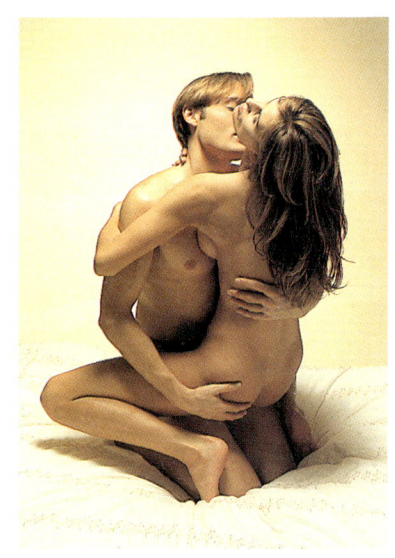

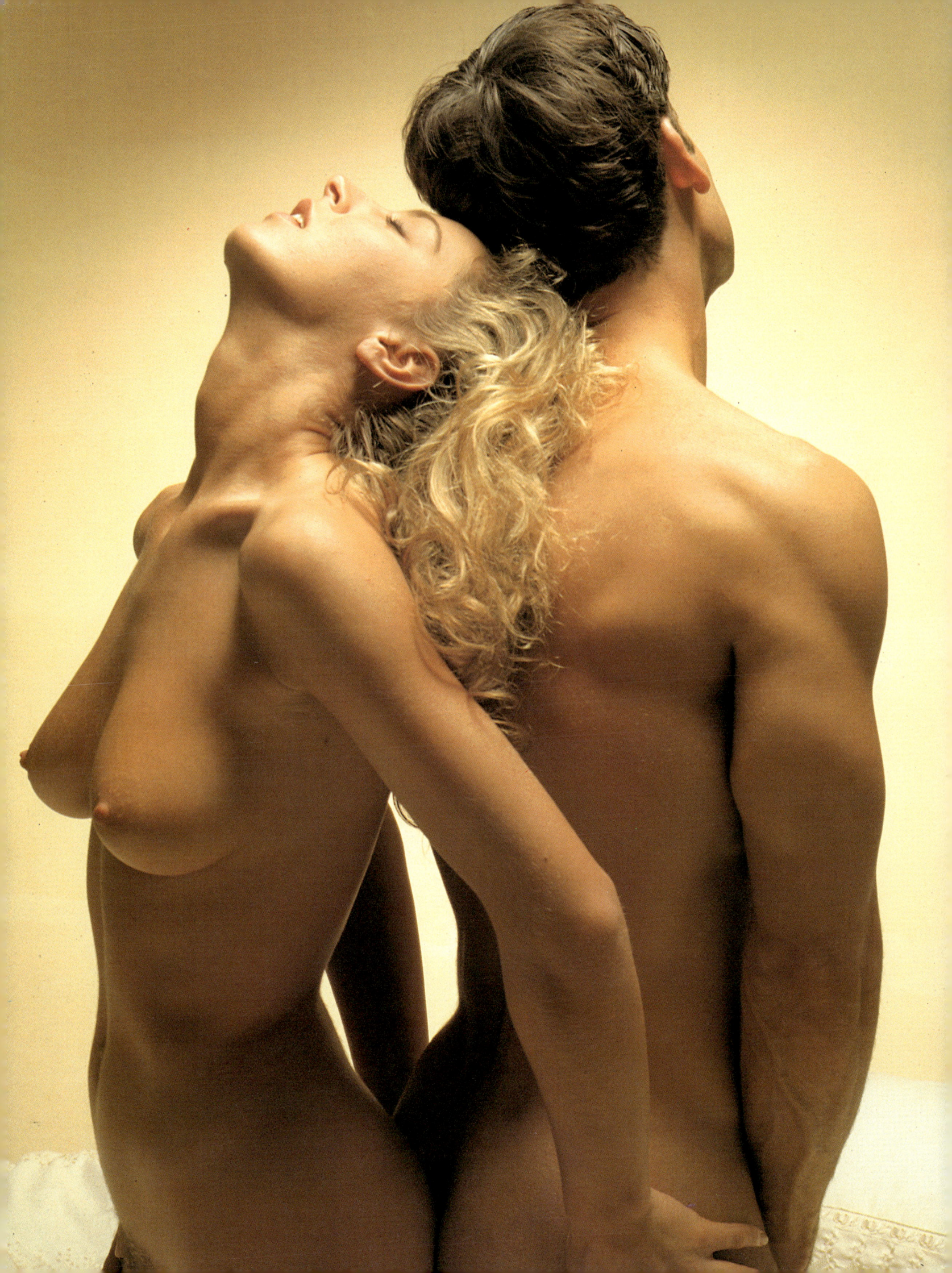

THE NEW GUIDE TO SEXUAL FULFILMENT

Nitya Lacroix

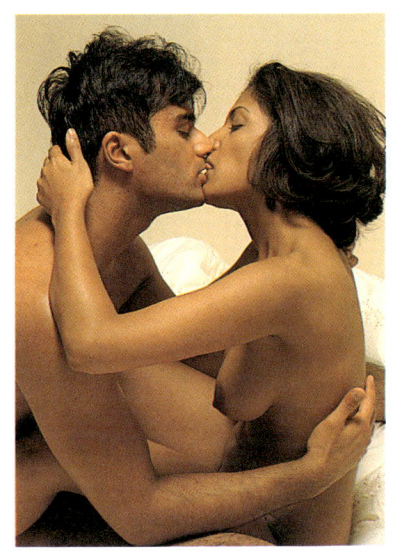

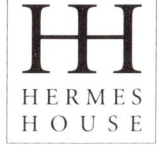

HERMES HOUSE

This edition published in 1998 by Hermes House

© Anness Publishing Limited 1996

Hermes House is an imprint of
Anness Publishing Limited
Hermes House, 88-89 Blackfriars Road, London SE1 8HA

All rights reserved. No part of this publication may be reproduced,
stored in a retrieval system, or transmitted in any way or by any means,
electronic, mechanical, photocopying, recording or otherwise, without
the prior written permission of the copyright holder.

ISBN 1 84038 113 2

A CIP catalogue record for this book
is available from the British Library

Publisher: Joanna Lorenz
Project editors: Casey Horton, Nicky Thompson
Design: Blackjacks
Special photography: Alistair Hughes
Hair and make-up: Bettina Graham

Previously published as part of a larger compendium,
Love, Sex & Intimacy

Printed and bound in Singapore

1 3 5 7 9 10 8 6 4 2

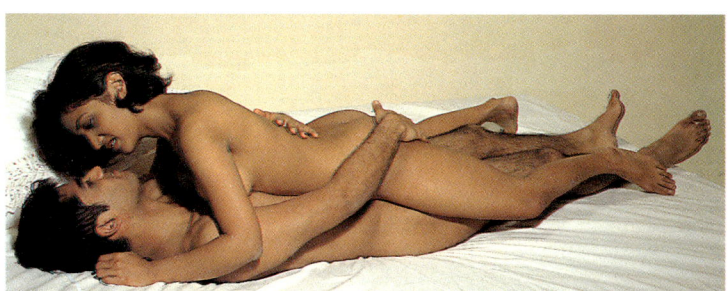

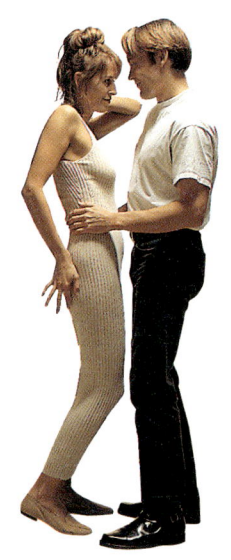
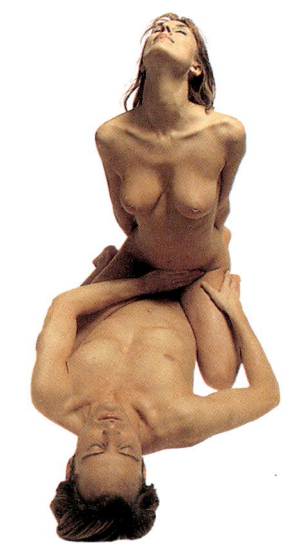

Contents

Safer Sex 6

Undressing Each Other 12

Sensual Play 16

Oral-Genital Sex 26

Compatibility 32

The Basic Positions 34

Expressing Our Sexuality 46

Orgasm 56

Adventurous Lovemaking 64

Masturbating Each Other 76

Sharing Sexual Fantasies 82

Getting Turned On 94

Spontaneous Sex 100

Overcoming Difficulties 106

Contraception 116

STDs / Sexually Transmitted Diseases 122

Index 126

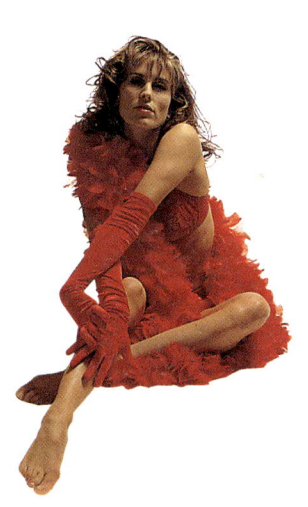

Safer Sex

Nowadays, the phrase "safer sex" is generally used wherever sexuality is written or spoken about. Safer sex practices help lovers to care for their own and each other's health while enjoying an exciting and joyful sex life. The term "safer sex" generally refers to all sexual activity which avoids the exchange of body fluids, such as semen, vaginal juices and blood, between partners. It is a way of modifying sexual practices to help prevent the risk of infection from the HIV virus and other sexually transmitted diseases (STDs). (See the section on Sexually Transmitted Diseases for information on HIV/AIDS and other STDs.) Safer sex practices apply to all members of the community, both homosexual and heterosexual.

Safer sex is essential to the art of love at the present time when the HIV/AIDS virus continues to spread through the world's heterosexual and homosexual population. HIV can remain in an otherwise healthy person for many years without causing symptoms, and any sexual acts that involve contact with the person's blood, semen or vaginal fluids can put lovers at potential risk of catching the disease.

Safer sex means taking adequate precautions against the exchange of these body fluids, and in abstaining from high-risk sexual activities which allow this to happen. For instance, the sensual and erotic massage programmes described in this book are examples of safer sex practices.

If you are making love with your partner in any way that involves penetrative sex, then you should consider using condoms. If used correctly, condoms reduce the risk of the spread of the HIV virus and other sexually transmitted diseases. Initially, you may feel that condoms inhibit the spontaneity of lovemaking, but by simply knowing they are the best method available of protecting yourself and your partner, you

Getting Attuned
▶ *Kissing, cuddling and hugging are safer sex practices through which new partners can discover if they are physically and sexually attuned.*

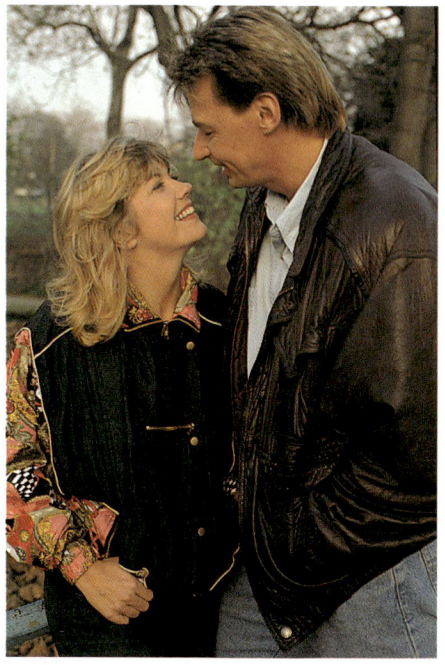

Return to Romance
◀ *Many men and women have longed for a return to old-fashioned courtship. As awareness grows around safer sex issues, romance is coming back into fashion. The wish to form monogamous relationships is popular again. Many couples now prefer to become better acquainted with each other before embarking on full sexual intimacy. Casual encounters or multiple sex partners are definitely not a good idea in terms of safer sex, and this provides an excellent excuse to modify sexual behaviour if you have previously allowed yourself to be pressured into casual sexual encounters.*

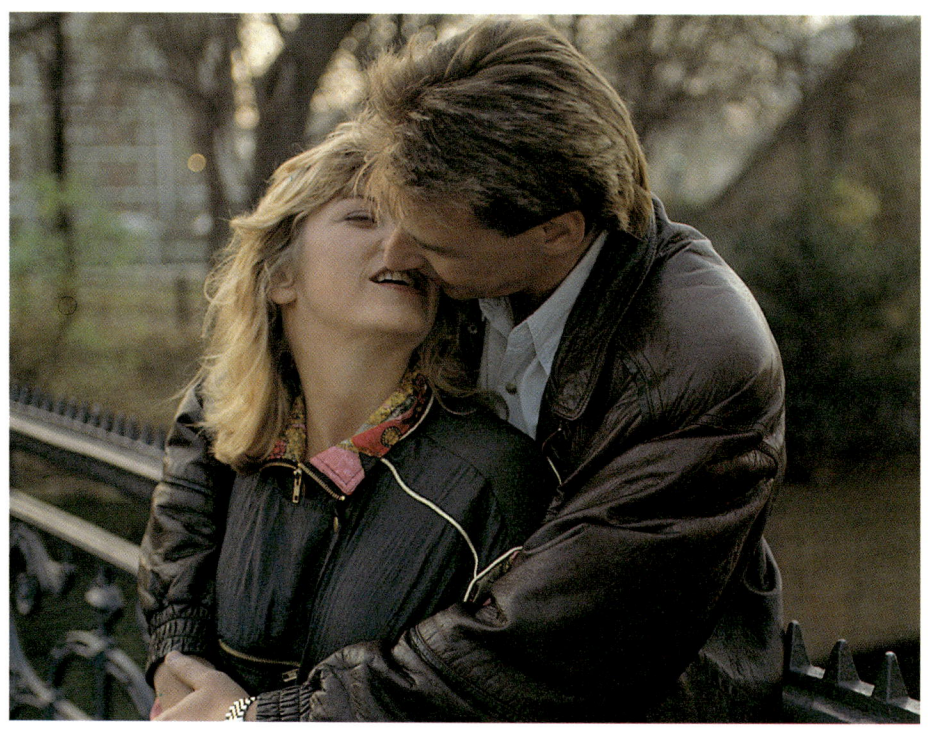

can begin to consider them as an integral part of the lovemaking. Safer sex, like massage, is a way of showing how much you care for the well-being of the body, mind and spirit of both yourself and your lover.

How To Discuss Safer Sex

Anyone who is contemplating a sexual relationship, or who is already involved in one, should consider safer sex. However, since sexual issues are invariably difficult to discuss, you may find it embarrassing to raise the subject of safer sex practices or to reach an agreement about it with a new partner.

The best way forward is to develop a clear and responsible attitude towards your own health and sexual practices, rather than relying on anyone else's responses. This clarity will enable you to stand firm on your decisions, and may also help your partner to resolve his or her own conflicts.

Adopt a clear but sensitive approach. You can affirm your attraction to your partner and add something like, "I would love to make love with you, but first I need to tell you that I always follow safer sex practices," and then outline what this means to you. Explain that, to you, safer sex is a way of showing a caring attitude.

If you meet a negative response, be patient but firm. Your partner may believe, mistakenly, that safer sex practices are relevant only to people who belong to high-risk groups. He or she may insist that they have had only a few sexual partners and, therefore, present no risk. The truth is, it is often impossible to know the sexual history of all the other people who have been linked in a sexual chain of partners.

For instance, a previous lover may have had a relationship with someone who, at another time, had sex, unknowingly, with a person from an HIV high-risk group. Making love only once with someone who carries the HIV virus can present sufficient risk of becoming infected yourself. People can be HIV infected without knowing it and remain in good health for a very long period of time, showing no outward sign of the infection. Also, there are other sexually transmitted diseases which need to be considered.

Some women, in particular, find it difficult to assert themselves over sexual issues. Old attitudes persist despite the dramatic changes in sexual mores and gender roles over the last few decades. Women are still generally more conditioned than men to please others, and often feel shy to take the initiative on safer sex issues, particularly if there is resistance.

As a woman, you may be worried that you will be deemed too sexually forward if you produce a packet of condoms at the opportune moment. Remind yourself that you have as much right to self determination over your sexual health as you would, nowadays, expect to have over your choices of contraception. If you are a sexually active woman, there is absolutely nothing wrong with your having a supply of condoms, or other barrier methods which protect you against sexually transmitted diseases, or with your decision to use them during lovemaking.

At the end of the day, however, both men and women have to make the decision for themselves on

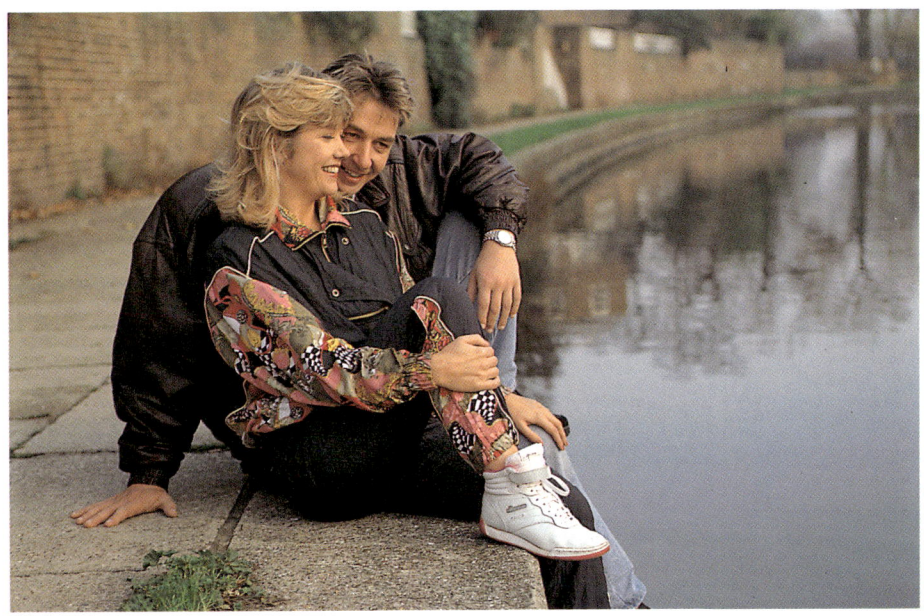

Find Time to Talk
▲ *Try to discuss safer sex issues at the point when you realize the relationship is going to become sexual, rather than leaving it to the last moment when passion and feelings are running high. Also, giving yourselves time to know each other better allows you to build up trust, discuss your past sexual histories honestly with each other, and to decide if you are ready to make this commitment.*

Basic Techniques

Caress with Confidence
▶ Close physical contact which does not involve the exchange of body fluids is perfectly safe. You can caress and explore each other's bodies with peace of mind.

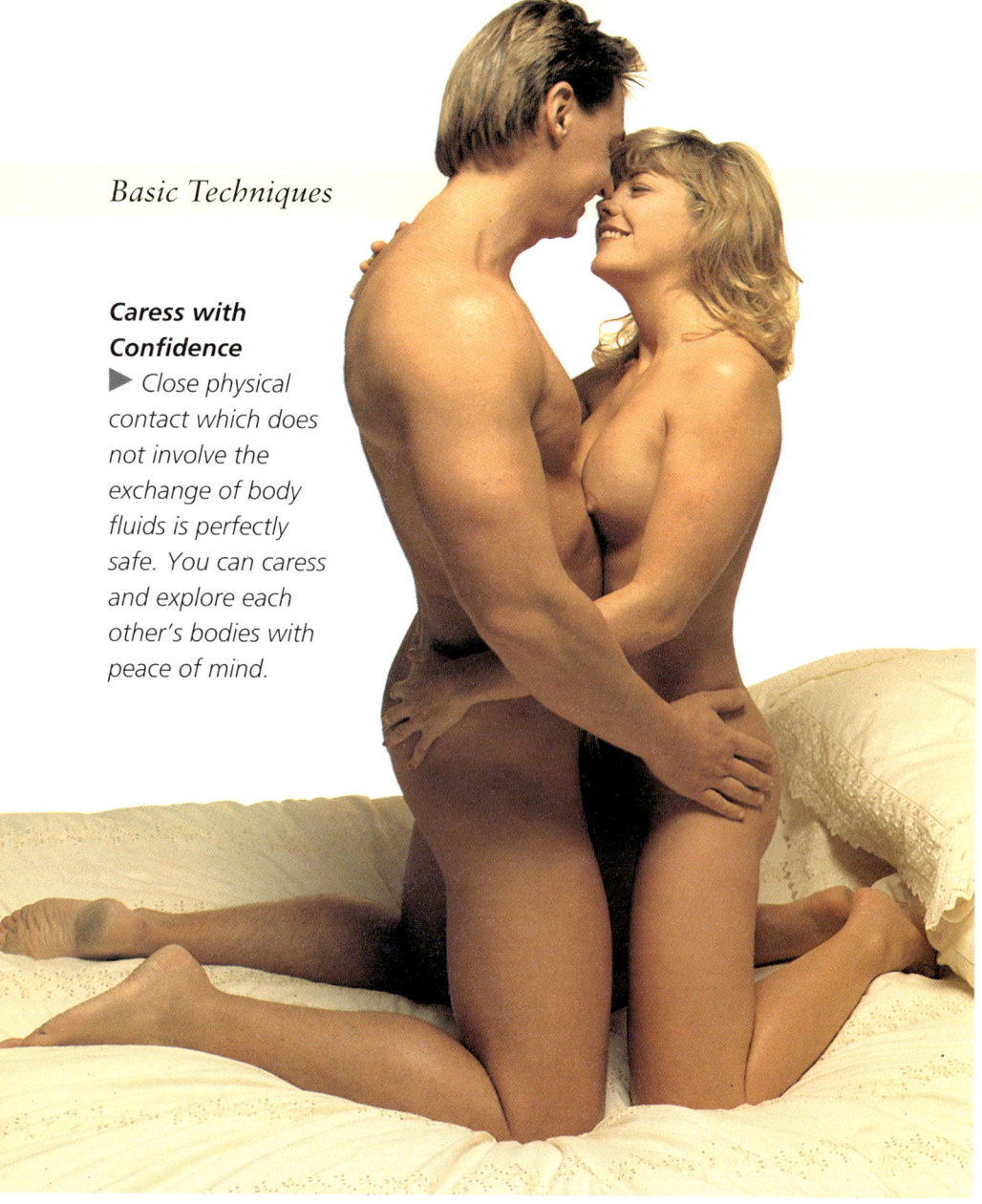

whether or not to use safer sex practices. This decision should be based, partly, on your own sense of self-worth and value for your health.

The bottom line is: if you want to use safer sex methods and your potential lover refuses, for whatever reason, you will need to delay any sexual activity involving the exchange of body fluids until you have reached a mutual agreement; or even be prepared to forgo a full sexual relationship with that person.

Long-Term Relationships

If you are already in an established relationship, you may believe that you do not need to consider safer sex issues. This is so only if the relationship is truly monogamous and you are both absolutely sure of the safety of each other's sexual and drug-related past. For the various reasons mentioned before, it is virtually impossible to know the whole truth because you can rarely vouch for the sexual history of all previous partners who have been linked by sexual activity. As a couple, you should examine and discuss all the implications involved before making a decision on whether or not to start or abandon safer sex practices.

The HIV Test

The HIV antibody can take up to three months to develop and be detected in a blood test after the virus has been transmitted. HIV testing is one possibility for couples who are willing to commit and be monogamous with each other and want a sexual relationship without using safer sex practices. There are, however, quite contrasting professional views as to whether this is an advisable or necessary step to take.

In any event, it is not a decision to be taken lightly, and all people testing for HIV should first receive proper counselling as to its advisability in their particular situation. This help can usually be obtained from health specialists attached to the STD clinics or specialized hospital departments. The decision to test for HIV must always be an individual one, and no one should allow themselves to be coerced into taking it.

Risky Behaviour

While considering safer sex issues, it is important not to become over anxious or alarmist. The HIV virus has a low infectivity rate, cannot survive long outside the human body, and is spread only when it enters the bloodstream through the exchange of body fluids. You cannot catch it from sharing utensils such as cups, knives and forks with an infected person, or from normal physical contact such as hugging or holding hands.

Transmission of the virus from sexual activity is only possible if either you or your partner are already infected.

However, it is essential for all sexually active people to become well acquainted with the facts of the disease and to put into practice safer sex methods whenever there is even the slight risk of infection.

The following activities are considered to present the highest risk:
Anal intercourse without condoms: The blood vessels in the rectum can easily rupture with the friction of sexual activity, creating a high

Safer Sex

risk of infection if one or other partner carries the virus.

Vaginal intercourse without condoms: Vaginal fluids and semen can both contain the HIV virus, as can the menstrual blood flow. Broken blood vessels, and small abrasions either in the vagina or on the penis can allow the virus to enter the bloodstream.

Multiple partners and casual sex: The more sexual partners someone has, the greater exposure to the risk of infection of all STDs, including the HIV virus. In the case of casual sex affairs, it is unlikely that you will know the full sexual history of that person.

Sharing needles: Although this is not a sexual activity, anyone who has been an intravenous drug user and has ever shared a contaminated syringe or needle with another person has a high risk of HIV infection. That person's sexual partners are also at risk if safer sex precautions are not used.

The following sexual activities carry less but some risk:

Oral sex: The HIV virus in semen and vaginal fluids will normally be destroyed by stomach acids if ingested. However, the risk of infection increases if the partner giving fellatio (when the woman gives oral sex to the man) or cunnilingus (when the man gives oral sex to the woman) has any small cuts, sores, or ulcers in the mouth, or bleeding gums. To minimize risk, condoms should be used during fellatio and latex barriers can be used during cunnilingus.

Intercourse with condoms: The use of condoms and other barrier methods reduces the risk of disease transmission by 98 per cent, so long as all the safer sex precautions are used. The risk lies in not following the proper procedures for barrier method protection, or in the accidental tearing of the rubber causing a spillage of semen or vaginal fluids.

Sharing sex toys: You should not share a sex toy with your partner because of the risk of cross-infection.

Safer Sex Activities

This term refers to all physical contact that does not involve the exchange of body fluids or create broken skin or bleeding. This still leaves many delightful ways to enjoy your sex life.

The following suggestions should present no risk so long as there are no open sores or cuts to the skin which could allow cross-infection. To be extra safe, cover any open wounds on the skin, however small, with adhesive plaster.

Cuddling, hugging and caressing: These are all perfectly safe and wonderful ways to make physical contact.

Kissing: Mouth to mouth or dry kissing is fine. Deep or "French" kissing and saliva exchange is only minimally risky if there are open

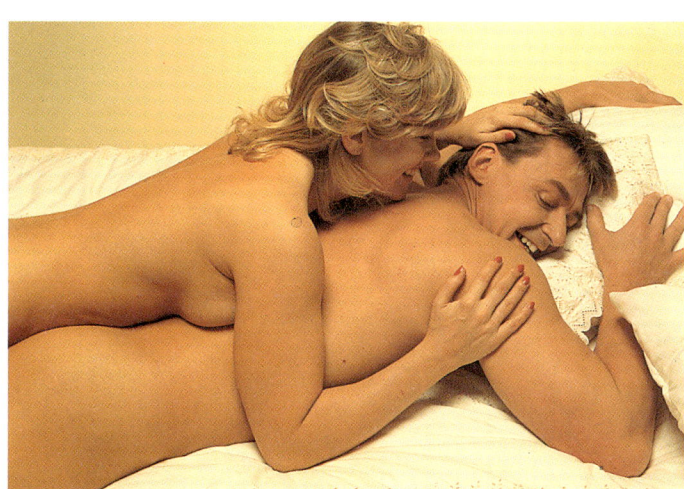

Safe and Exciting
▲ Safer sex need not mean boring sex. Couples can explore and enjoy a whole range of exciting sensual and sexual practices. By stroking, massaging and caressing each other you will become more familiar with your partner's body and its unique erogenous responses.

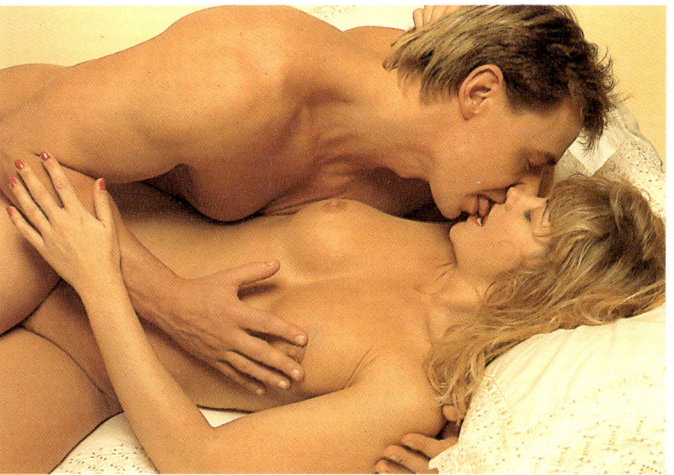

Enhance Your Pleasure
▲ Kissing, licking, nuzzling and touching are all safer sex practices which can only add greater pleasure to your sexual relationship as well as extending your range of foreplay techniques. As your relationship develops, you will learn how your lover likes to be caressed.

Basic Techniques

cuts, bleeding gums or ulcers in the mouth.

Licking, nibbling and sucking: Go ahead and enjoy yourselves, but ensure that you do not bite so hard that you break the skin.

Masturbation: Self-masturbation is fine. So is mutual masturbation, so long as you take care that body fluids, such as semen and vaginal fluids, do not penetrate the skin. Keep all skin abrasions covered.

How To Use Condoms

Learn to regard the use of condoms as a natural addition to your lovemaking techniques. There are a few tips to make this easier. Don't wait until you are too fired up with passion before debating whether or not to use a condom. Discuss and agree on this issue as soon as you know you are going to make love. Keep the condom packet on you, close to the bed, or under the pillow, so you know where to find it at the crucial moment. The suggestions listed below can ensure that your condom usage will bring you maximum safety and pleasure.

❖ Open the packet carefully and ease the condom out, taking care that you do not snag it on your jewellery or fingernails.

❖ At this point, do not start to unroll the condom. Make sure you have the condom round the right way, with the rolled up ring on the outside, and just squeeze its tip between your index finger and

In Place Before Penetration
▼ *The condom should be in place on the man's penis before any kind of penetrative sex takes place as pre-ejaculation seminal fluid can also contain the HIV virus.*

Choosing Condoms

Condoms are also popularly known as "rubbers", and "French letters". Once you and your partner decide that safer sex is caring sex the use of condoms can have a really positive place in your lovemaking. Condoms are about 98 per cent reliable when used as a barrier method during penetrative or oral sex to protect against infection of sexually transmitted diseases, including herpes and HIV.

Nowadays, there are many varieties of condoms to choose from, and you can experiment with different brands. Flavoured condoms can make protected oral sex more enjoyable and palatable, and coloured ones add to the fun. Some condoms are already lubricated and covered with spermicide, while others are not.

You should always use a water-based lubricant, such as KY jelly, and not an oil-based one, such as petroleum jelly, which can interact with the rubber and damage it. Lubricated condoms are less likely to tear with friction. Always check that you are using a suitable condom and lubricant. Look for the use-by date on the condom packet as the rubber can deteriorate with age, and always store condom packets away from direct sunlight, heat, perfumes and sharp objects.

In the United States, condoms from certified manufacturers will have an expiration date and lot number. They will have passed stringent tests by the International Standards Association. In the United Kingdom, check for the Kitemark guarantee on the packet, though it is important to be aware that this is usually a statement of suitability for vaginal sex rather than anal sex. Especially strong condoms are now made for anal sex.

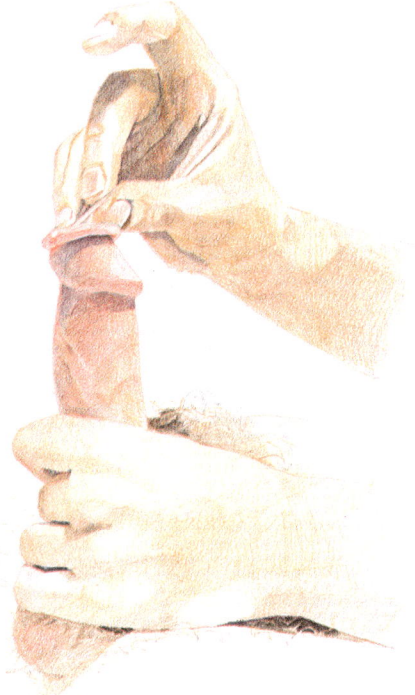

Penis Must Be Erect
▲ *Wait till the penis is erect before putting on the condom, otherwise it can easily slip off.*

Safer Sex

thumb to dispel air. (Most condoms have a teat at the tip to collect the ejaculated sperm.)

❖ The man can either put the condom on by himself, or his partner can do it for him as part of their foreplay. Ensure the penis remains erect while putting it on.

❖ Unroll the sheath down to the end of the penis. If there is no teat, then leave about 1cm/½in spare at the top to collect the semen.

❖ The vagina should be moist before penetration, for the woman's comfort and to avoid tearing the condom with dry friction. You can smear a little water-based lubricant over the outside of the rubber, or either of you can carefully insert extra lubricant inside her vagina, if necessary.

❖ While making love, check to see if the condom is still in place, as it can sometimes slip off. After ejaculation, the man should hold the base of the condom securely with his fingers while he withdraws his penis from the vagina before he loses his erection. This will prevent the condom coming off and causing a spillage of semen in or around the vagina.

❖ Wrap the used condom securely in tissue and dispose of it safely. It is advisable not to flush it down the toilet. Never re-use a condom.

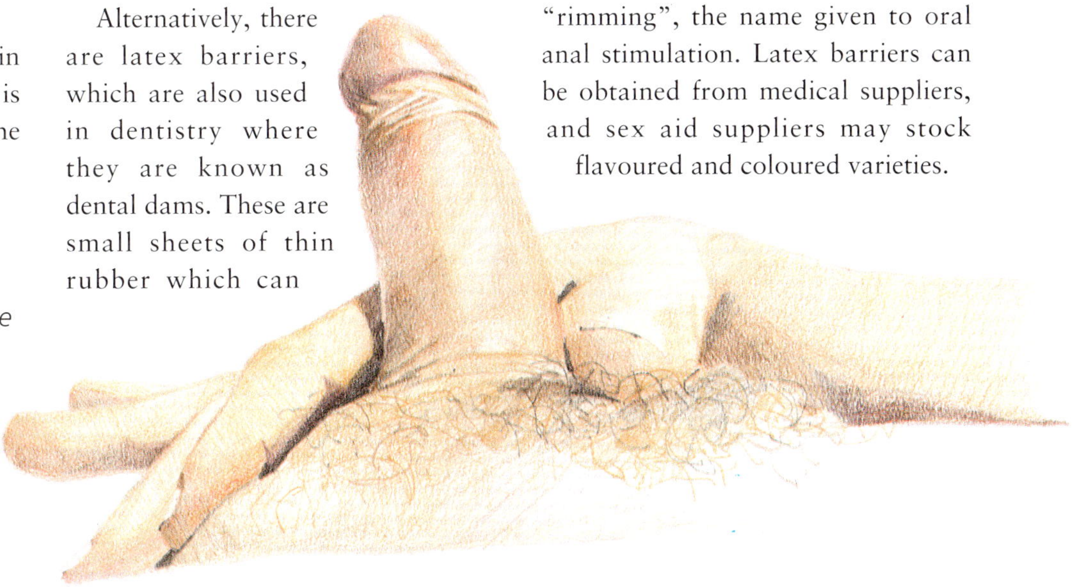

Keep It In Place
▶ Once in place, the ring of the condom should fit comfortably at the base of penis and remain there during the whole of the lovemaking session. If the penis becomes soft during lovemaking, hold the ring of the condom with your fingers to keep it in place until the full erection has resumed.

Ways to Stay Aroused
▼ The woman can keep her man in a state of arousal by manually stroking the shaft of his penis, and saying sexy things about him, as he rolls down the condom. If the female partner is putting the condom on her partner's penis, he or she can stroke it so that he stays erect.

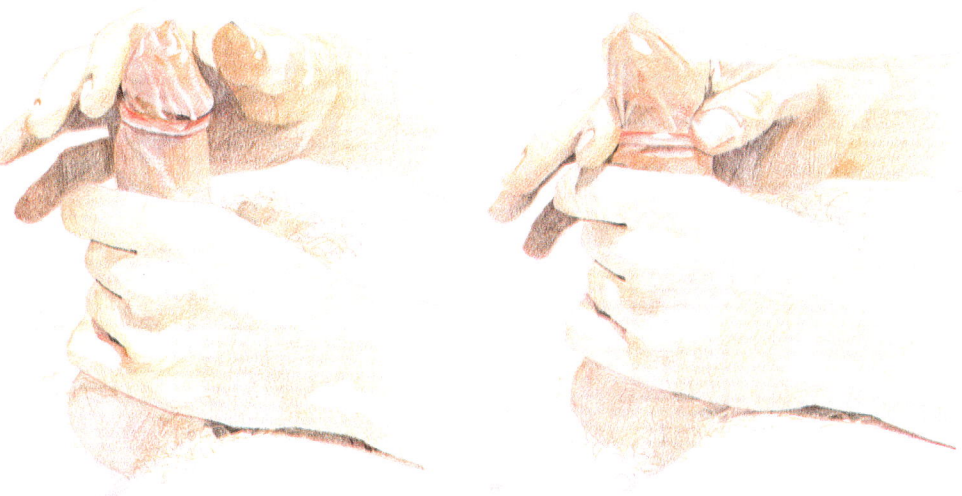

Other Barrier Methods

In addition to the male condom, there are other barrier methods that can be used for safer sex practices. The female condom, which lines the vagina, is claimed by its manufacturer to be 98 per cent effective against the transmission of sexually transmitted diseases, provided it is used correctly.

Alternatively, there are latex barriers, which are also used in dentistry where they are known as dental dams. These are small sheets of thin rubber which can be placed over the vulva to make oral sex or cunnilingus safer. They act to prevent vaginal fluids or menstrual blood from passing into the mouth which can present a risk to your partner if he has open cuts, sore or bleeding gums, or mouth ulcers.

Latex barriers can also be placed over the anus to prevent the spread of disease if either of you enjoy "rimming", the name given to oral anal stimulation. Latex barriers can be obtained from medical suppliers, and sex aid suppliers may stock flavoured and coloured varieties.

Undressing Each Other

Whether your relationship is new or well established, there is always a delicate moment of transition when it moves into a more intimate and sexual dimension and you both know that you want to make love. Men and women have developed all sorts of signals, both subtle and overt, to convey to their partners that they are ready for sex. So now is the moment to get undressed, to expose and reveal your bodies to each other, to explore one another and to become naked in body and desire.

Getting undressed with your lover is an important part of foreplay, an art in itself, a vital scenario in the theatre of love. Of course, you can tear off your clothes, or each other's, throw them into a heap and leap into bed. Sometimes, when passions are running high, that uninhibited approach is all part of the fun. Or you may be shy about your body, have judgements about it, and end up trying to get undressed surreptitiously in the bathroom or under the bed clothes. Getting undressed and being naked in front of a lover can be very traumatic for some people.

You may prefer to take off your own clothes and present yourself naked in front of your partner. But if you are shy, and your relationship is new, then you could choose to get undressed alone, and slip on an attractive dressing gown before returning to the bedroom.

Dressing For Undressing

For the bold and uninhibited and for couples who like to bring fantasy into their love lives, why not try a tantalizing strip-tease for your partner. However, undressing each other, slowly and lovingly, letting each part of the body reveal itself when the moment feels right, is a romantic way to become unclothed in your prelude to making love.

If the love scenes in movies are anything to go by, undressing your partner is guaranteed to be a smooth and graceful operation. Clothes slip like silk off the skin, buttons undo themselves and, most certainly, the bra fastener pops open with the greatest of ease.

It is rarely like that in real life, and most people have had embarrassing moments of fumbling and fiddling with fasteners, zips that stuck, or jeans and skirts which simply refused to budge past the thighs. If any of these situations happen then you may need to give your lover a hand or take off the awkward item of clothing yourself.

You do not always know when you are going to make love but if you have a suspicion that sex is on the agenda, dress with undressing in mind. Simplify your clothing so it can be removed easily, and avoid wearing items which leave marks on your skin. Don't be caught out wearing your oldest and most ragged piece of underwear, your woollen thermals, baggy Y-fronts, string vests, socks with holes, or immovable bra. What you have on next to your skin should add to your allure, and that applies both to men and women.

If you have time to prepare, put on soft lighting. Low-light lamps or candlelight will spread a more flattering and romantic glow in the room, softening your skin tones and body shape. Background music can help you to relax, so have your favourite tapes close at hand.

Strip-teasing

▼ *Try to make the act of undressing part of your love play. Slowly undressing each other and allowing your mutual nakedness to reveal itself, stage by stage, will intensify your desire for one another. As each item of clothing slips from the body, pay your partner a compliment, mentioning not just the obvious sexual areas, but also the eyes, hair, mouth, skin, hands, feet and so on.*

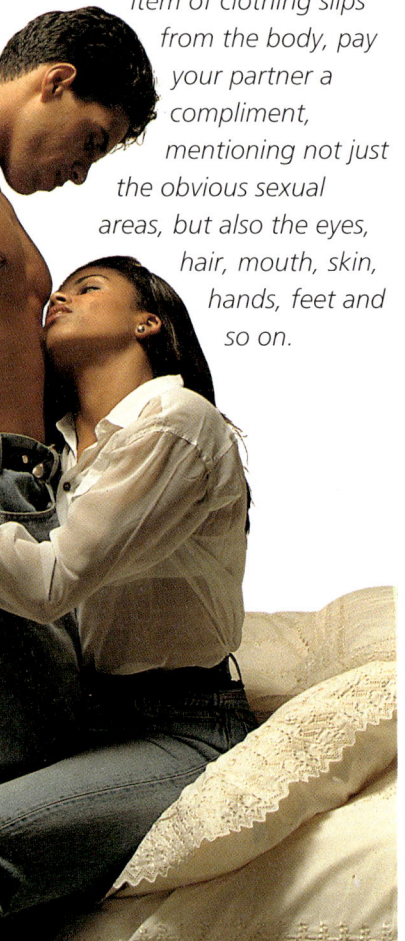

Opening Moves

▶ If you have been petting, hugging and kissing each other, you may need to signal that you are ready for more. It is sometimes a relief for the man when the woman decides to take the initiative, giving him signs that she wants to go further. Slowly undoing his belt buckle and trouser zip should really do the trick!

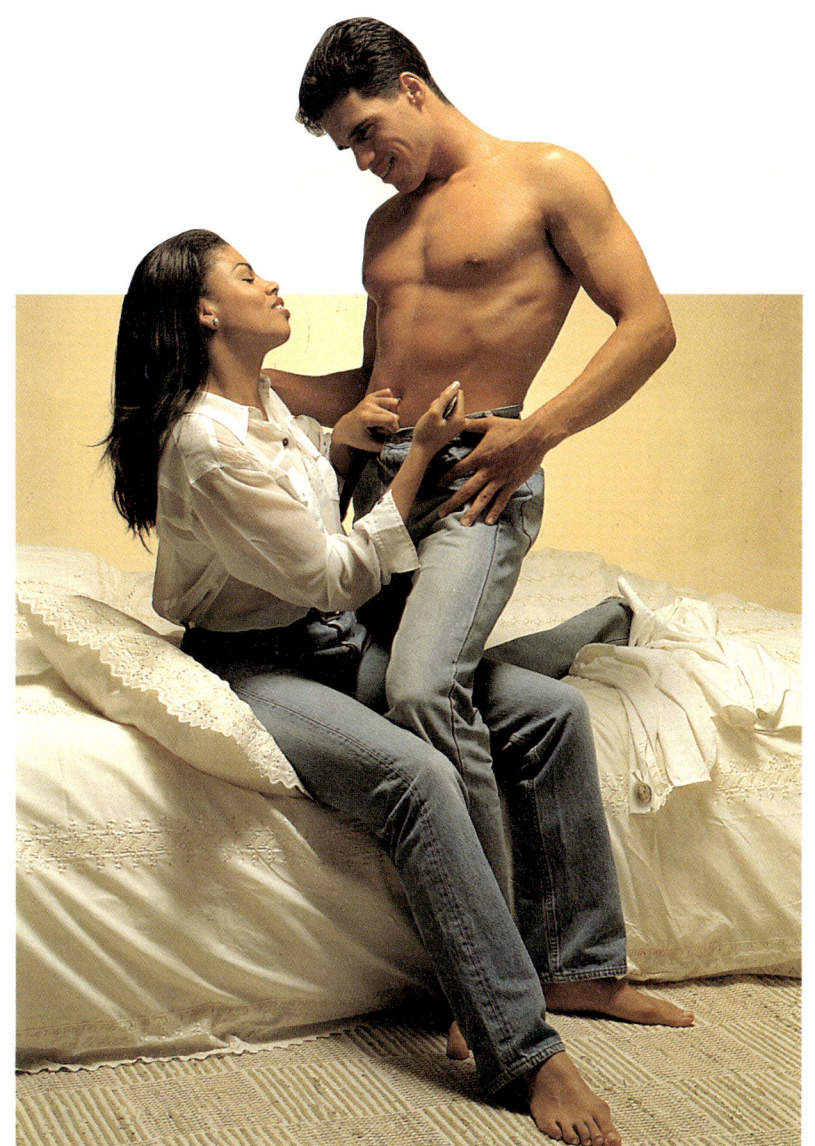

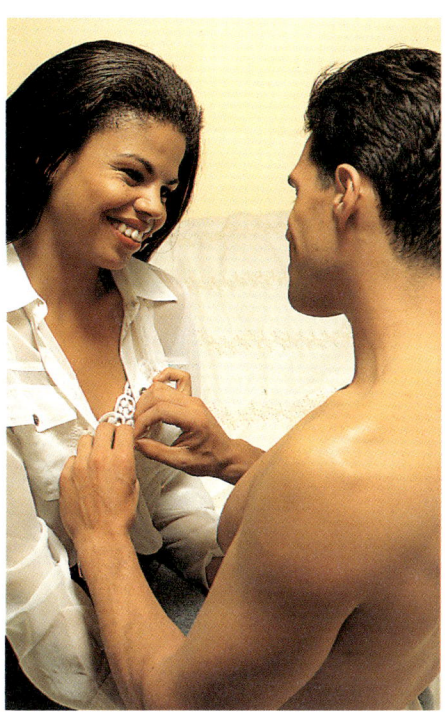

Slow and Steady

▲ Now it is his turn to make a move. Take things slowly and let your mutual anticipation of pleasure build up gradually. Open the buttons carefully one by one, and joke about it if one gets stuck. Telling her just how much you have been looking forward to this moment of love will help to put her at ease.

Touching and Kissing

▶ Getting undressed should be part of the whole lovemaking experience rather than a means to an end. As the clothes begin to slip from her body, continue to touch and kiss her.

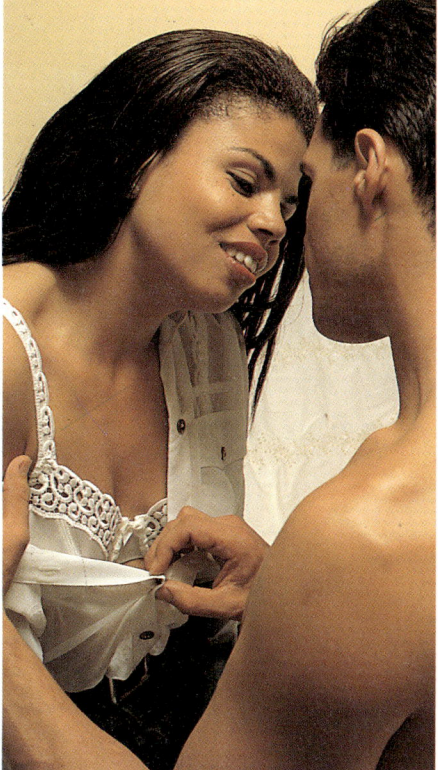

Keeping Active

▼ She is going to need to move around so that you can remove her outer clothing with ease. Part of the fun of undressing each other is to constantly exchange the active and passive roles. As her body becomes more exposed, stay sensitive to her signals so that she feels happy and relaxed about what is happening.

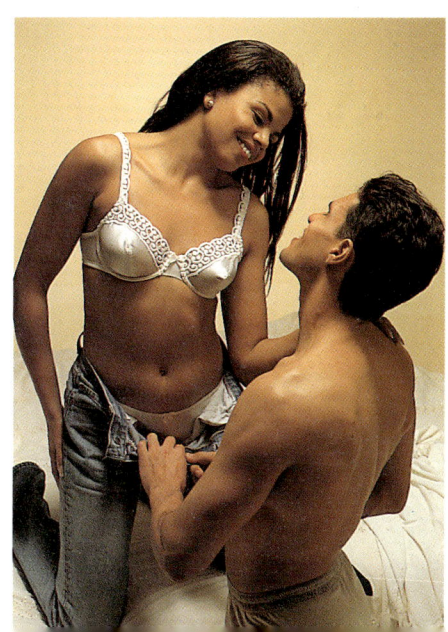

Basic Techniques

Baring It All

Removing the top layer of clothing is an art to master, but even more sensual skill is needed when you start to take off each other's underwear. You are going to be naked and vulnerable and also, very turned on. There is something very erotic about starting your foreplay with your underwear still on. At this point, you know you want to make love, but the presence of this scant clothing against your skin makes the whole situation more tantalizing. It creates an exciting sense of seduction as if you are saying to each other: "I want you and I know you want me but let's not take anything for granted."

Some couples like to make love while still wearing an item of clothing because a half-exposed body is more exciting to them, or they find certain types of underwear or lingerie inspire their sexual fantasies and hot up their sex lives.

The Esquire Report, *Men on Sex* reveals that many men find it more arousing to see their partners partially clothed rather than totally naked. The reason given was that it added to the air of expectation and anticipation even in a long-term relationship.

Also, keeping some clothes on encourages you to extend your time of foreplay, allowing you to embrace, kiss and caress longer before intercourse which gives your bodies more time to warm up and tune in to each other's mounting sexual feelings. If either one of you is shy or nervous about being seen naked or of making love, the lingering presence of these clothes will give you the extra time you need to relax.

Fun of Unfastening
▲ Wearing a front-fastening bra will make the undressing manoeuvres easier for him. If it closes at the back, lean into his body and snuggle up to him, whispering some sexy words while he focuses on the job in hand.

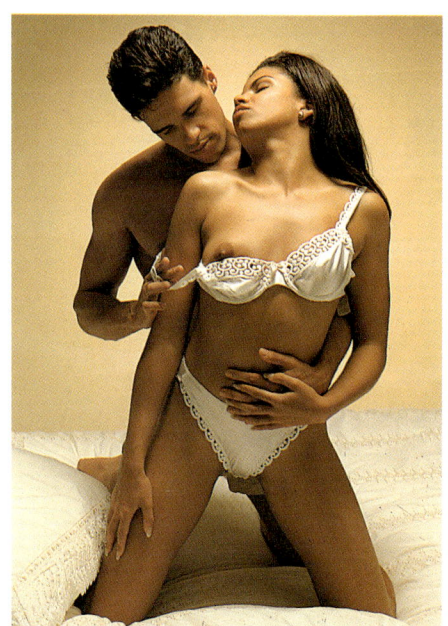

Sexy Texture
▲ As you stroke and touch one another, the brush of the cloth against your breasts and genitals can be very arousing. Only you will know the point when you are ready to remove all your clothes.

Getting Undressed

Jane, aged 42, a nurse: "I've always been a little shy about undressing in front of a man, and I prefer to make my appearance in the bedroom already undressed but covered with a slinky, silk kimono. I feel most relaxed about it when I'm involved in a deeply trusting relationship, then somehow, if I feel relaxed, sensual and sexy enough, my skin just seems to have a special glow and I lose my inhibitions."

Lucy, aged 26, a production assistant: "I'm all for the bodice-ripping stuff and getting on with it the first time around. If I undress too slowly, then I'm afraid the man is going to be checking out my body too much. My fantasy, though, is to find a relationship with a man I trust enough, and who knows my body well enough, that I can undress for him by doing a slow strip-tease."

Ernie, 32, a photographer: "I prefer mutual undressing because it is less threatening. It's more playful and the power is shared. I find it very sexy."

Don, aged 28, a courier: "When I am going to have sex with my girlfriend, I like it best if we undress slowly and start doing it with some of our clothing on. I think it adds something 'naughty but nice' to the whole thing. It adds a bit of extra excitement as if we shouldn't really be going the whole way – though we both really know that we are."

Undressing Each Other

Voyage of Discovery
▶ As her bra falls from her body, and her breasts are exposed, cradle them in your hands to acknowledge their soft, sensual beauty. Touch and stroke her naked belly, letting your fingers slip under the panty line with just a hint of exploration.

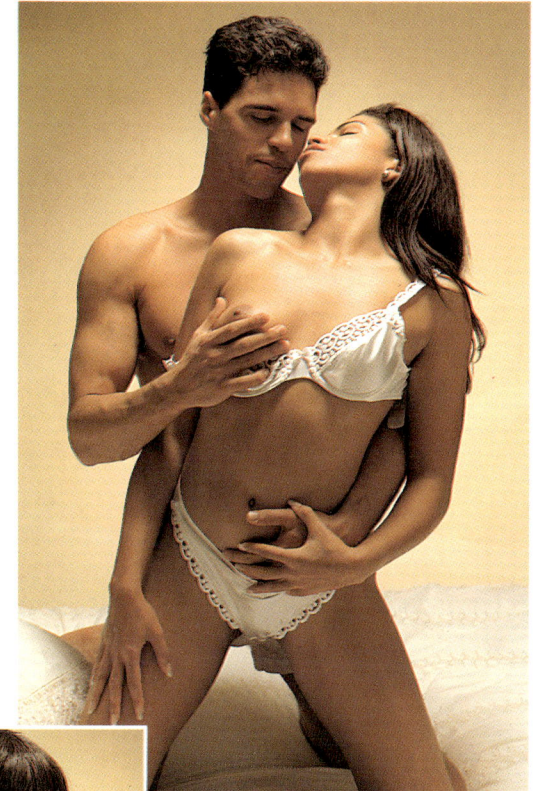

Brief Encounter
▼ Your man will be thrilled if you show your desire for him by removing his underpants. Roll them down slowly over his buttocks, allowing him to touch you while you do so.

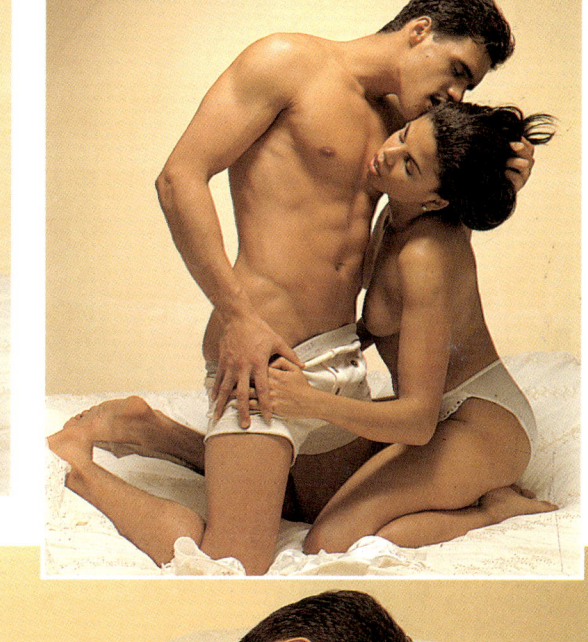

Unpeeling Her Panties
▲ When you remove her panties, try not to do so with indecent haste! She'll enjoy the feeling of having them peeled away from her like the skin of a forbidden fruit. Edge them down little by little, stroking and squeezing her buttocks gently. In certain positions, you can pull her close to your body to kiss and caress her at the same time.

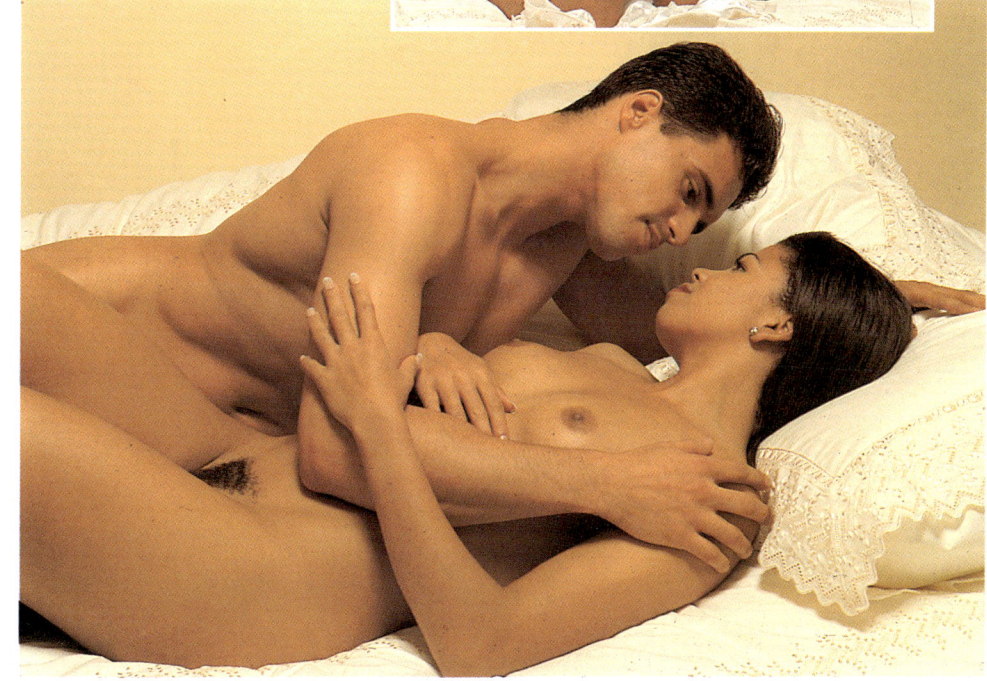

Naked Passion
▲ Once the clothes are removed and there's nothing more to hide, your foreplay enters into a new and exciting stage. The whole body is available for all the touches of love that you can lavish on each other. Take some moments just to be there with each other, savouring and enjoying your own and your lover's nakedness.

Sensual Play

The term "sensual play" is probably more apt than "foreplay" to describe all the many wonderful, caring, romantic, sensual and sexual activities that a man and woman can engage in to express their attraction and love for each other. "Foreplay" usually refers to those sexual techniques that lovers can use to arouse each other to ensure satisfactory intercourse and orgasm. As such, it implies an activity with a goal in mind, something that comes before the real thing, a little like the hors-d'oeuvres before the main meal – a nice taster but not quite substantial enough in itself.

While this section mostly focuses on sensual play in the context of lovemaking, it can actually start from the moment two people become attracted to each other. It manifests in body language signalling a desire to become more intimate with each other. It includes holding hands, cuddling, hugging, kissing and the exchange of sweet words.

It plays a part in the way partners choose to spend time together – dancing to music, going to the theatre, walking in the woods, arranging candlelit dinners, and the exchange of small but meaningful gifts. Sensual play acknowledges the special relationship, both sexually and emotionally, that you have developed with your chosen partner, whether that person is a new or long-term lover. It is not a set programme of techniques but more a response to, and an acknowledgement of, the whole person – body, mind and spirit – which makes you and your partner unique and special to each other.

It is important to give it the time and space it needs, both outside and inside the bedroom, for it will nurture and enhance your relationship, so that it remains caring and sensual, warm and erotically alive.

Comforting Contact
▼ *Sensual contact may be as simple as a cuddle for comfort and closeness, a massage for relaxation, kisses to show affection, caresses to soothe or pamper, or moments spent looking tenderly into each other's eyes. All of these can be the start of a sexual journey, but they can also be relished purely for their own sake.*

Kissing
Kissing is one of the most intimate aspects of sensual foreplay and lovemaking because, in addition to being sexually arousing, it reveals the degree of affection and tenderness which exists between you and your lover. Attitudes towards kissing change from culture to culture, and in some parts of the world it plays a very small role, if any, in the sexual relationship. Most of us, though, regard it as a highly personal part of our lovemaking which reflects emotional closeness. From our earliest memories, kissing is associated with warm and caring contact, and some people find it easier to have full penetrative sex for purely physical sensation and release than to kiss mouth to mouth without a certain depth of loving feeling.

Kissing usually plays a big part in the early stages of romance as a way of exploring sexual compatibility and expressing attraction and tenderness. However, it can become a sadly neglected activity once the relationship has become firmly established and is taken for granted. One of the most common

Sensual Play

Kiss and Tell

Jacqueline, aged 28, a secretary, has been married for four years: "To be honest, kissing is the best part for me. If my husband doesn't kiss me enough, I just don't get that turned on. When he takes the time to kiss me properly, I feel he is appreciating me rather than just my body."

Roger, aged 27, unemployed, has a long-term girlfriend: "I used to be an action man, you know, straight to the point. When I met Louise, she was keen on lots of kissing and foreplay. I started to really enjoy it too, and sometimes now we just kiss and cuddle for ages before going on to anything else. It's great."

Avril, 31, a model, is currently single: "I love kissing, but I hate it when I've just met someone and he tries to stick his tongue in my mouth straight away. I prefer to be seduced into a full French kiss, and even then, only after the first few dates. How a man kisses me tells me a lot about how he is going to make love to me."

Fred, 62, a taxi driver, has been married for thirty-two years: "We are from the old school, and we didn't have a full sexual relationship until we were married. We were courting for several years and it was very romantic, but all we did was pet and kiss. Those kisses were lovely and so full of promise. Even now, we make sure we kiss each other every day."

complaints made by women in long-term relationships is that their men do not kiss them often enough, either as a purely romantic and affectionate gesture, or as part of their sexual lives. Too often, a sexual relationship can settle down to the basics, where arousal techniques are focused purely on intercourse and orgasm, while the subtler expressions of love and tenderness, such as kissing, are regularly overlooked. Let kissing remain an important part of your physical interaction outside the bedroom, as well as an integral part of your foreplay and lovemaking.

Tender Touches

▶ Kissing during a sexual episode can change from being tender and sweet to deep and passionate. It can start with the gentle brushing of the lips over the face. Kissing the forehead is an especially caring and affectionate gesture. So is planting little kisses on her nose and cheeks.

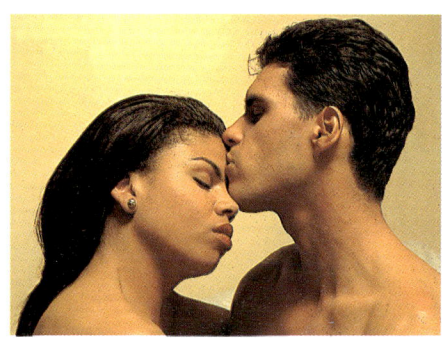

Tease with Kisses

▶ Playful kisses are also exciting. You can lift his face towards yours and teasingly kiss him all around his chin and jaw, moving down to the erotically sensitive areas of the neck and throat.

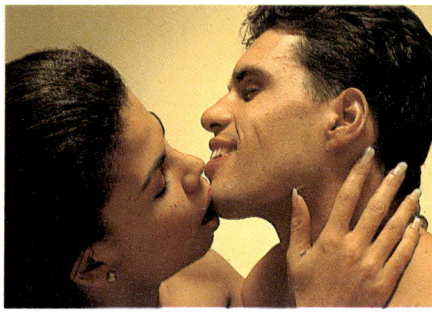

Savour the Moment

▼ Having taken your time to enjoy the sensuality of lip-to-skin contact, let eager anticipation grow as your mouths come closer together. As your lips meet, close your eyes to savour this deliciously intimate moment.

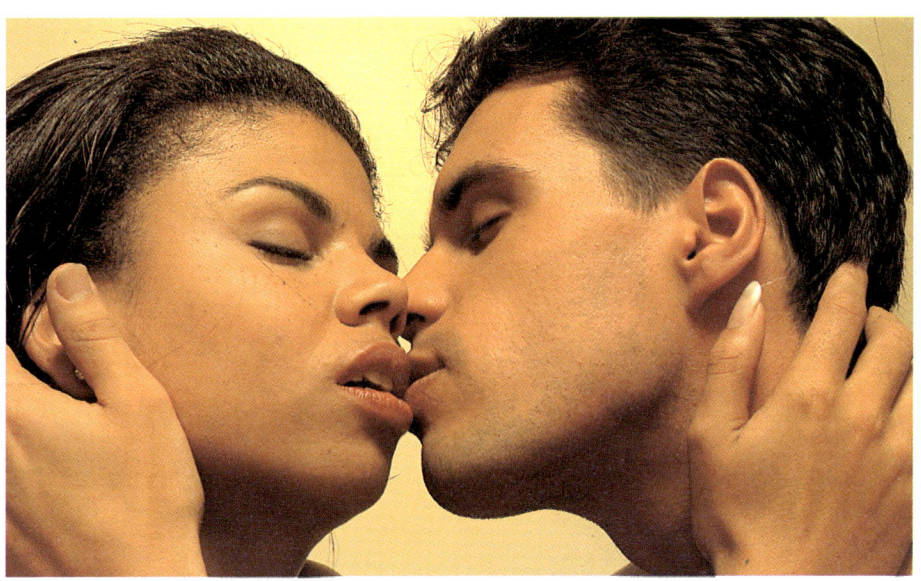

Basic Techniques

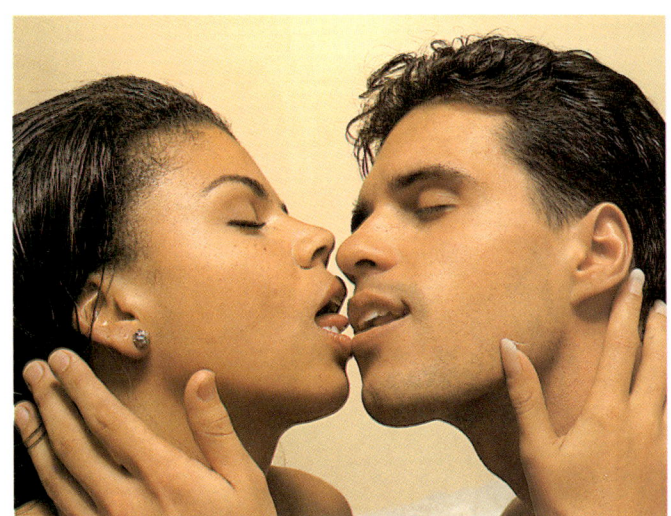

Gentle Kisses
◀ When you first begin to kiss, let your mouths and lips relax together so that they become soft and yielding to one another. Don't rush into a deep, passionate kiss too soon. The longer you can delay before inserting your tongue into your partner's mouth, the more sensual and stimulating the kissing will be as it slowly begins to build up into an erotically charged embrace. Try kissing all around the edges of the lips, then run the tip of your tongue over them, as this can also be very sexy.

Passionate Embrace
▶ The chemistry between you both will heat up once the tongue enters the mouth – but don't thrust it immediately towards the throat. Instead, roll it languidly over the teeth and trace the moist contours of the mouth's interior. Then, let your tongues move and dart together to initiate a sexual rhythm, setting the pace for what is to follow. The act of kissing each other, gently and slowly, or passionately, can involve you both so deeply that you can begin to feel as if you are dissolving together. It can keep you attuned and responsive in both body and mind, while increasing your sexual arousal.

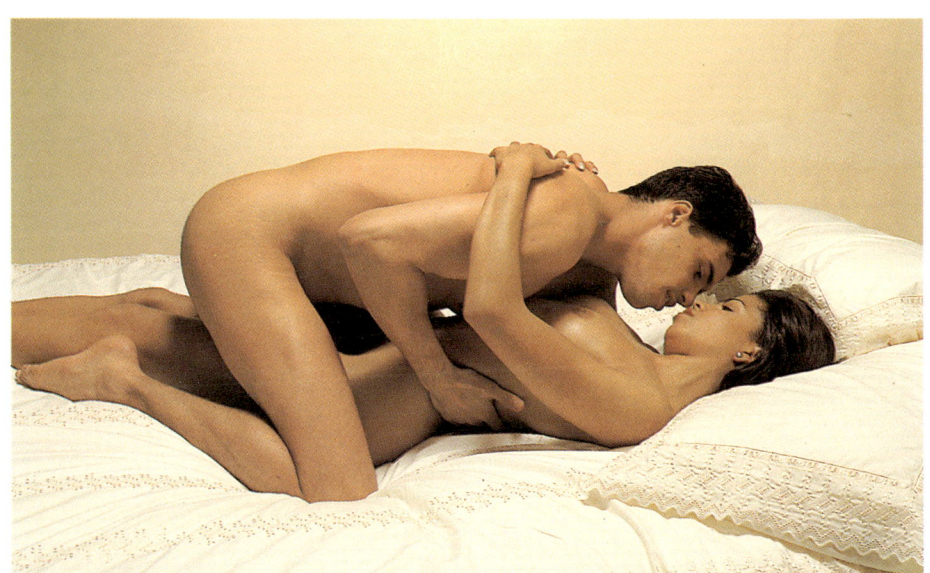

Thrusting Tongues
▶ During intercourse, kissing can become very exciting if it imitates the movements of coitus. As you hold each other tight, your lips may meet with a new sense of urgency and your tongues will seek each other to dance together to the tempo of the pelvic thrusts.

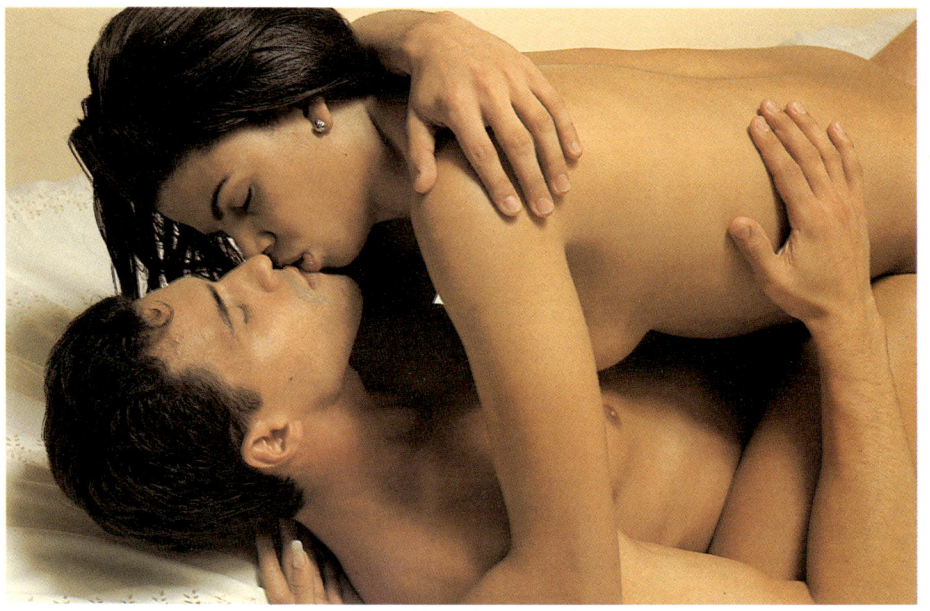

Sensual Play

Be Spontaneous

Sensual play is tremendously important to your emotional happiness and your sexual life. Forget the pre-conditioned programmes and learn to pleasure each other's bodies in ways that acknowledge the needs of the heart, mind and emotions of your partner at any particular moment. Also, become more aware of your own physical and emotional needs which will require different degrees of tactile stimulus depending on your own shifts in mood.

Acknowledge that there are times when either of you may want to be hugged and held, kissed and stroked, but may not necessarily be ready for full sexual intercourse. Couples often hold back from comforting physical contact because they are afraid it will lead to sexual intercourse for which they are not ready. If either you or your partner are under stress and simply not in the mood for sex, or if you have an infection or disability that would make intercourse unwise or undesirable, there is no need to abstain from loving physical contact. In its broadest sense physical contact answers a huge spectrum of human needs, sexual and non-sexual, as well as a certain sensual state which exists between the two.

Becoming Sexually Alive

Play with each other's bodies in such a way that you enjoy each touch for its own sake, and try not to worry about achieving an orgasm, because that will create a subtle tension. Every person has different sexual responses, so explore with each other what turns you both on.

There is no specific programme of foreplay techniques that will be able

> ### Hygiene Matters
>
> Sensual foreplay means close physical contact with every part of your body, so take special care of your hygiene so that your body is fresh, clean and smelling good. Nothing is quite such a turn-off as unpleasant body odours, bad breath, smelly feet or dirty nails. Bathe or shower beforehand, alone or – even better – together, and try adding a few drops of luxuriant aphrodisiac essential oils, such as jasmine, ylang-ylang, patchouli or sandalwood, to the bath water. If you have eaten a spicy meal, garlic or onions beforehand, smoked a cigarette, or drunk alcohol, make sure that you clean your teeth and rinse out your mouth.
>
> Some people enjoy "rimming" in foreplay, the term used for anal stimulation. If you do practise this, make sure you wash your fingers before inserting them into the vagina as you risk spreading bacterial infection to its delicate tissues. Taking special care about your hygiene is a statement of your self-esteem and also shows you care about your partner.

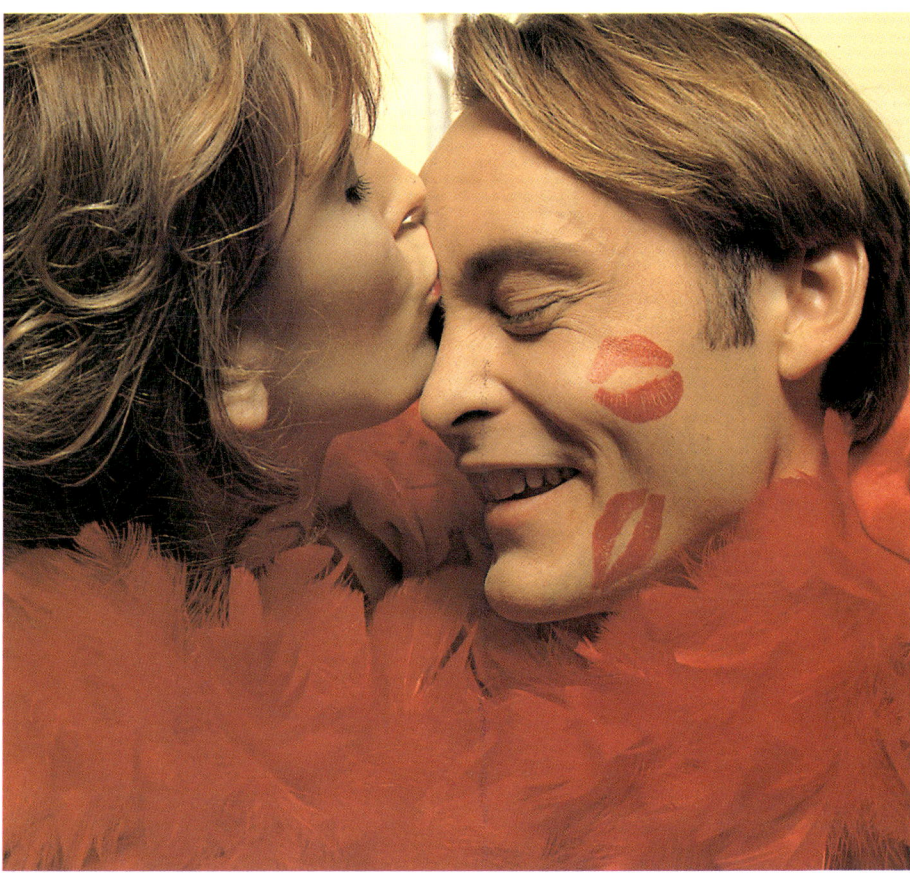

Sensual Celebration
◄ *Sensual play can achieve something greater and more holistic than foreplay. It can be a wholly satisfying experience in itself, an expression of love, and a celebration of the playful, sensual and erotic capacity of the human body.*

Basic Techniques

to guarantee sexual success. What pleased and thrilled a previous partner may not be as exciting or acceptable to a new one. Also, sexual responses vary, not just from person to person, but at different psychological and biological stages of life and even day to day.

Learn to recognize your own sexual needs and those of your partner, and enjoy experimenting so you do not fall into boring patterns. It is not always easy to guess what a partner wants at any particular time, so be prepared to talk to each other about your likes and dislikes.

When something feels good, say so or make appreciative sounds. If it does not feel good, there is no need to criticize. Just say to your partner something like: "I would really like you to do this to me," and then be prepared to explain or demonstrate exactly how you want to be touched. Rather than focusing your whole attention on the most obvious sexual areas, such as the genitals or breasts, read the section on erogenous zones to appreciate how the whole body can be responsive to erotic touch. Enjoy the exploration so that you can turn your foreplay into a delightful variety of sensual play.

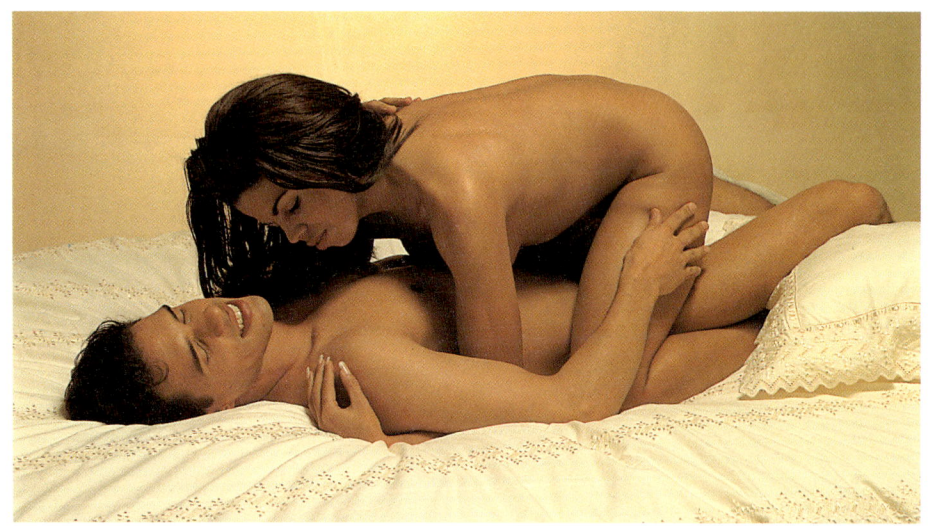

Making it Last
◀ Take time to include sensual play as foreplay so that lovemaking lasts longer and is more luxurious, making every cell of your body come alive and more responsive while letting yourselves become emotionally open and relaxed with each other. In this way your sexuality can envelop your whole being.

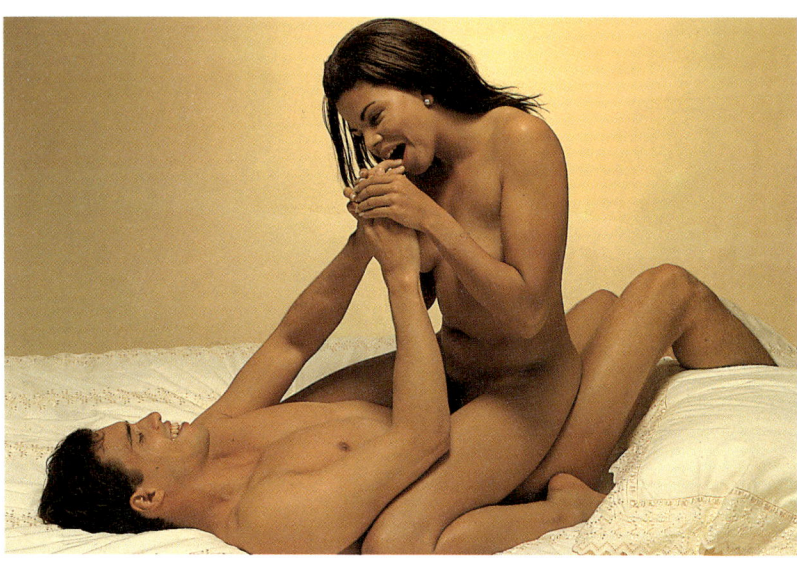

Stoking the Fires
▲ Sensual play includes all forms of touch, such as stroking, caressing and holding, or oral contact, such as kissing, nibbling, sucking and licking. It can involve every part of the body. Sucking on his fingertips or rolling your tongue around them will certainly fire up his imagination.

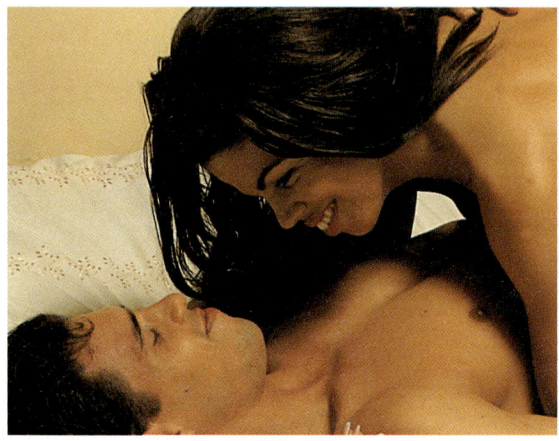

Fun and Foreplay
▲ Humour is an important part of foreplay. It takes away the seriousness of performance-related sex and helps you both unwind and relax so your bodies feel completely at ease with each other. Play fighting, gentle bites, giggling, making sounds, rolling on the bed together can all be part of the fun.

Sensual Play

Touching the Whole Person

There are no rules to sexuality except what feels good or right to the people involved. There are times when the passion is high and the "quickie" way of having sex is exciting and welcome to both parties. More often, though, extended loving foreplay is important to a sexual relationship, because it enhances the emotional bond, and helps the man and woman become sufficiently aroused so that the ensuing lovemaking is compatible and deeply satisfying to both people.

This is particularly important for a woman, who needs more time than a man to become sexually aroused, and whose sexual responses are heightened when she feels emotionally and physically cherished. Also a woman's whole body is erotically sensitive to loving touches, not just the most obvious erogenous zones, such as her genitals and breasts.

It would be a great mistake, though, to believe that foreplay is primarily a "woman's thing", and that it is something a man should learn to do just to satisfy his partner and be deemed a good lover. Men are sensual beings too, and can also enjoy full body stimulation, loving and playful strokes, kissing, licking and all kinds of erotic tactile contact.

A man who is relaxed in his sexuality will enjoy extended foreplay for its own sake, for his pleasure as well as his partner's. It will help him to be less genitally orientated so that he can feel all kinds of wonderful sensations throughout his body. He is then more emotionally in tune with his partner.

If he relaxes into full body sensuality, a man can be more spontaneous and less programmed to performance. He will be less anxious about all the sexual pressures to which men are invariably subjected, such as performing well, maintaining an erection, fear of a premature ejaculation, fear of emotional vulnerability, concern about whether his woman will have an orgasm before he ejaculates, and so on. Sensual play will be an emotionally nourishing experience for him too.

Text-book lovers, male or female, may achieve the sexual responses they seek from their lover, but the partner will know that the touches and techniques are more mechanical than loving, and geared to an ulterior motive. He or she may feel personally abandoned or used, even while being turned on. Most women dislike the experience of having a man zone in on their breasts or clitoris, and having them rubbed or stimulated purely to achieve sexual stimulation.

Similarly, a sensual man may not be keen on having a woman grab for his crotch as a way of achieving an instant turn-on. Bodies are not separate from the feelings of the person within them. They are not machines to be geared to results, regardless of their intrinsic emotional and subtle responses. Sensual play gives time for both men and women to warm up and tune in to each other, on both somatic and psychic levels.

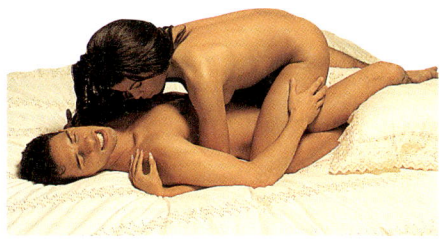

Tools of Arousal

▲ *Any part of the body can become a sensual tool in foreplay. The sweep of your hair, the soft brush of your nipples and breasts against his body, or the warmth of your breath on his skin will be extremely arousing to him. Trailing your fingertips or nails lightly over his skin will heighten its sensitivity. Try to involve your whole body in sensual play, so that even while kissing one part of his body, you are aware of the impact of your thighs, belly, and pubic area as they press gently against him.*

Body Worship

▼ *A woman's whole body, not just her most obvious sexual areas, is an erogenous zone. Take time to let your kisses and touches worship her total sensuality. Focus your attention not just on the front of her body, but on her arms, legs and back. Cover her back with a carpet of kisses, following its sensuous curves and lines. Then stroke and gently squeeze the muscles in her buttocks and thighs so that they become warm and erotically alive.*

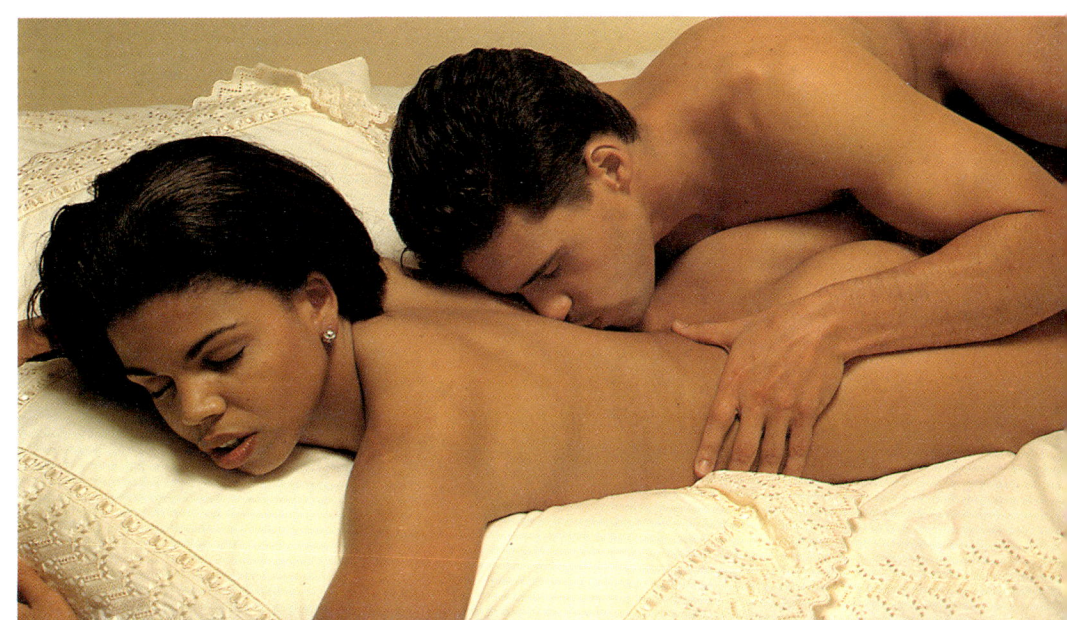

Basic Techniques

Loving Touches
▶ Your man will also enjoy having your touches and kisses on the back of his body. This can include massaging the legs, kissing and licking the highly sensitive soft skin at the back of the knees, stroking, pummelling and squeezing the buttocks, and lightly scratching your fingernails over his skin to excite sensory nerve endings. In this way, the whole body will be suffused with sensual feelings.

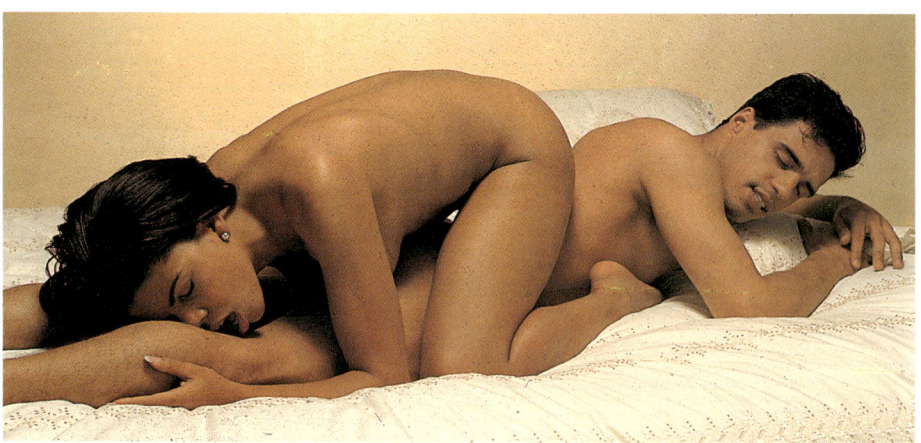

Tongue and Toe
▼ The feet and toes are remarkably sensitive to tactile stimulation if your partner is not too ticklish. Rubbing and massaging the feet can be followed by deliciously erotic toe sucking. Run your tongue around her toes, sucking on them playfully one by one. Special attention can be given to the big toe which, according to zone therapy, has a special connection with the pituitary gland, which regulates the sex hormones.

Wave of Passion
▶ Your extended foreplay should give you time to relax together emotionally, as well as becoming sexually aroused. If you enjoy it for its own sake, rather than proceeding headlong

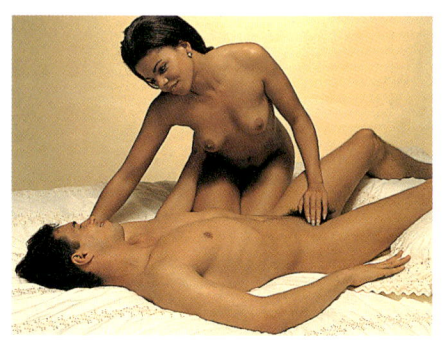

towards a goal, you can savour moments of tenderness and touching purely to enhance your intimate connection. Do not be afraid to let your states of arousal rise and fall like waves in the ocean. Once you are in harmony, both physically and emotionally, you can ride those waves together, letting one peak of excitement ebb to give way to another. Touching, stroking, caressing and eye contact will keep you closely attuned to each other.

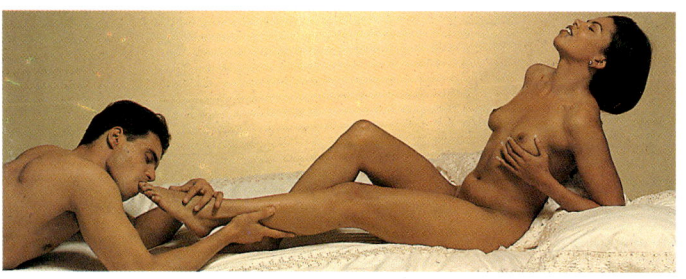

Sexual Arousal
Extended foreplay allows the whole body to become flooded with sex hormones so that the correct physiological changes can occur to ensure harmonious lovemaking. For a woman, sufficient arousal will allow her vagina to undergo changes which enable successful and comfortable penetration during intercourse. The outer and inner lips of her vagina will swell and secrete lubricants, to give off her own special sexual scent. The shape of her vagina will change, so that the outer third becomes narrower and better able to grip the penis to ensure adequate friction, while the inner two-thirds of the vagina expands. It, too, will secrete a sexual lubricant as she becomes excited. Her clitoris also enlarges, as it becomes engorged with blood, and its nerve network becomes erotically sensitized.

As a woman's arousal increases, her breasts may increase slightly in size, and her nipples become erect. If the sensual play which has preceded intercourse has acknowledged her whole person, then physically and emotionally she should feel vibrant and receptive and ready to receive her man.

Loving and sensuous foreplay benefits the man because it can take the sexual charge away from his genital area so that it streams through his whole body, enabling him to become more relaxed and better able to enjoy full body pleasure without the fear of ejaculating too soon. If intercourse is to be the result of the foreplay, when the excitement grows the right tactile stimulation will enable him to achieve a full erection. As his arousal increases, the scrotum skin thickens, and the testes draw up closer to his body. In some men, nipple erection during arousal is also common.

Sensual Play

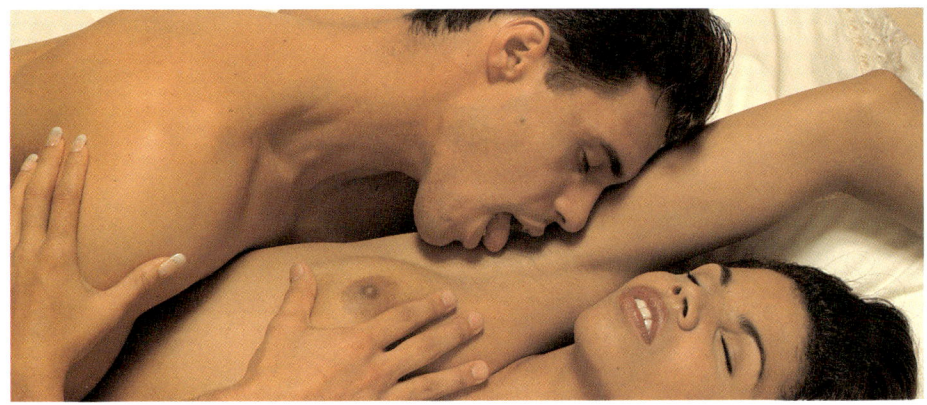

Secret Zones
◄ A woman's body has many surprising and hidden areas of sexual sensitivity. Sensual play allows you to unravel its mysteries, so that you both can discover new and exciting pleasure places. The underarm and armpit can be very responsive to your loving attention. Try rolling your tongue languidly over its soft skin while gently stroking her breast.

Breast Care
► A woman's breasts are one of her most erogenous areas, but their responsiveness to tactile stimulation may vary, depending on her mood or the phase of her menstrual cycle. Always be sensitive to them and to her responses, and do not zone in on them before she is ready for such intimate contact. Gentle palpation of the breasts can feel great, but remember her breasts are glands and not muscles, so handle them with care.

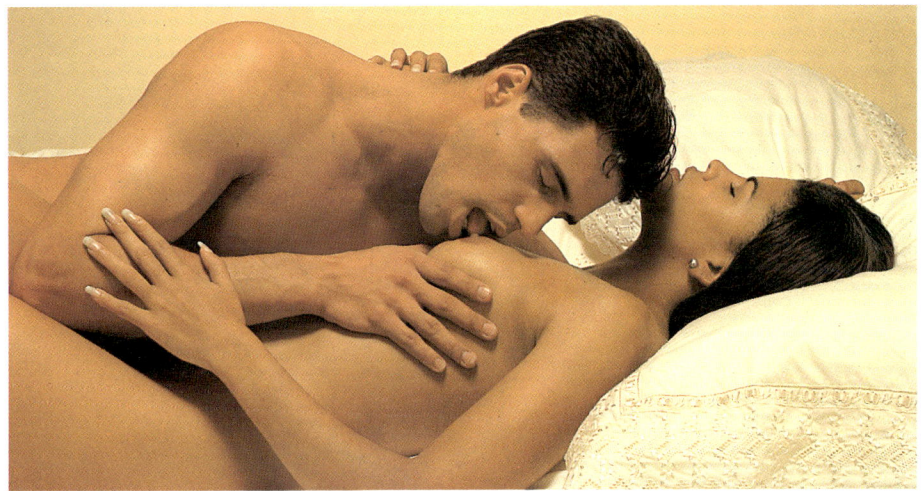

Increase Arousal
▼ When your woman is sexually aroused, you will notice changes to the shape of her breasts as they begin to swell; the areola darkens and the nipples become erect. Licking and trailing your tongue around the areola at this point will be highly exciting to her, increasing her eager anticipation as your lips move closer to her nipple.

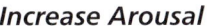

Peaks of Pleasure
▲ When sexually excited, the nipples seem magically connected to her whole nervous system, sending waves of pleasure down through her body to her genitals. Kissing, licking, sucking and flicking your tongue over the nipple will bring her to a peak of arousal. Pay loving attention to both breasts, moving from one to the other, and tell her how beautiful and special they are to you.

Chest Massage
▼ Many men love to have their nipples kissed, licked and stroked during foreplay. In some men, just as in women, the nipples will also become erect when they are sexually aroused. Stroking, kissing and massaging his chest can help him contact his more emotional and vulnerable feelings as well as increasing his whole-body sensuality.

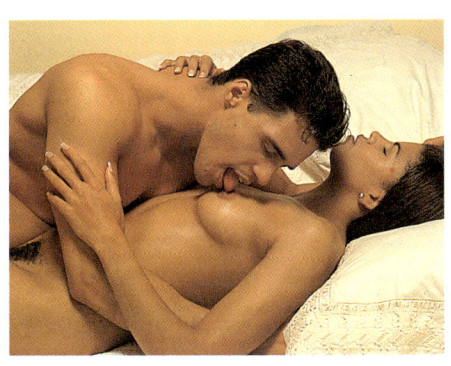

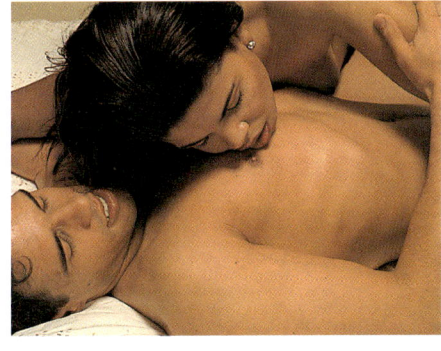

Basic Techniques

Warm and Welcoming
▼ The soft roundness of her belly will welcome your loving kisses as your lips move down her body. This vulnerable area needs your attention so it can become charged with sexual energy. Kiss it tenderly all over, run your tongue teasingly around the navel, and warm the skin with your breath. Work slowly down to her pubic area. Stroking and rubbing her mons with your fingers and tugging gently on the pubic hair will enhance clitoral stimulation. Kissing along her groin can also produce wonderful sensations.

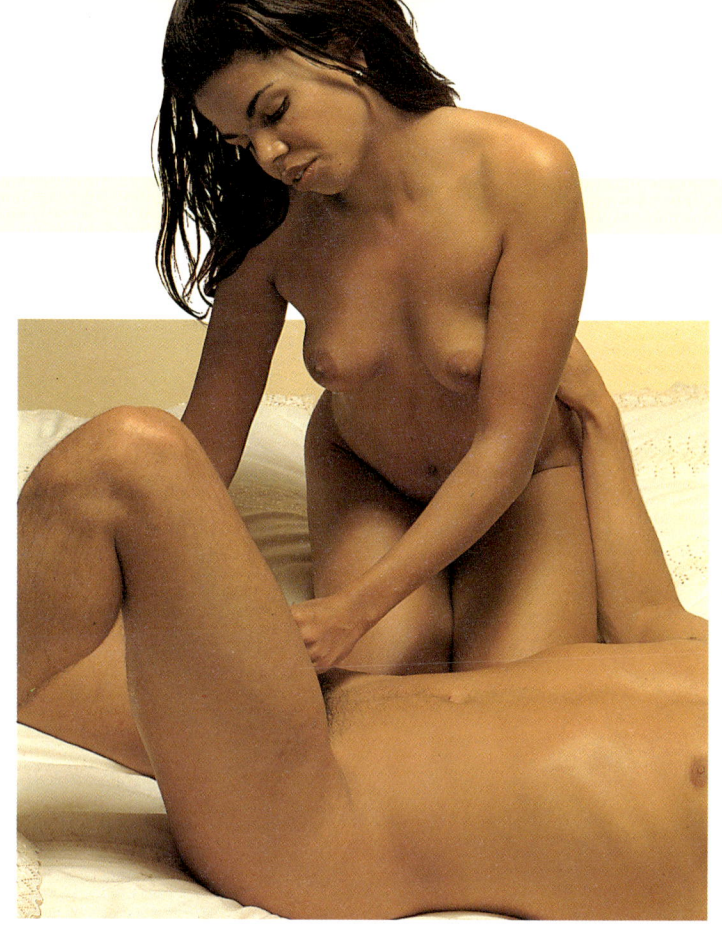

Guiding Hand
▲ Ask your man to show you exactly how he likes his penis to be touched. Stroking, rubbing and kissing his penis is all part of your sensual play. Being comfortable about touching this important part of his body will enhance your mutual satisfaction in lovemaking.

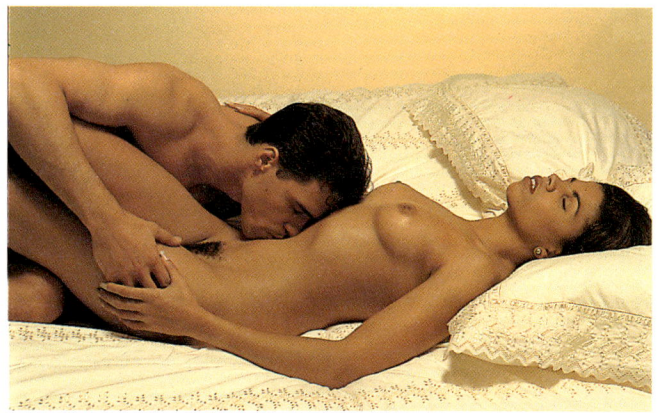

Understanding Each Other

Even in close relationships, both men and women can be remarkably shy about discussing their sexual needs with each other, including what turns them on and what turns them off. This is partly because the sexual ego is very fragile and it is easy to feel rejected or to take any comments, other than highly positive ones, as criticism.

Talking about sexual issues requires delicate negotiation, being able to choose the right moment, a willingness on both sides to experiment and explore new methods, and a readiness to change old patterns. The latter can be particularly difficult if your methods have worked perfectly well on previous occasions or with another partner.

However, by not disclosing your sexual needs and preferences, there is a danger that you may become resentful and gradually withhold your sexuality altogether from your partner, or deaden your sensory responses so that your sexual life becomes more of a functional duty rather than a joyful celebration of your relationship.

Sexuality should not be imposed on the other person regardless of how he or she may feel. Much of the pleasure can be in the mutual exploration of each other's bodily responses. It is a two-way interaction, involving many subtle nuances and variations. You can jangle along together, or you can compose a symphony of love, touch, sensuality and eroticism which will always hit the right note, depending on your changing needs and moods.

How most men and women touch and want to be touched in their most erotically charged areas – the penis and clitoris – reveals quite opposite male and female needs. A man will often long to receive firmer touches to his penis during manual stimulation, while a woman generally prefers a more subtle approach to the stimulation of her clitoris, usually after she has become aroused. You can help each other by showing exactly how you like to be touched.

Many men and women experiment with genital touching during masturbation and usually perfect their technique in doing so. (See Self-Pleasuring, and Mutual Masturbation.) Watch each other masturbate, or guide your partner's hand or fingers with your own, showing the different pressures and strokes that you most enjoy and that are most likely to help you reach your peak of arousal.

Sensual Play

Thighs and Sighs
▼ Don't focus your attention solely on her clitoris, but regularly return your sensual touches to other parts of her body, especially the areas close by, so that the erotic sensations can stream through her body. The insides of her thighs are a very erogenous area. Cover the soft skin with kisses, bringing your lips a little closer each time to this most intimate part of her body.

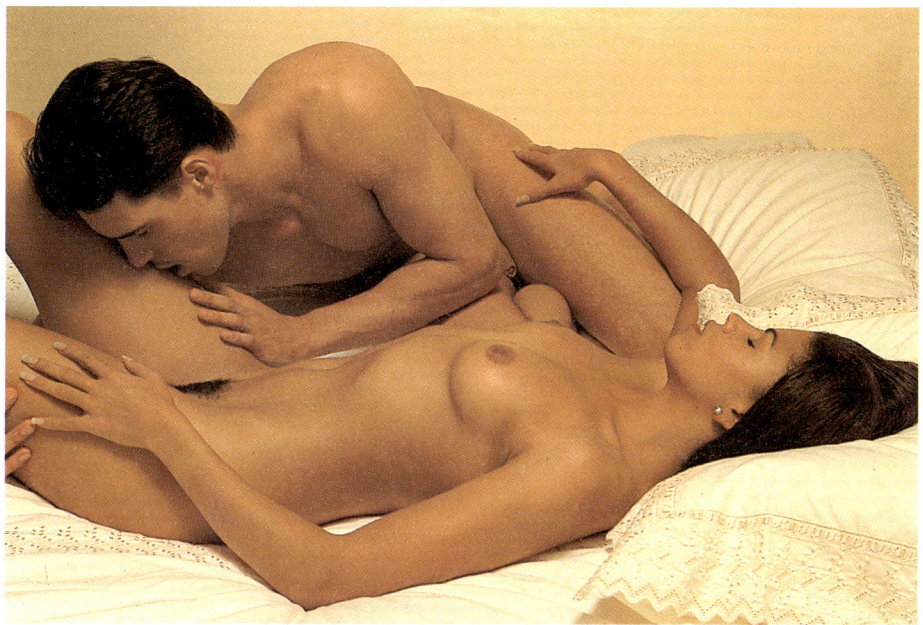

Just Connect
▼ Foreplay can bring you both to a state of arousal, where intercourse is the desired conclusion. As sensual play, it can also be complete in itself without penetrative sex. Just pleasuring each other, exploring every part of the body with loving oral and tactile stimulation, can create a deep and mutual sexual and emotional connection, whether or not it eventually leads to orgasm or sexual intercourse.

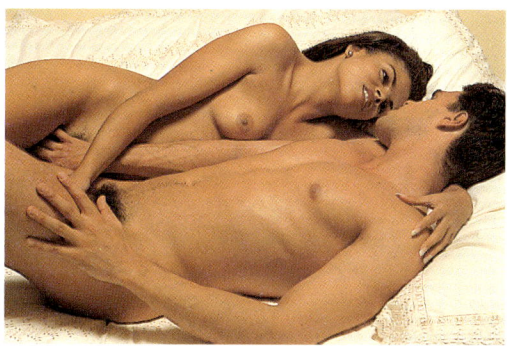

Clitoral Stimulation
Most women dislike having their clitoris roughly handled; it is an exquisitely sensitive part of their sexual anatomy. Correct stimulation of the clitoris is very important to a woman's sexual satisfaction and to her achieving an orgasm. Too much, too soon can be irritating and even painful.

Once your woman is aroused by more loving and sensual foreplay, and she is naturally producing her vaginal secretions, stroking, rubbing, licking, flicking the tongue back and forth and gentle sucking on the clitoris can create euphoric sensations throughout her whole body. However, she may not want you to focus stimulation directly onto her clitoris for a prolonged period of time, but would prefer if you also touched and palpated the surrounding areas, such as the vaginal lips and mons. Also, from time to time, return your attention to other parts of her body which will be pulsating with pleasure and demanding your caresses.

If you are using your fingers to stimulate the clitoris, then lubrication is important. It is best to spread some of the sexual juices from her vagina onto her clitoris. Otherwise, use your own saliva, or, if necessary, an appropriate cream, gel or oil (make sure it is hypo-allergenic as the tissues here are very sensitive and delicate – scented creams should never be used).

Vary your rhythm, vibrations and movements, but remain alert to her responses, which she will indicate by the movements of her pelvis, and her sighs, moans, and words of encouragement. Do not be afraid to ask her what, exactly, she likes best.

Penile Stimulation
A man most definitely wants his penis to be handled with care, but he may well prefer firmer pressure and strokes than he is actually getting from you. Many women err on the side of being too timid in the way they handle their lover's penis. Ask your man to show you exactly what he likes. Watch him stimulate himself, and then let him put his hand over yours to move it up and down the glans and shaft. This way you can learn whether he likes short or long strokes, rapid or more sensual ones.

Remember, though, if you want to extend your foreplay, do not overstimulate his penis at this point, or you can bring your man to orgasm too soon. During sensual play, kissing and licking the penis and testicles tenderly, flicking your tongue over them, and saying appreciative things about this treasured part of his body, will make him feel especially good.

Oral-Genital Sex

Oral-genital sex can be one of the most enjoyable and sexually arousing options available to people who seek pleasure and fulfilment from a sexual relationship. The term refers to the sexual activity in which men and women stimulate each other's genitals by use of the mouth and tongue. When a woman receives this from a man it is called cunnilingus, and when a man receives this from a woman it is called fellatio. The degree to which a couple may include oral sex in their lovemaking will vary from one sexual episode to another and between one couple and another.

Many people like to include oral sex as a special intimacy to aid arousal in their foreplay, but prefer to attain orgasmic satisfaction through coitus. Others like it to be a complete sexual experience in itself, through which both sexes are able to achieve a deeply satisfying orgasm and emotional and physical intimacy, with or without intercourse.

A woman, who is more inclined to reach orgasm through clitoral and vulval stimulation rather than vaginal stimulation from the penis alone, can find it particularly beneficial to her arousal and subsequent sexual satisfaction. The soft moistness of the tongue and its sensual movements suits the delicate clitoral area very well, and is more likely to excite her and less likely to irritate than having a dry finger rubbed against the area during manual stimulation. If her partner is prone to ejaculate before she has reached her own peak of arousal, he can use his tongue to help her reach an orgasm.

The majority of men take special pleasure in receiving fellatio from their partners. Depending on the particular situation, a man may enjoy it purely as a method of arousal and then want to proceed towards full penetrative intercourse, or he may hope that his woman uses her mouth to bring him to orgasm.

Although oral sex is highly arousing, some men who have a tendency to ejaculate prematurely find that oral stimulation gives them greater control over their orgasmic processes than if they had vaginal sex without it. In other circumstances, the very thought or sight of seeing a woman performing fellatio, or the erotic sensations created by her tongue and mouth on his penis can very quickly bring a man to the peak of arousal. In this case, if the couple are looking forward to an extended period of lovemaking, it would be better to avoid overstimulating his penis through oral sex methods.

One of the most delightful aspects of oral sex is that it provides the opportunity for lovers to take it in turns to surrender themselves totally to simply giving or receiving loving and highly erotic attention. Some couples save oral sex for a special treat, perhaps only on a birthday, or on holiday, or to mark a romantic

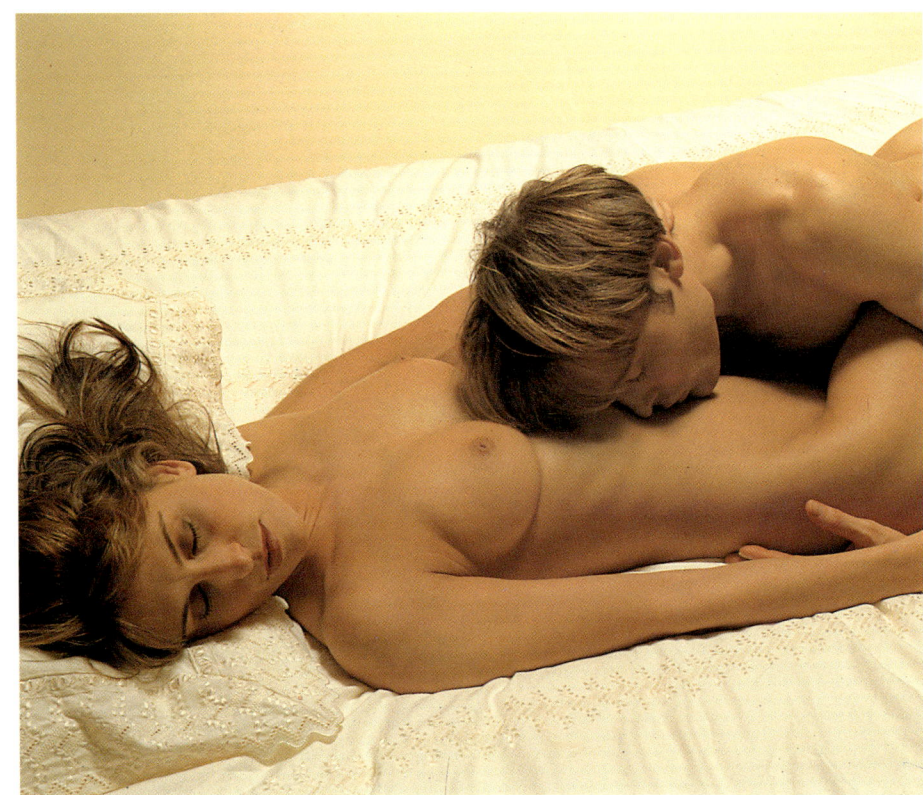

Spread Your Loving Touch
◀ *She will be more receptive and eager for oral sex if she feels able to trust in your love for her and is already aroused by your mutual sensual play. Don't let her feel as if her clitoris and vagina are the only areas of her body you are interested in. Before, during and after cunnilingus, acknowledge her whole body and pay special attention to the areas surrounding her genitals, such as the belly, mons and thighs.*

Oral-Genital Sex

anniversary. In a relationship that includes oral sex, only the couple involved will know from experience, when and how to use it to enhance their love life.

Cunnilingus

Your sexual partner is the best teacher in showing you exactly how to please her. Woman all have different responses, so experiment together and let her guide you with soft sighs, encouraging words, and pelvic movements to discover how your mouth and tongue can thrill her.

Most women would prefer to be aroused through sensual play, loving strokes, kisses, and whole body attention before they receive any direct stimulation of the clitoral area. This gives a woman time to produce and secrete her own love juices, so her vulva becomes receptive, warm, wet and welcoming.

Women often complain that men either neglect the clitoris or they zone in on it before they have become aroused, which can be irritating and painful. Before you begin to perform cunnilingus, kiss and excite all the areas adjacent to her genitals, then gently nuzzle and lick over her mons and vulva.

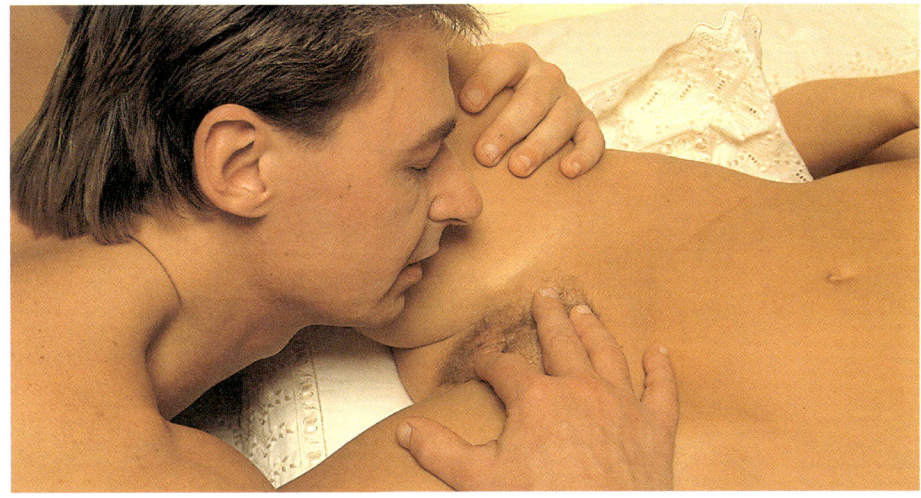

Her Arousal Blossoms
▲ Nuzzle into her mons and vulva, seducing it with the warmth of your kisses. As she relaxes and becomes increasingly aroused, her vaginal lips will begin to swell and lubricate and produce her exotic sexual scent. When she is ready, this area will begin to open to you like a flower in the morning sun.

When she is aroused, her clitoris will swell, as will the lips of her vulva. You can gently part her lips, and begin to thrill her with your tongue. Change your strokes and pressures and pay special attention to the areas surrounding her clitoris as this can be even more arousing. Let your tongue playfully stroke around the vagina, even thrusting a little into it. (Never blow air into her vagina. This can cause an air embolism and may be dangerous.) Change the rhythm and action of your tongue, as too much sustained pressure can be irritating. You can also suck gently on her clitoris, and flick your tongue over it from side to side.

Be alert to her signals so that you can judge whether she wants you to take her all the way to orgasm, or would prefer to change to another activity. She might want to return the favour, or to take your penis into her vagina so that you can both orgasm in coitus. Cunnilingus can bring some

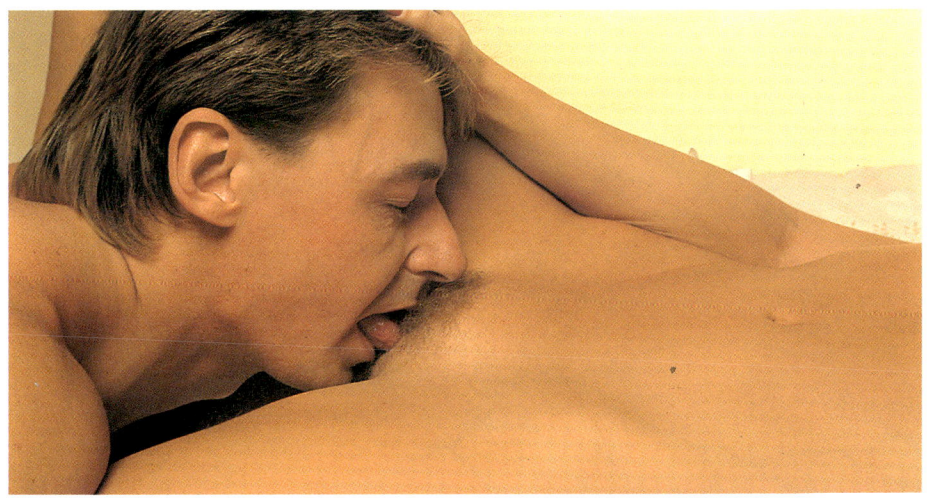

The Pleasure Builds
◀ She will treasure you as a lover if you really learn to love this intimate part of her. Apply stimulation to her clitoris only after she is fully aroused, but don't focus directly on it all the time. She may find it more pleasing to have the areas surrounding the clitoris stroked by the moist softness of your tongue. Slowly build up the pressure, or speed up your strokes, but let the tempo vary. Be alert to her signals of pleasure.

Basic Techniques

women into a multi-orgasmic state, so she may just want you to continue.

For other women, the clitoris becomes extremely sensitive after an orgasm. In that case, she probably won't want you to continue to stimulate it and may even move your head away. If you are sensitive to her cues, you can take her all the way to a state of ecstasy.

Fellatio

If you are performing fellatio on your man, it is probably a good idea to place one hand around the shaft of the penis so you can control his thrusting movements. In this way, you can overcome the fear that you might inadvertently choke. Your man should always let you remain in control of the movements, and he should refrain from thrusting deeply into your mouth, no matter how excited he is.

Begin by nuzzling, fondling, kissing and licking his pubic area, penis and scrotum and stroking his perineum so he becomes more aroused and his erection increases. Then run your tongue over the most erotically sensitive parts of his penis – the top and around the ridge of its tip (the glans) – and along its shaft, flicking your tongue from side to side or up and down. Focus special attention on the underside of the penis as this part is particularly sensitive to stimulation.

Experiment with the movements of your tongue, changing its pressure and rhythm, and encourage him to tell you what he likes. Men generally prefer a strong, firm pressure on the penis, and sometimes complain that a woman's touch is too light and timid. He will enjoy you fondling his scrotum too, but remember that here you need a light touch as this is his most delicate area. Once you have taken his penis into your mouth, ensure that your teeth don't make contact. Cover them with your lips – remember, his greatest fear is that you will bite or nip it by accident.

Prolonged fellatio may make your jaw ache, so rest your mouth if you need to, continuing the stimulation by hand in the meantime. Try to put yourself in your man's body and imagine what sensations he must be feeling and let your imagination guide you. (Despite the fact that fellatio is commonly referred to as a "blow job", never blow into your man's penis as this can be harmful.)

Ask him to let you know if he is going to orgasm – or be alert to his signals. It is up to you to decide whether you want him to ejaculate in your mouth, or would prefer to move on to another stage of lovemaking. You may be very willing to go all the way during fellatio, feeling that you are imbibing the very essence your man into yourself if you swallow his semen. It can bring you great pleasure because you know he will feel loved and totally accepted by you and that, in itself, can be deeply arousing.

You may, however, be willing to do this only if you feel secure and very much in love with your partner. It may be that you simply cannot stomach the idea of swallowing seminal fluid, even though you may feel fine about performing fellatio, or even of having your man ejaculate in your mouth. In that case, keep some tissues close at hand so that you can discreetly dispose of the seminal fluid from your mouth.

If you don't want him to ejaculate in your mouth, you can manually stimulate him to orgasm. Let him

Teasing Touches

▼ *Work your way slowly and sensuously down his body towards his genitals, bringing the whole surface of his skin alive with your breath, lips, tongue and touches. Linger over his belly, kissing teasingly around the pubic area, and moving inch by inch closer to his genitals.*

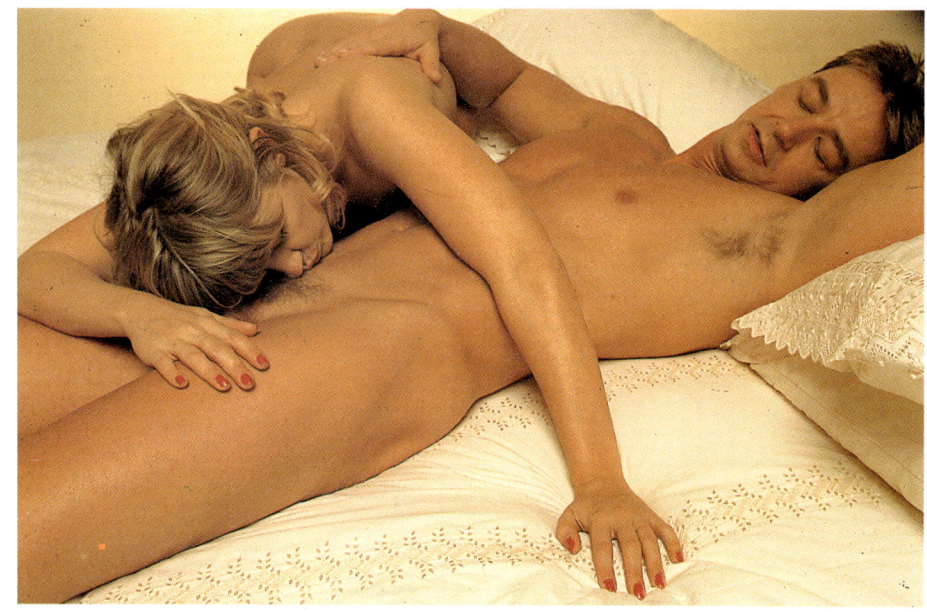

come on another part of your body, rub his penis between your breasts until he ejaculates, or guide it into your vagina so you can carry on to intercourse.

Concerns and Objections

Many couples feel that oral sex is an integral and natural feature of their sex lives and, for some, it is the best part of it. Oral sex has always been an option for men and women in sexual relationships and the practice is recorded in ancient texts such as *The Kama Sutra*. However, at different times in history, and in different cultures, it has been considered deviant behaviour. In the early part of this century a request for oral sex could be considered grounds for divorce. In some states of America it was outlawed.

Research now shows that the majority of sexually active people have participated in oral sex at some point in their lives, though statistics indicate that more men than women enjoy it or put it at the top of their list of favourite sexual practices. This may have something to do with the fact that men are not always so skilled in performing oral sex to their women's satisfaction.

Women, too, can have deep anxieties about the smell, taste and appearance of their vaginal area. They may be against the idea of putting the penis into their mouths for fear of choking, or repulsed by the idea of swallowing seminal fluids if the man ejaculates.

Oral sex is a normal, healthy activity in an intimate relationship. However, if you do not want to do it, you should not consider yourself lacking or abnormal in any way. It is a very personal choice. You should never try to pressurize your partner, or be forced against your will into performing or receiving oral sex, or any other sexual activity, if either one of you objects, even if you participate in it on some occasions but are just not in the mood right now.

It is an extremely intimate activity, and should only be performed with total mutual consent. A partner's refusal to participate in oral sex may be rooted in deep moral or religious convictions and is not necessarily a rejection of the other person. Everyone has their own sexual boundaries and limits, and while many loving couples feel secure enough to abandon all or most of their sexual inhibitions, some individuals may genuinely need to set rules.

Discuss these issues honestly with each other because understanding and accepting each other's truths is an important part of a loving and intimate relationship. Some people, particularly women, can only participate in oral sex activities if they are deeply in love and feel the relationship is a committed one. They may come to enjoy oral-genital contact once the sexual relationship has become established and secure. Patience can often be rewarded.

Some of the objections people have to oral sex may be based more on fears, misconceptions and misinformation, such as that it is "dirty" or harmful, or they may have anxieties about the genitals being ugly, or smelling or tasting unpleasant. Such

Good Vibrations

▶ When you are ready, take his penis into your mouth, to whatever depth you feel most comfortable. You can suck on his penis or vibrate your tongue over the shaft.

Sexual Exploration

▼ Many men love the sensation of having their scrotum gently stimulated by loving licks and kisses. Move his penis gently to one side and explore the whole area with your tongue, while stroking his thighs and buttocks and perineal region with your other hand.

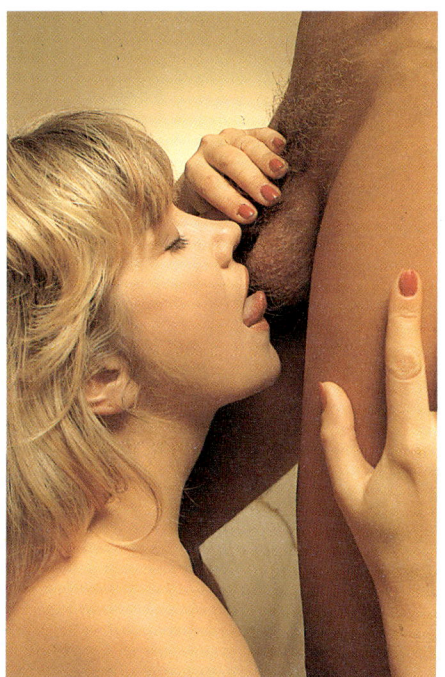

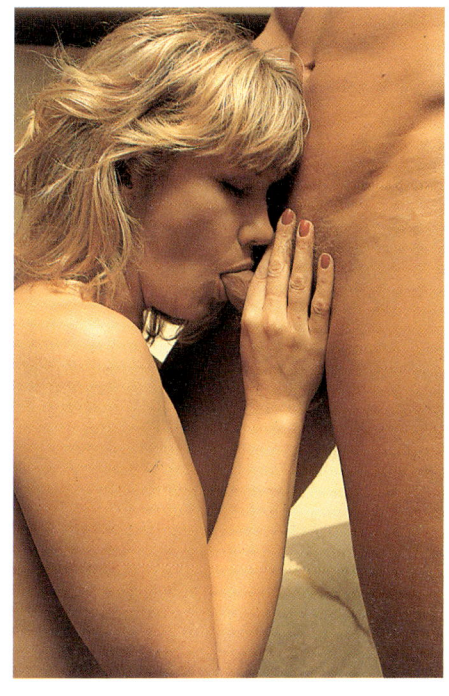

Basic Techniques

anxieties can usually be alleviated with gentle understanding, exploration and support. Reading sex manuals like this one, or speaking to a psycho-sexual counsellor can also help to alleviate unnecessarily inhibiting anxieties or phobias.

Smelling and Tasting Good

As a woman, probably your biggest concern about receiving oral sex is whether those intimate parts of you are going to taste and smell good to your man. Normally, your natural, special, musky, and earthy sexual scent and taste will be very appealing to him. Those men who are squeamish about vaginal secretions and smells will probably avoid oral sex altogether, or move on quickly. The taste and smell of your sexual secretions can be affected, however, if you have eaten lots of spicy or garlic-flavoured food.

The secretions sometimes become more acrid or metallic tasting just before a menstrual period. Try sexual honesty, and ask your partner to let you know if the taste suddenly changes and he would rather abstain. If you notice a strong smell or discharge from your vagina, you may have an infection. In that case, put oral sex on hold and seek a medical check-up.

The normal amount of seminal fluid in each ejaculation is about a teaspoonful, and for those who are weight conscious, it contains about five calories. It has the constituency of raw egg white and tastes a little salty. Except in the case of infection or sexually transmitted disease (in which case oral sex should be avoided), there is no evidence to prove that swallowing semen is harmful in any way to a woman, providing she is a willing participant in the act.

Sixty-Nine

The name sixty-nine refers to a form of oral sex in which the man and woman take up a head-to-tail position to mutually pleasure each other. It is sometimes known as soixante-neuf – which is French for sixty-nine. It can be performed with one person lying on top of the other, but facing the opposite direction, so that both mouths are close enough to the genitals to apply simultaneous oral stimulation. In this position, it is usually preferable for the woman to be on top of her man because of the probable weight difference.

Another more comfortable position to take is with both partners lying on their sides, facing each other, but in opposite directions. The upper leg should be opened away from the genital area. Each partner can then place his or her head on the other's lower thigh so that mouths and tongues are close to the genitals.

Soixante-Neuf
▼ *The sixty-nine position is worth experimenting with and adding to your sexual repertoire.*

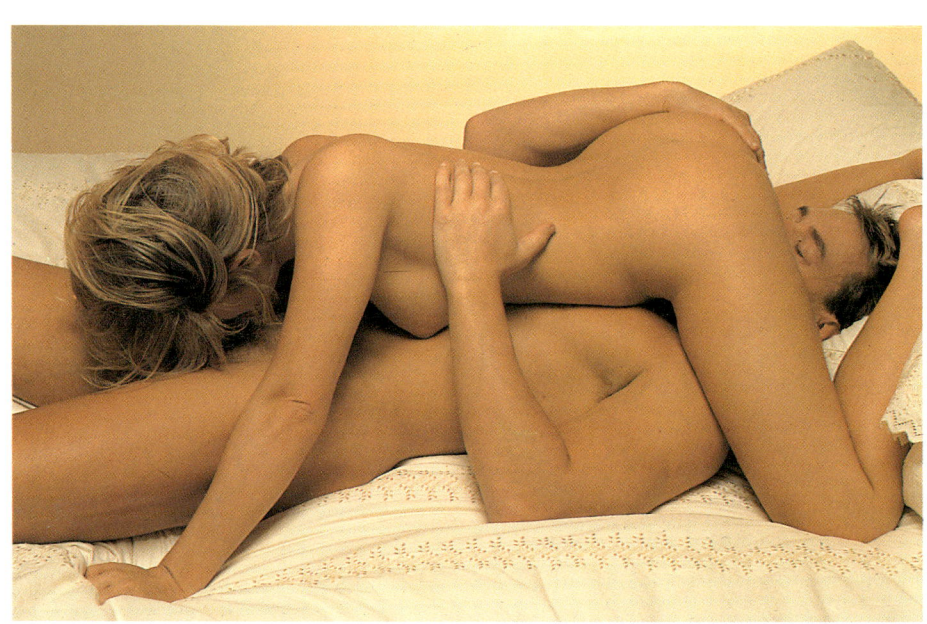

> ### When To Abstain From Oral Sex
>
> The chapter on Safer Sex explains the risks involved in HIV/AIDS transmission during oral-genital sex practices. If you are unsure about your own or your partner's health, or know little about each other's sexual history, then fellatio should be performed only when using a condom or, in the case of cunnilingus, a dental dam.
>
> You should not participate in oral sex if you have an active cold sore around your mouth, or a genital herpes sore, or any other kind of infection or sexually transmitted disease, until it has been treated and cleared up. Oral sex is not advisable during a menstrual period because of the risk of blood-transmitted infections.

Oral-Genital Sex

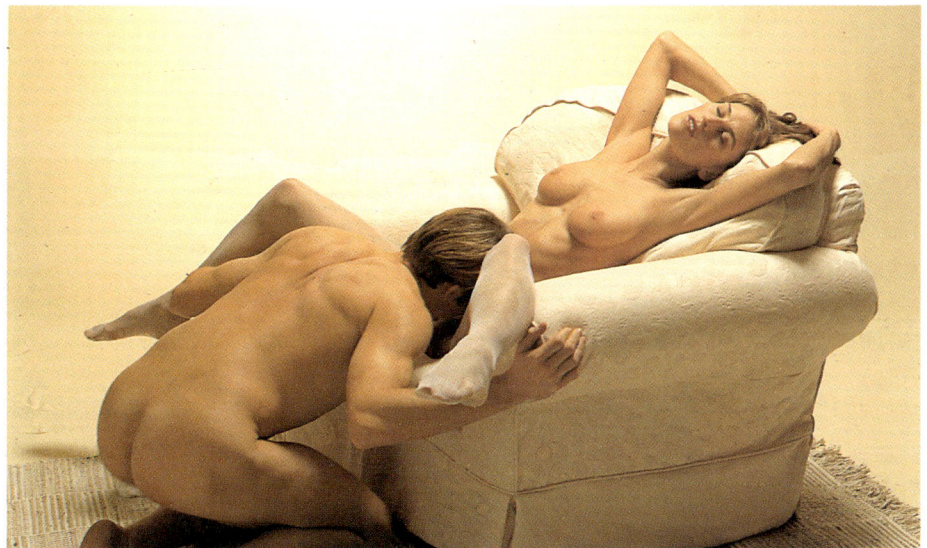

Kneel and Play
▲ *She can sit on an armchair with legs spread over the arms while you kneel in front of her and adorn her vulva with succulent kisses, licks and all manner of exciting forms of oral play. In this position, she can relax completely, abandoning herself to overwhelming whole body sensations.*

While the sixty-nine position in oral sex can lead to wonderfully erotic sensations, and can be taken all the way to mutual orgasm, it is often preferred as a part of foreplay, rather than as a full orgasmic experience in itself. One disadvantage of the practice is that it is quite difficult to really relax and enjoy the sensations you are receiving at one end of your body, while being actively involved at the other. You may also climax at different times.

If you do achieve an orgasm while receiving this kind of oral stimulation, you won't necessarily be able to control your responses or muscle contractions, and it is highly unlikely in these moments that you will be able to continue returning the favour.

Other Positions

Couples can be fantastically inventive with sexual positions once they feel relaxed about each other's bodies and are in the full flow of arousal. Here are some other suggested positions for giving and receiving oral-genital stimulation – though the chances are, you will create some more that are uniquely your own.

One partner can lie down with the other partner kneeling over the face, so that the genitals are close to the mouth. From this position, the active person can also stroke and squeeze the buttocks to give added stimulation. If a woman is performing fellatio from this position, she should ring her man's penis with one hand so she can have full control over how much enters her mouth. The man should be careful not to thrust too hard.

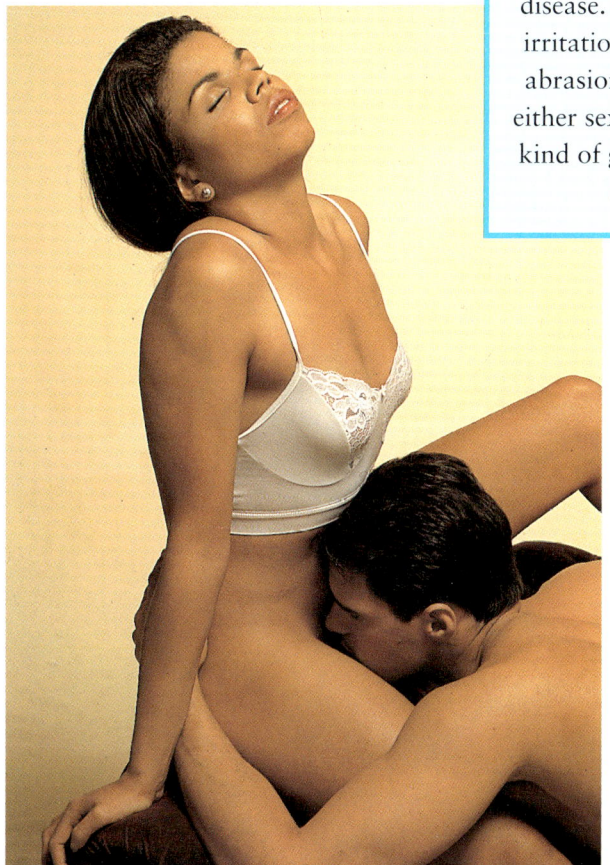

Armchair Arousal
◀ *She can support herself while sitting back in an armchair or on the edge of the bed, while you arouse her with your mouth, and stroke her buttocks and thighs at the same time.*

> ### Sexual Hygiene
> Careful hygiene precautions should be taken by both men and women before intimate sexual contact but there is no reason to believe that the genital area is a dirty, taboo or unclean part of the body just because it is "down there". Adequate bathing, or even washing each other's genitals in the shower before making love, should suffice. Special care should be taken to ensure the anal area is also clean before any intimate contact to avoid the risk of spreading infection or passing on a sexually transmitted disease. If there are any signs of irritation or discharge, sores or abrasions in the genital area of either sex, then abstain from any kind of genital contact and seek medical advice.

Compatibility

There are no rules about the positions you take or the things you do while making love, except one – that both of you should feel physically and emotionally satisfied by the experience. Often, at the beginning of a relationship, you need time to gauge what gives pleasure and feels good, which movements work harmoniously and what pace and rhythm feels right. Lovemaking tends to improve as you get to know one another's preferences and responses. You then begin to fall in tune with each other in much the same way that musicians or dancers do when they continually practise their art together.

What will increase your sexual compatibility is not an array of impressive techniques, nor a unique sexual position, but intimacy and tenderness, and the willingness to learn from, and be open to, each other. The way you make love may change from one episode to another because the act of intercourse should reflect the mood and feelings of the moment, rather than following a preconceived pattern. Passionate lovemaking may feel exhilarating on one occasion, yet on another, a vulnerable and tender approach will suit your needs better.

Well tried and tested formulas of lovemaking may need to be jettisoned if new lovers are to remain spontaneous with each other. What worked well in a past liaison may simply not be appropriate to a new sexual relationship. Everyone's timing, arousal levels and bodily responses are unique – unravelling those mysteries together is the key.

Sharing and Caring
▶ *Sexual intercourse is not just about body positions and movement, or skills and techniques – it involves the heart, mind and emotional being of each person concerned. Love and intimacy, and a sense of comfort, appreciation and sharing, are the main ingredients necessary to ensure that coitus satisfies and nurtures both parties.*

Compatibility

Time to Explore
▼ With a new sexual relationship, allow plenty of time for sensuality, exploring your partner's body during foreplay, so that you get to know each other's physical responses. Being in tune with one another leads to compatible lovemaking.

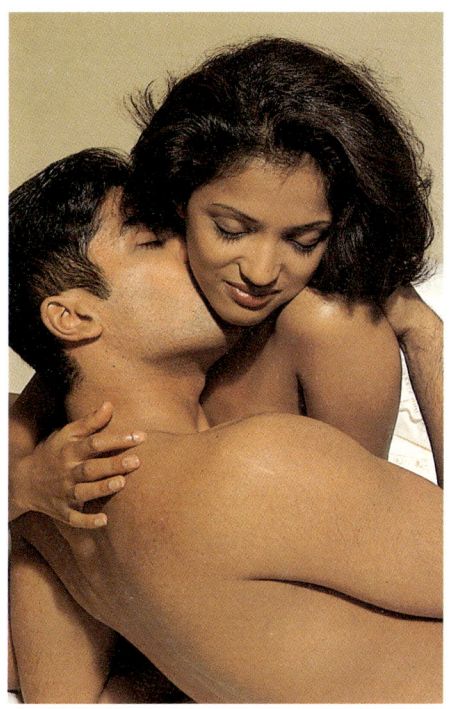

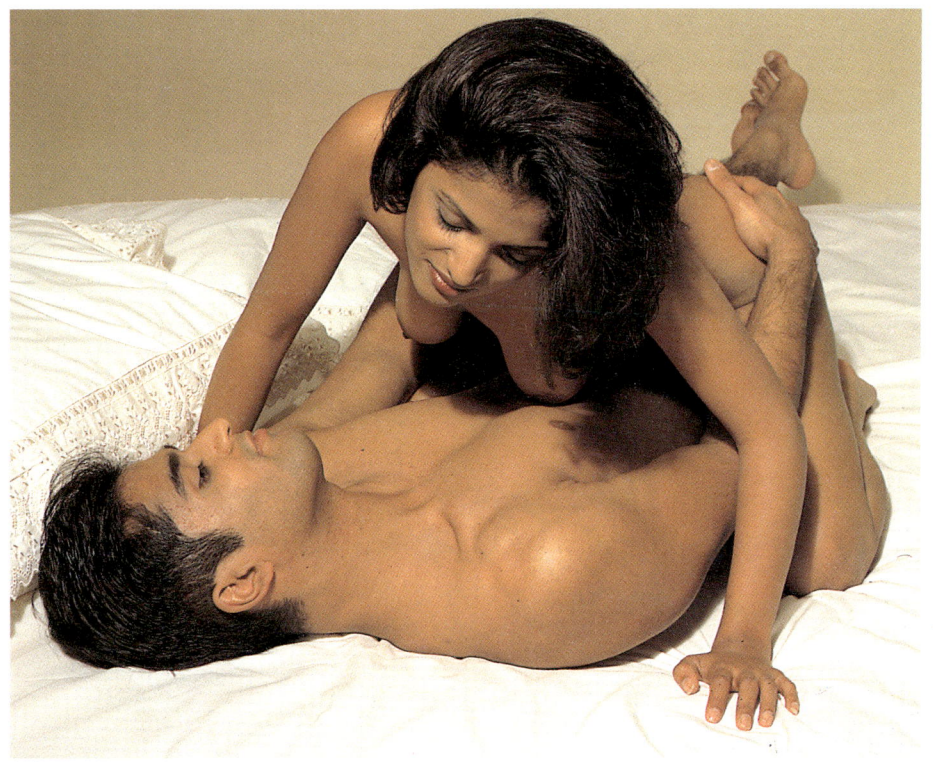

Whole-Body Contact
▲ During intercourse, tactile contact should not be confined to the genitals alone. For example, the female partner can use her breasts and hair to caress the man's chest as she sensually sways her body from side to side. Continue touching and kissing the whole body throughout lovemaking.

Enjoying the Afterglow
◄ After making love, you can lie in each other's arms, bathed in a glow of contentment, rested, relaxed and nourished by the experience. For some people, these are the happiest moments of all.

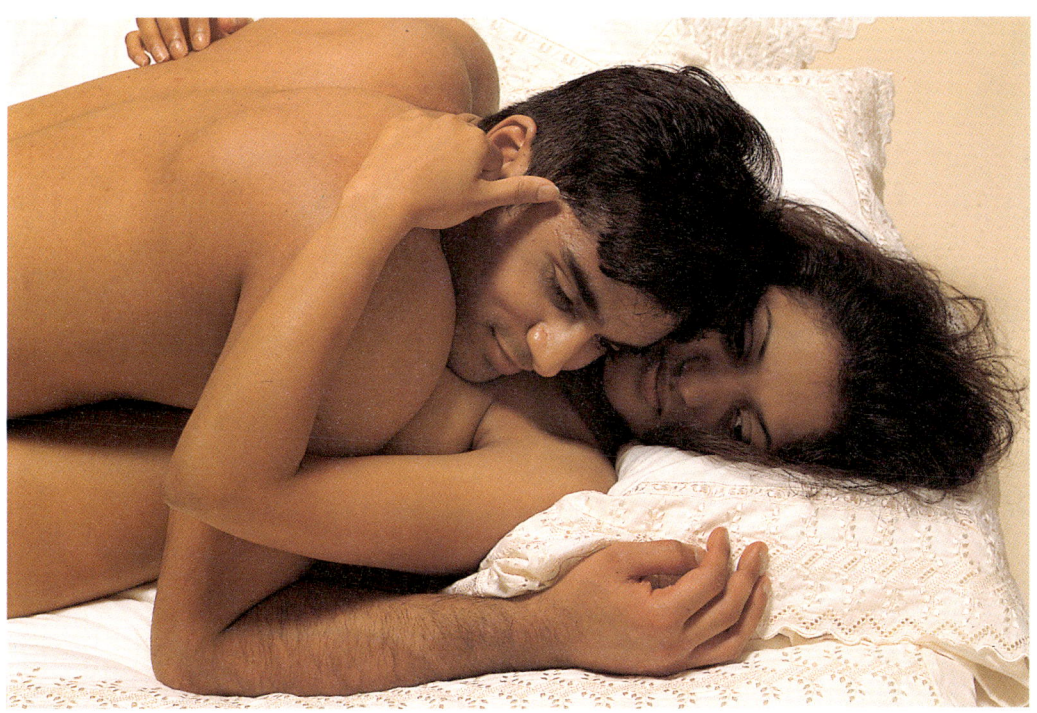

The Basic Positions

There are a number of lovemaking positions in common practice that most couples feel comfortable with. These allow both the man and woman to express themselves sexually in different ways by taking more active or passive roles in the lovemaking, and thereby eliciting a variety of physical and emotional responses. An equal and balanced sexual partnership is capable of sharing the more dominant and submissive roles quite easily, allowing a natural transfer between the two, either within one episode of lovemaking, or on different occasions.

Exploration, experimentation and a sense of humour are important to keep a sexual relationship interesting and alive. Once you feel comfortable and secure with each other, it is worth trying something new to add variety, fun, and excitement to your lovemaking.

Here, we sum up the basic lovemaking positions, and then on the following pages of this chapter, some of the more popular sexual positions assumed by couples in coitus will be discussed in greater detail. In other sections of this book you will find more adventurous positions that you can add to your lovemaking repertoire, as well as ideas on spontaneous and fun lovemaking.

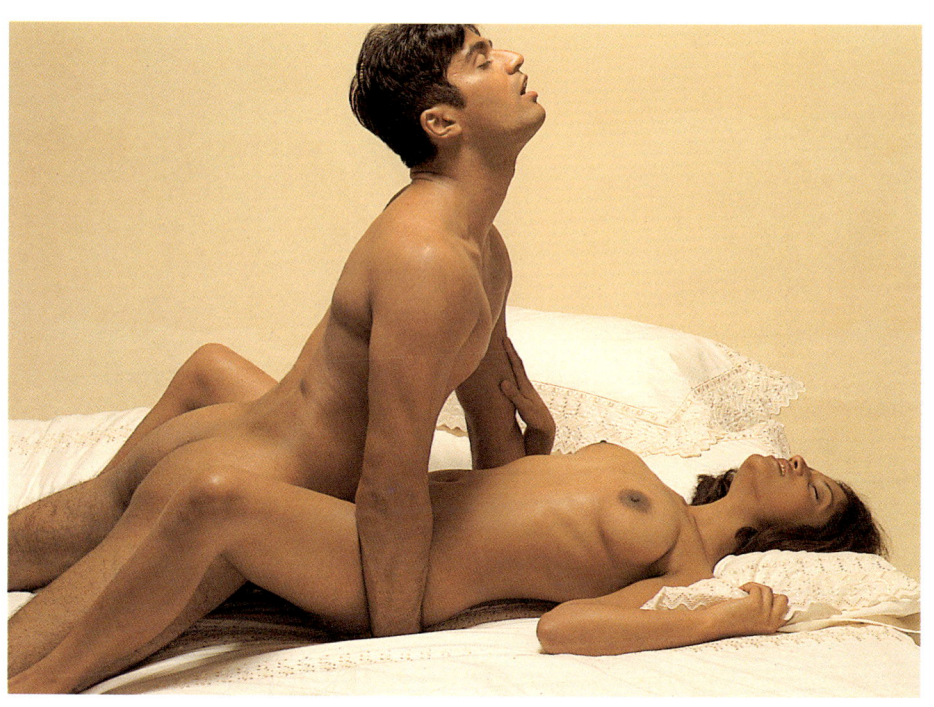

Man on Top
▲ The most commonly practised position for lovemaking is when the man assumes the more active role and moves on top of his partner. This allows face-to-face intimacy and full, front-of-the-body contact. The nature of this position means the man takes the more dominant role, while the female role is more submissive.

Woman on Top
◄ The woman-on-top position enables the couple to swap the more active and passive roles and allows them to experience and express other aspects of their sexuality. The woman has more freedom to move and is better able to control the depth of the man's thrusts and the stimulation she may need to reach orgasm.

The Basic Positions

Sitting Position
▶ In this sitting position, the couple can feel equal in their sexual roles as it allows them to embrace each other closely and feel intimately bonded. While their movements are somewhat limited, it is a perfect lovemaking posture for more meditative intercourse.

Kneeling Back to Front
▼ This is a variation of the woman-on-top position in which she kneels astride the man's hips with her back turned to him. While it does not have the intimacy and contact of a face-to-face position, it can allow both partners time to surrender deeply to their own sensations of sexual pleasure. The man can also stroke the woman's back and buttocks, or squeeze the buttocks gently to give her extra erotic stimulation.

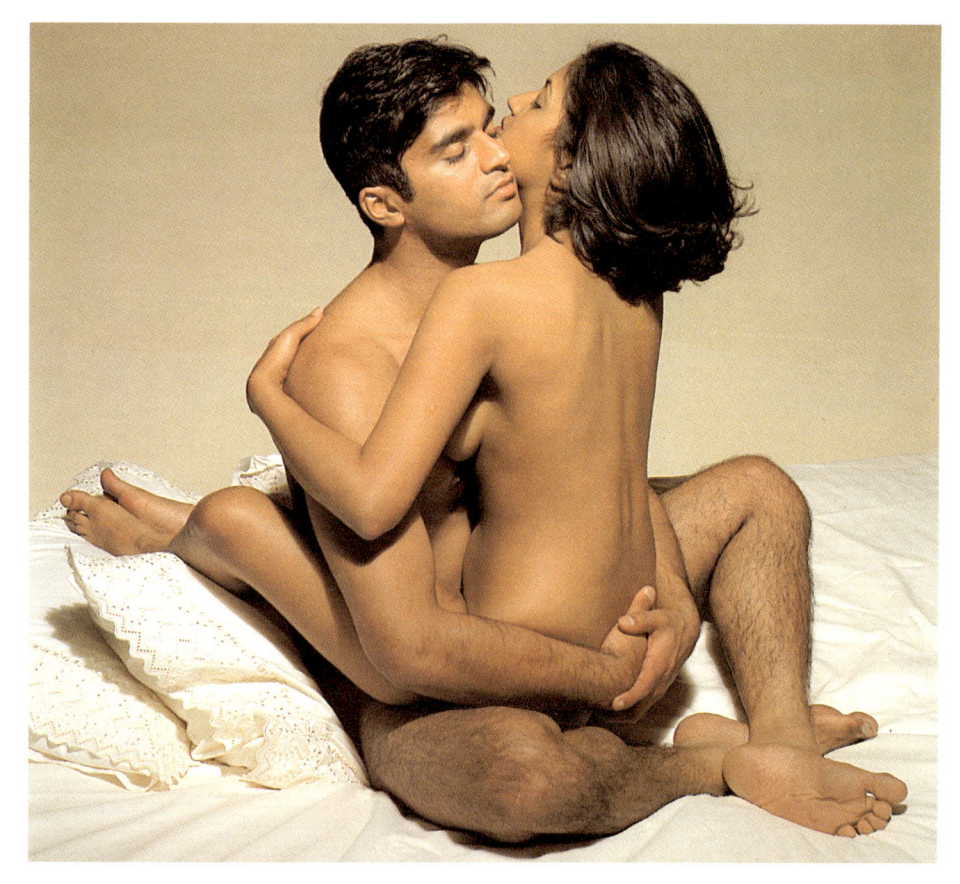

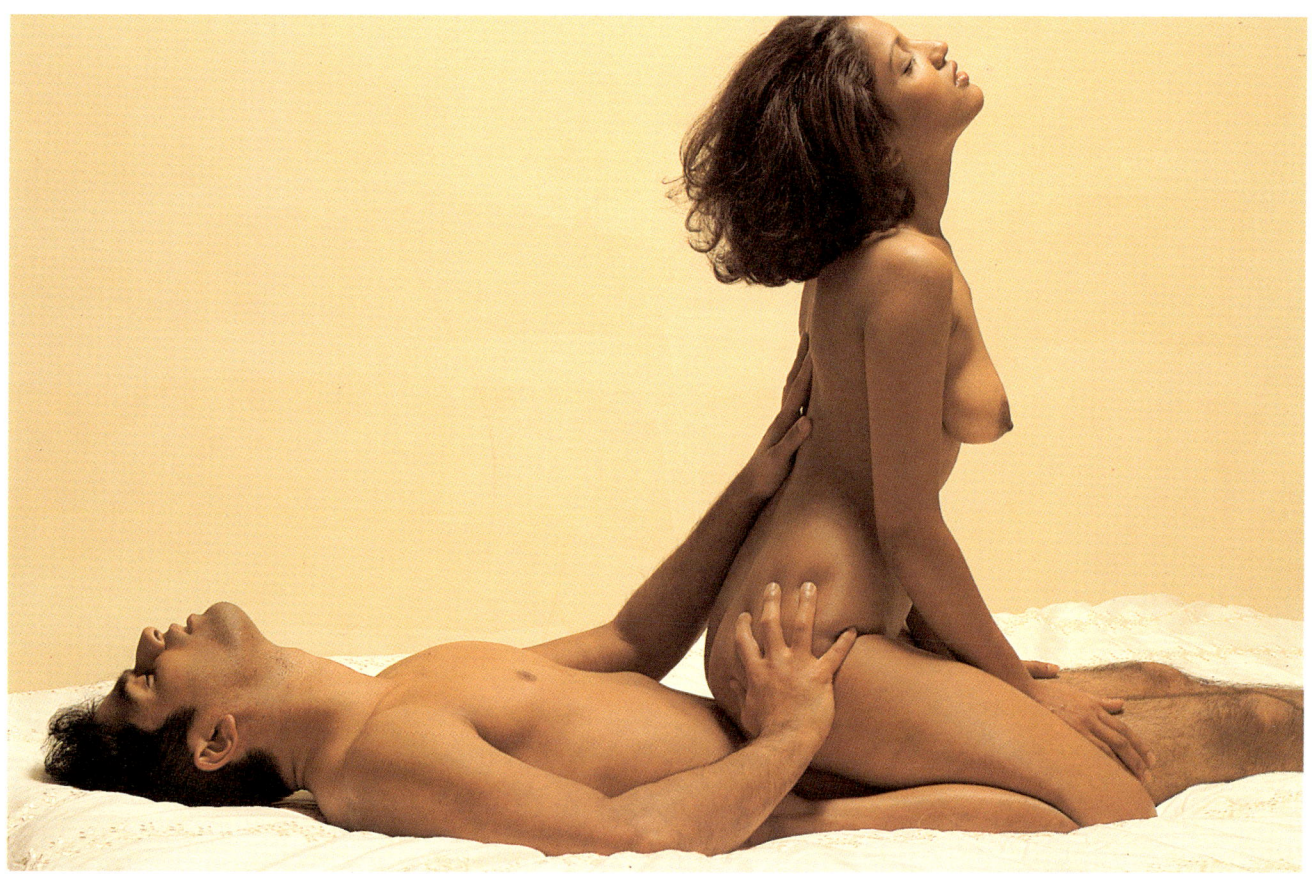

35

Basic Techniques

The Man-on-Top Position

Intercourse in which the man assumes the more dominant role, on top of the woman, is one of the most commonly adopted sexual positions. However, as an automatic choice it has been challenged in more recent times because sexually liberated women are just as eager to share the active role in sex.

It is popularly known as "the missionary position", a name first given by Pacific Islanders who witnessed the "strange" marital activities of white missionaries – the wife on her back with her husband on top. The islanders preferred to make love with the woman squatting over her man – a position which allowed her to express her sexuality fully. Certainly the "missionary position" would have been the obvious choice whenever the man assumed the dominant role in the partnership, or the woman regarded her sexual role purely as a duty.

That it still remains a popular choice for sexually emancipated couples is probably because it is a very intimate position, in which partners remain face to face and in eye contact, allowing the exchange of tender and arousing kisses, and words of love. In addition, it offers close physical contact between the most erogenous and vulnerable parts of the body, the pubis, abdomen, chest and breasts.

A woman who, on other occasions, enjoys exploring and expressing the more active part of her erotic nature may also enjoy relaxing sexually into the more submissive role, and letting her man take charge. While this position obviously suits a man who prefers to be the active sexual partner, he should also be prepared to explore other postures if his partner so desires.

The advantage of this position for a man is that he has more command over his pelvic movements. His penis is at a comfortable angle to enter the woman's vagina, and he has better control over the depth of its thrusts, which enables him to regulate his pace and rhythm so that he is able to gain the maximum stimulation needed to reach orgasm.

Preparing for Penetration

▼ *When sensual play progresses to intercourse it is a moment of physical and psychological transition for the man and woman. Both need to be ready in body and mind for this deeper level of intimacy and penetration, so it is important to stay in touch with your own and your partner's responses. Don't rush into penetration if either of you is not quite ready for it. If both are fully aroused by the touches, kisses, words and embraces of foreplay, the woman's vulva will have swelled, and her vagina will be secreting its juices, in readiness to receive the penis; the man's penis will be erect and firm, and able to enter her. Emotionally, both should be open and available to each other, as they enter into coitus. To check that the woman is sufficiently lubricated to accept his penis, the man can stroke his fingers over her vulva and vaginal opening, or simply ask her if she is ready for penetration. She may indicate by words, sounds or touch that she wants him to enter her. He can then guide his penis into her vagina.*

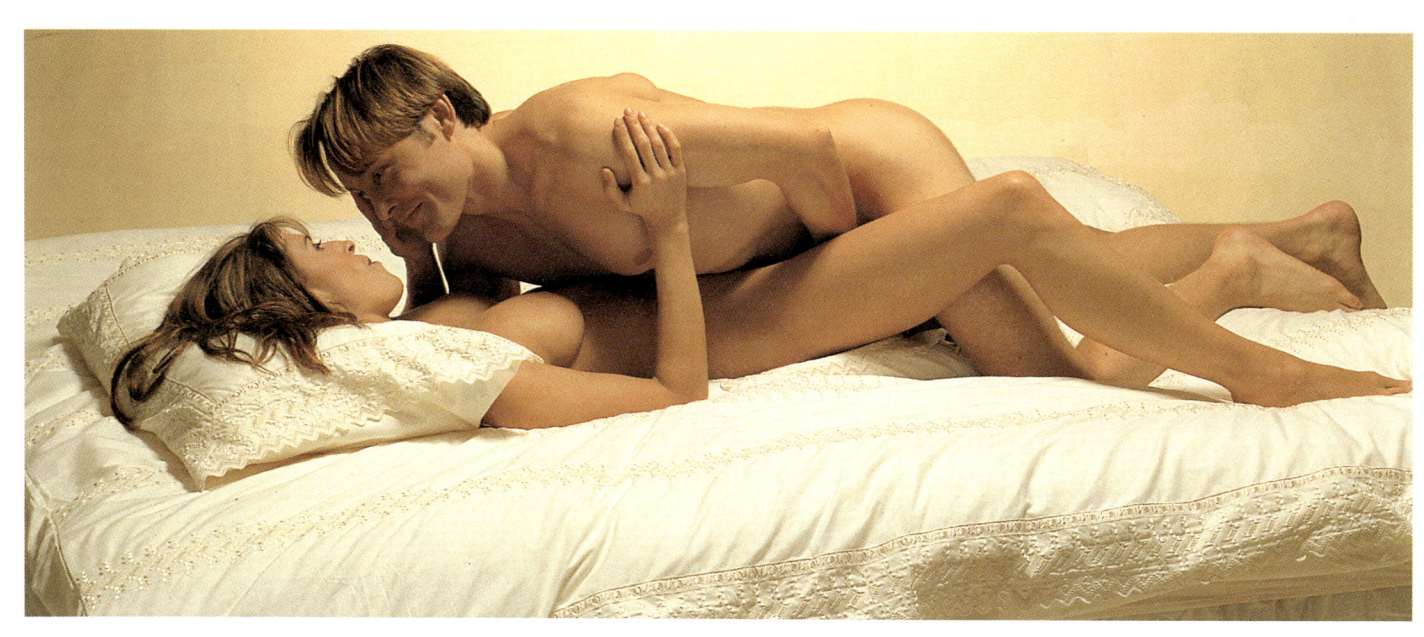

The Basic Positions

Slow Entry

▼ In this basic man-on-top position, the man is between the woman's legs as his penis begins to penetrate her vagina. She lies on her back, and opens her legs wide to give him room to enter her. Slow and careful manoeuvring will ensure the penis remains in the vagina and does not slip out, which can happen if either tries to move too rapidly before both bodies have adjusted their fit to each other. Many women love a slow entry, when the tip of the penis enters and lingers teasingly just within the vaginal orifice. This can give her further time to relax, emotionally and physically, so that her vagina is flooded with the total desire to be filled. She can also reach down to caress his scrotum and the shaft of his penis, which is waiting to enter.

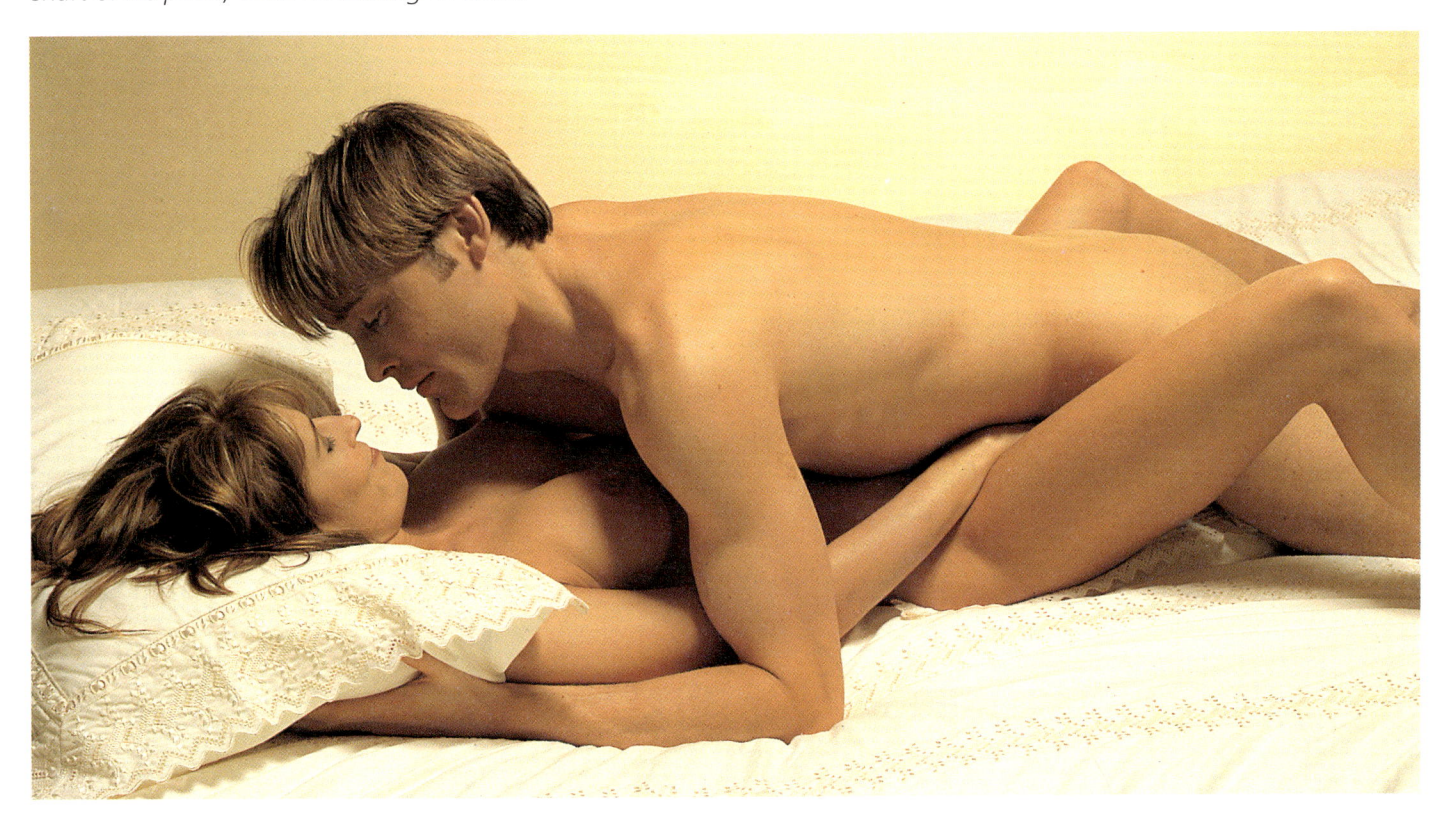

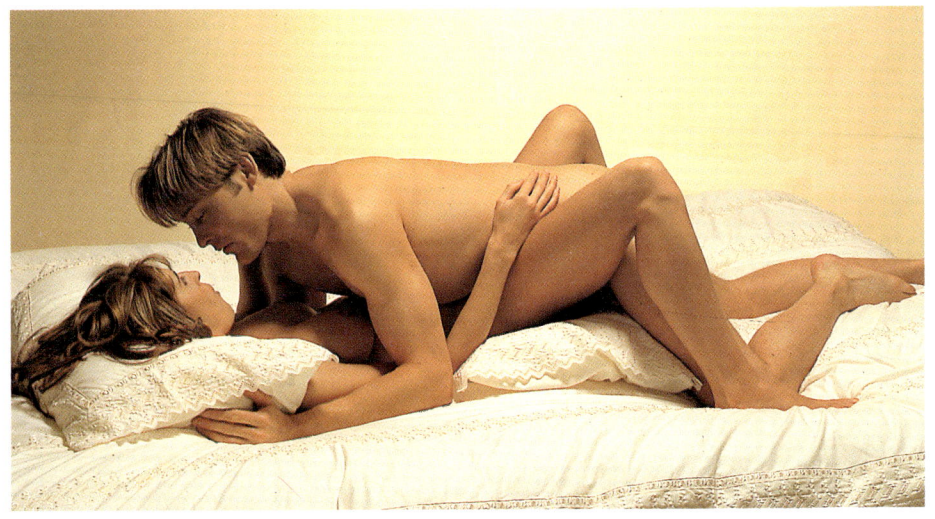

Slow Motion

◀ The man can begin thrusting with shallow actions, moving his pelvis slowly and gently back and forth, and allowing more time for attunement. On arousal, the first part of her vagina constricts, enabling it to grip the penis securely, adding to the pleasurable sensations of friction. However, if the man is in a state of high arousal, he needs to be careful not to overstimulate the erotically sensitive tip of his penis if he is prone to ejaculating too quickly.

Basic Techniques

Making it Comfortable

For the woman, the main disadvantages of the man-on-top position are the restrictions to her own pelvic movements and, unless her partner is particularly aware of his actions, the inadequacy of the clitoral stimulation – an important factor if she wishes to be aroused to orgasm.

Other situations can make this position an unsuitable choice. If a woman is suffering from a back condition, she may find that making love in this position will add to the strain. If her partner is much heavier than her, she may feel confined and burdened by the size difference.

A pregnant woman can feel anxious and uncomfortable about having any weight bearing down on her abdomen. Her breasts may feel particularly sensitive to pressure and, in the later stages of her pregnancy, this position may simply be impossible. In all of these cases, if the man is on top of his partner, he should take care not to put all his weight on her.

The man-on-top position puts the onus on the man to perform, and this may not suit him if he is tired or under stress. While he may desire physical intimacy with his partner, at a time like this it is usually preferable if the woman takes the more active role. Also, if the man is prone to premature ejaculation, he would do well to experiment with the woman-on-top positions which may slow him down and give him greater control over this process.

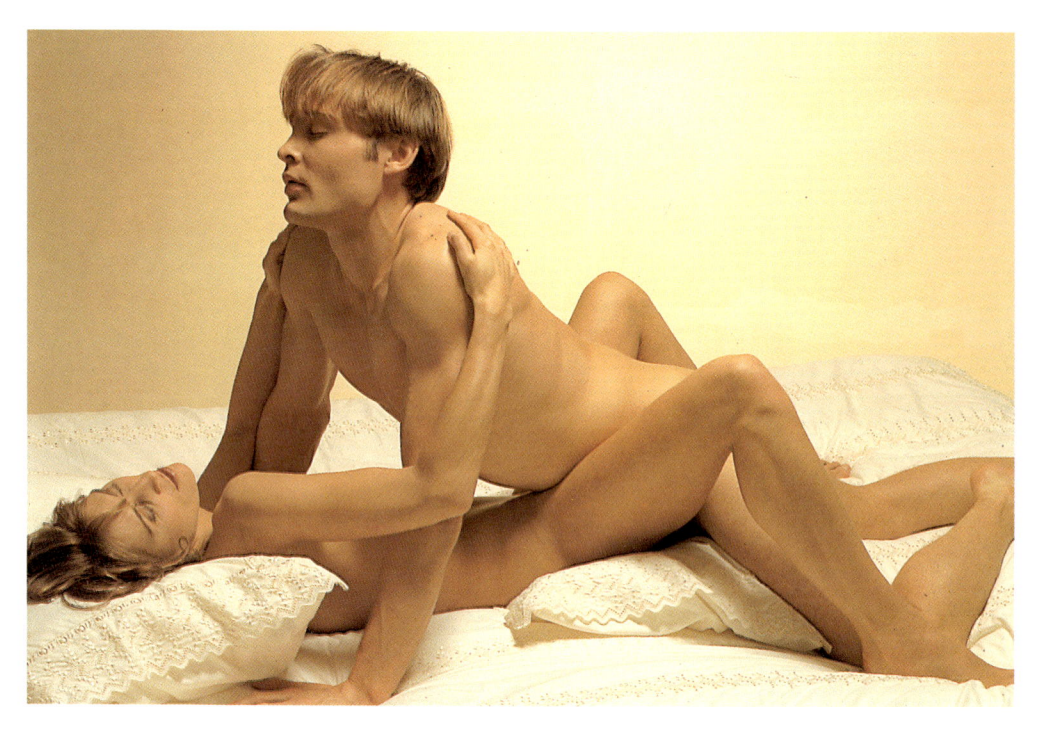

Aiding Mobility

▲ *For a woman, mobility is more difficult when making love in the man-on-top position. She may find it helpful if a pillow is placed beneath her buttocks to tilt her pelvis. This will give her more freedom of hip movement and take the strain away from her lower back. By placing her feet firmly against the mattress, she can use her leg muscles to add leverage to her pelvic motions, to increase sensation for both of them, and to allow greater clitoral stimulation as it rubs against his pubic bone. To avoid pinning her down with his body, the man should support his own weight with his arms and hands, keeping the trunk of his body slightly lifted above her.*

Intimacy in Intercourse

The man should always remain aware of his partner's sexual responses, and ensure that the shared intimacy which inspired the lovemaking is not suddenly abandoned in the heat of arousal. Unfortunately, some men see penetration as a green light to go, and start thrusting away intent on an orgasm regardless of what is happening to their partners. In other scenarios, a man may be conscious of the woman's needs and start performing a series of mechanical manoeuvres aimed at giving her an orgasm so that he can go ahead and achieve his own. Neither type of behaviour is particularly desirable nor likely to please the woman, because intercourse is not a race or a gymnastic show, or a question of pushing the right buttons to gain an end result. It is all about two people meeting and merging, breathing and moving together, feeling and responding, and abandoning themselves equally to the sheer physical and emotional pleasure of the moment.

Fortunately, recent research shows that most sexually active men, while still considering female sexuality to be something of a mystery, believe that their partner's satisfaction is as important as their own. For many men, giving sexual joy to their women is the best part of making love. According to the studies, the majority of men do believe that intimacy and affection during lovemaking are very important factors in a woman's sexual happiness.

The Basic Positions

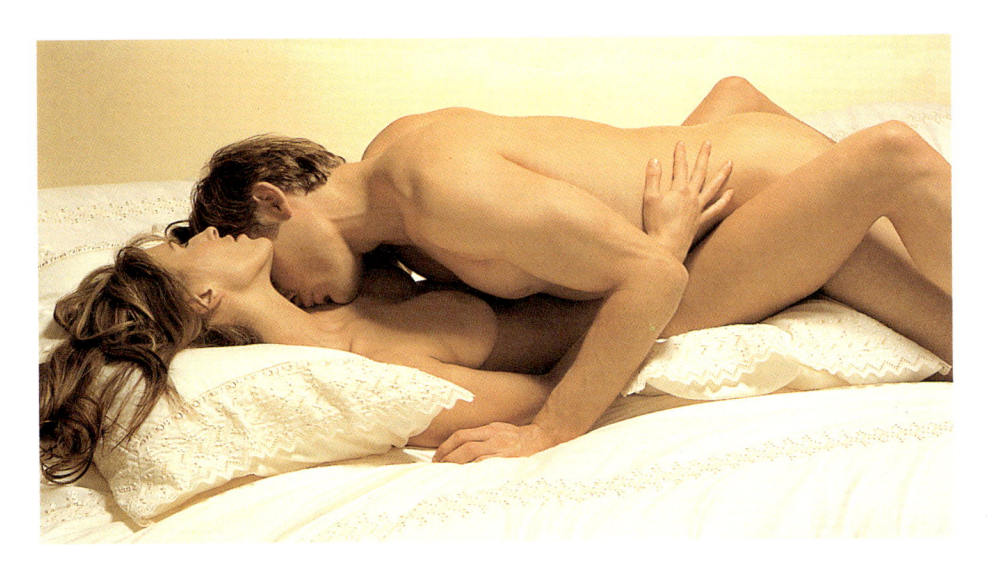

Penetration with Care
◀ Full penetration can create feelings of vulnerability as well as physical pleasure. These feelings need to be experienced and there is no need to rush ahead into immediate thrusting. It is important, too, that the man thrusts deeply only when his partner is physically and psychologically ready to receive him, or it may cause her discomfort. Initially, she can place her hands on his hips to help control his pelvic movements until she is ready.

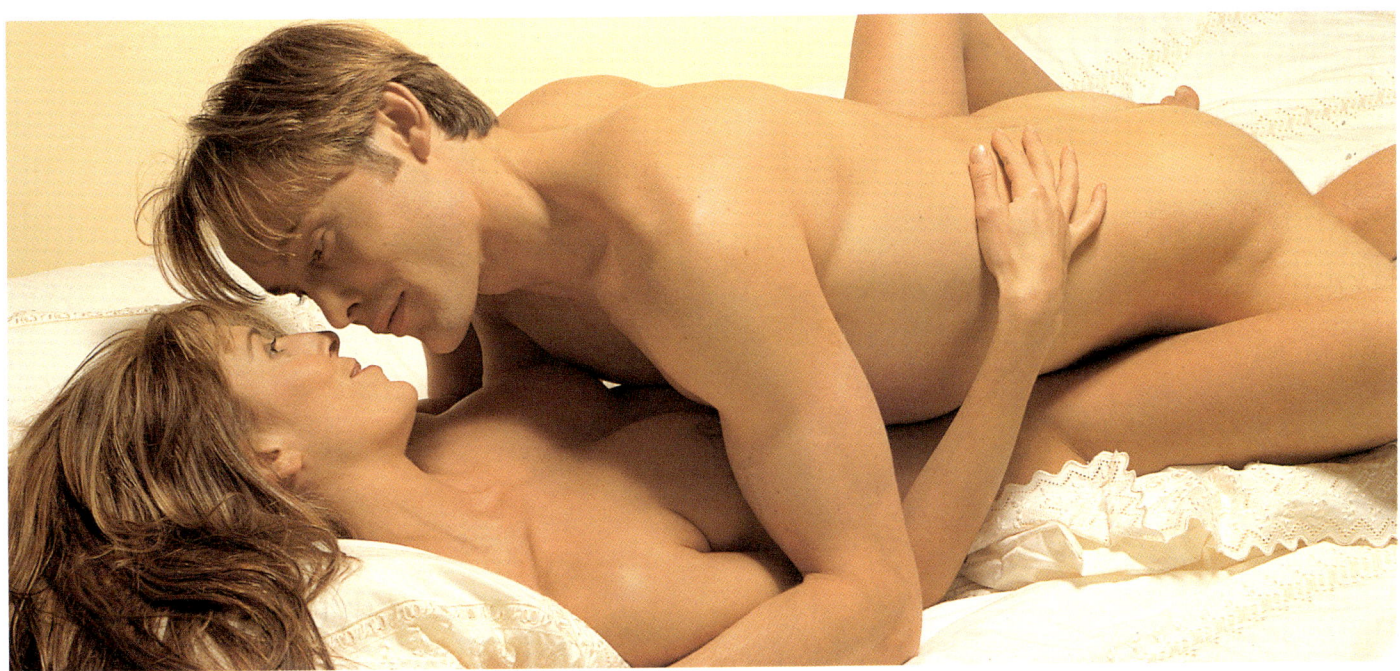

Sex with Sensitivity
▲ It is important to stay in touch on an emotional level throughout intercourse. Slow down once in a while, and look deeply into each other's eyes. By allowing the intimacy you feel to be expressed, silently or with words, your lovemaking will become deeply satisfying. Women need to feel emotionally nourished as well as physically aroused during the sexual act. Men benefit too if they try to get in touch with their softer and more vulnerable feelings.

Focusing Inwards
▶ Some lovers like to keep their eyes open during lovemaking, while others prefer to keep their eyes closed. If your eyes are open, you can take pleasure in looking at your partner's body and watching his or her arousal and responses. Closing your eyes while making love takes you into a different dimension of sensual feeling because you are able to focus on and enjoy the exquisite bodily sensations arising within you. To savour both experiences, switch from one to the other, so that sometimes you have a total awareness of your partner, and at other times you have complete awareness of yourself.

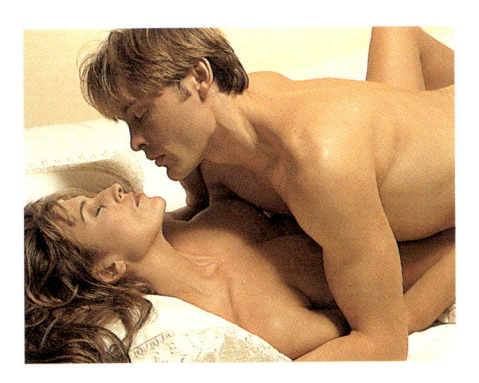

39

Basic Techniques

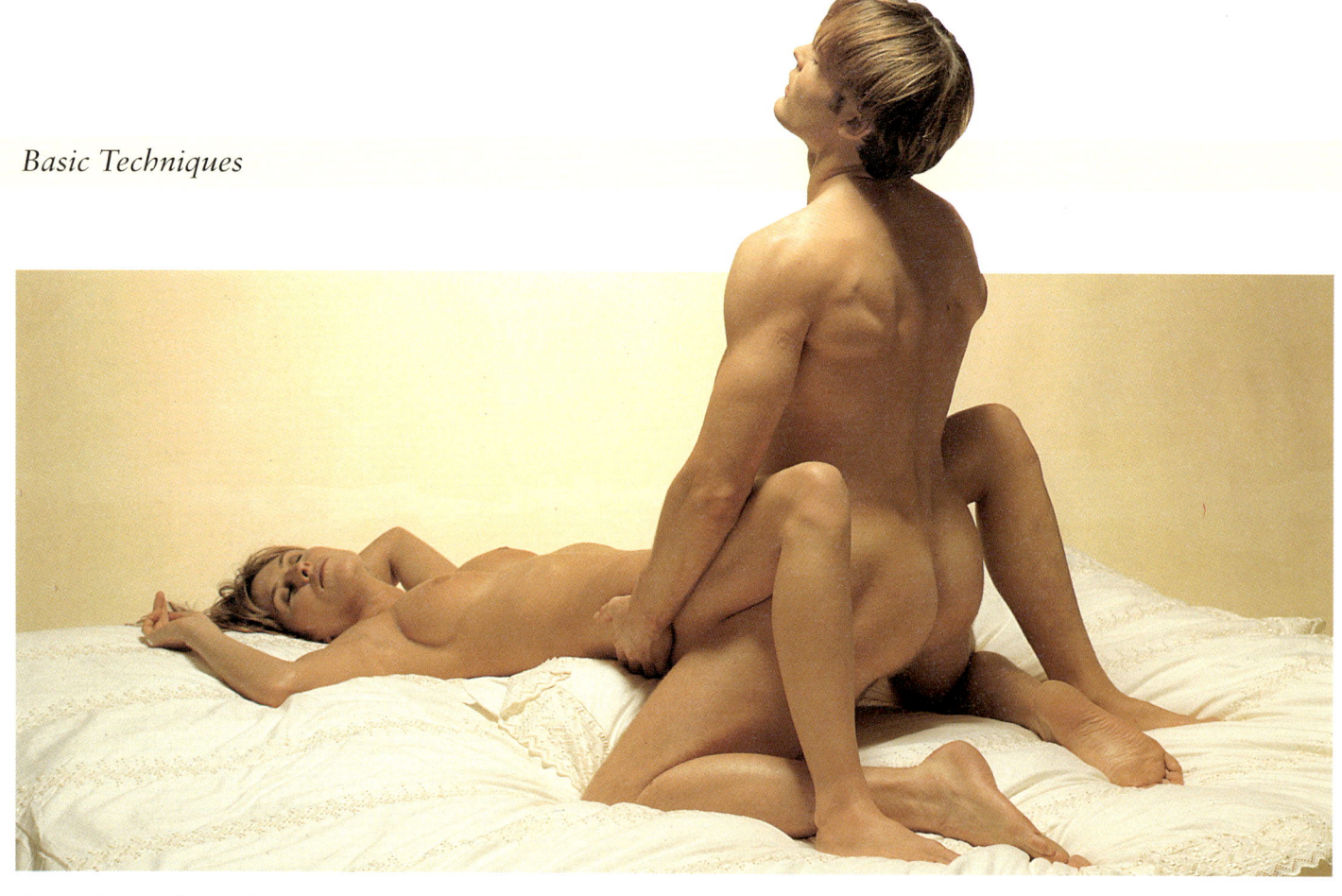

Varying the Movements

When lovers are sexually compatible, their rhythm and movement seem to flow from one beat to another without orchestrated effort. This harmony arises when a couple have allowed sufficient time in foreplay for full sexual arousal, or because they are familiar and comfortable with each other's bodies and share a deep sense of mutual trust.

To experience a whole range of pleasurable sexual sensations when the man is on top, it is important to change the position and angle of your bodies occasionally, and to vary your pelvic movements. The man should take care not to thrust his penis in and out of the vagina with a monotonous regularity of rhythm and motion. This can make the whole experience very unsatisfying for his partner, not only because she may be unable to receive the clitoral stimulation she needs, but also because the

Deeper Penetration

▲ *Deep penetration can be achieved from a position in which the woman arches her back slightly so that her vagina is raised and open. The man can help by lifting and supporting her pelvis, while pulling her slightly towards him. Many women find it very exciting to have the cheeks of the buttocks parted slightly while in this position, so the anus is exposed and gently stretched. Thrusting in this position creates intense vaginal sensations and by taking the weight of her pelvis with one hand he can use the fingers of his other hand to stimulate her clitoris at the same time.*

Varying Direction

◀ *Angles of thrusting should be changed throughout intercourse to produce a variety of sensations, and to stimulate different areas of the vagina. The man can use his hand to lift and tilt the woman's pelvis in one direction, so that his penis strokes along the side of her vaginal wall. Deep thrusting should only occur when the woman is fully aroused as her cervix and uterus will then have become elevated. He must also avoid thrusting too deeply into the side of her cervix.*

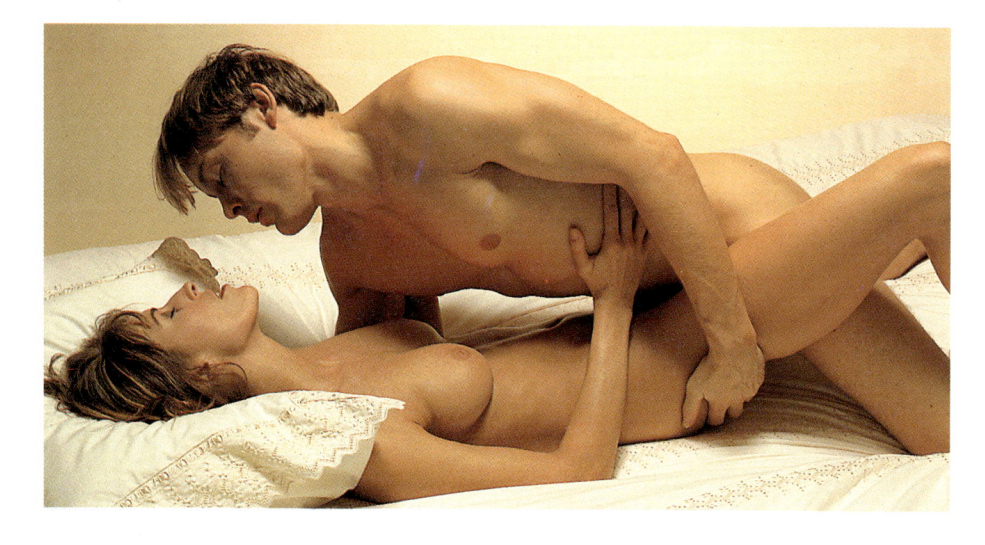

The Basic Positions

sex act itself can begin to seem automatic and boring. When this happens, and unfortunately it sometimes occurs in even the best sexual partnerships, the woman may start thinking about something else altogether. She may mentally vacate her body, beginning to wish the whole episode was over.

Pelvic motions can be wild, passionate and thrusting, or they may be deliciously subtle, depending on the intensity of sexual energy at any given moment of lovemaking. The man obviously has more freedom of movement in this position, but both partners should try to reach a synchronicity and fluidity in their motions to avoid the "bump and grind" effect. You can try moving your hips from side to side to create a sexy wiggle, or circulate both pelvises simultaneously to produce some highly erotic sensations and to add a touch of variety to the more usual back-and-forth rocking motion.

If your movements do fall out of rhythm, don't hesitate to tell your partner you need to slow down for a while. Relax and breathe together and make eye contact so you regain harmony. You can remain like this for quite a long period of time, just moving your hips enough to ensure the penis receives sufficient stimulation to remain erect inside the vagina. Let the sexual feelings rise again, and focus on these inner sensations, letting them move you gradually into a new and easy flow of movement.

Enjoy the range of depth to which the penis can penetrate the vagina. Play teasingly between shallower and deeper thrusts. Shallow penetration can be very exciting to both sexes because it produces friction on the tip of the penis and stimulates the outer reaches of the vagina, both regions that are richly served with erotically charged nerve endings.

Deep penetration produces more powerful emotional responses, creating a profound sense of fulfilment and connection between the partners. So do add spice and vitality to your love life by enjoying and experimenting with varying thrusts, positions, pressures and angles to create maximum pleasure for you both. Let sex be adventurous and fun.

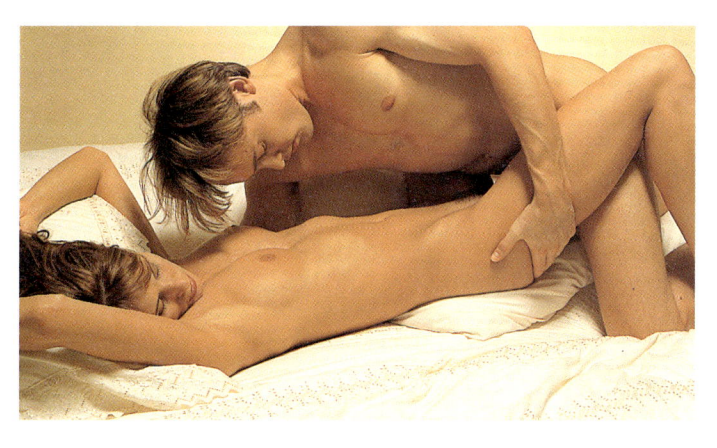

Watch and Enjoy
▲ Watching the motions of the penis thrusting in and out of the woman's vagina can be highly erotic for both partners. By lifting his body a little way from hers, they are able to enjoy this visual stimulation. To make it more arousing, vary the speed and depth of the penile thrusts. For the man, having his woman watch his actions can make him feel very potent.

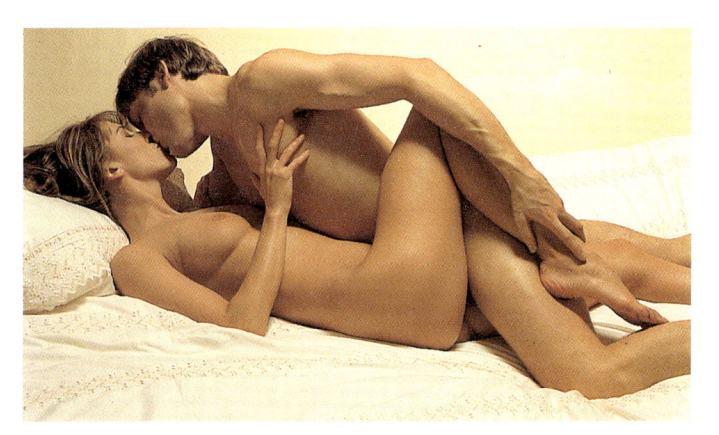

Angled Approach
▲ In this position, the man shifts his weight to one side, using one arm for support, and inserts his penis into the vagina from a slight sideways angle. This allows the woman to use more of her body and she can caress his thigh with her leg and foot, while he, in turn, strokes them. Men also enjoy being touched and stroked during intercourse, especially on the chest and nipples.

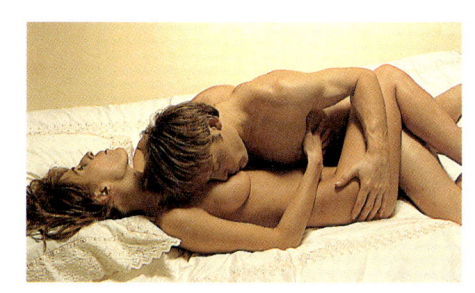

Caress Her Body
◀ Whole body sensuality should not finish just because intercourse has begun. This is especially important to a woman because every part of her body is sensitive to erotic stimulation, not just her genitals. While making love, you should continue to kiss, lick and caress her body and not just concentrate on thrusting movements. When she is aroused, the sensation of your lips and tongue on her breasts and nipples can drive her wild with excitement. She may also enjoy having her buttocks held, squeezed and stroked.

Basic Techniques

The Woman's Satisfaction

Even though the woman assumes a more passive role in lovemaking when her partner takes the on-top position, it is important that she receives the right kind of stimulation to achieve sexual satisfaction. What constitutes satisfaction will be different for each woman. For many it will mean being able to reach their full orgasmic potential, while for some it may be the need to feel as equally involved as their partners. Others would say that emotional and physical intimacy is the most important aspect of lovemaking, whether or not they reach orgasm.

Sexual performance is as much subject to mood and change as any other function in life. It can be ecstatic, passionate and mutually orgasmic, or it may be comfortable and cosy – more like a cuddle. Most couples do take a realistic view of their sex lives, and do not expect to "feel the earth move" on every occasion. However, when a man is in the more dominant on-top position, he needs to exercise a certain amount of conscious control over his movements and arousal level. He may need to slow down from time to time, so the duration of lovemaking and the involvement of his partner provide fulfilment for them both.

How long it should last is a matter for the couple concerned, but the answer will probably lie in whether each person feels sexually and emotionally fulfilled during and after a session of lovemaking.

Side and Rear Entry

◀ *This is an exciting lovemaking position, and one which adds to the woman's pleasure because of the pressure of his body against the back of her thigh and vulva. The man enters his partner partly from the side and partly from the rear of her body, so that her leg is drawn up and wrapped around his waist. He will need to support his weight with both hands.*

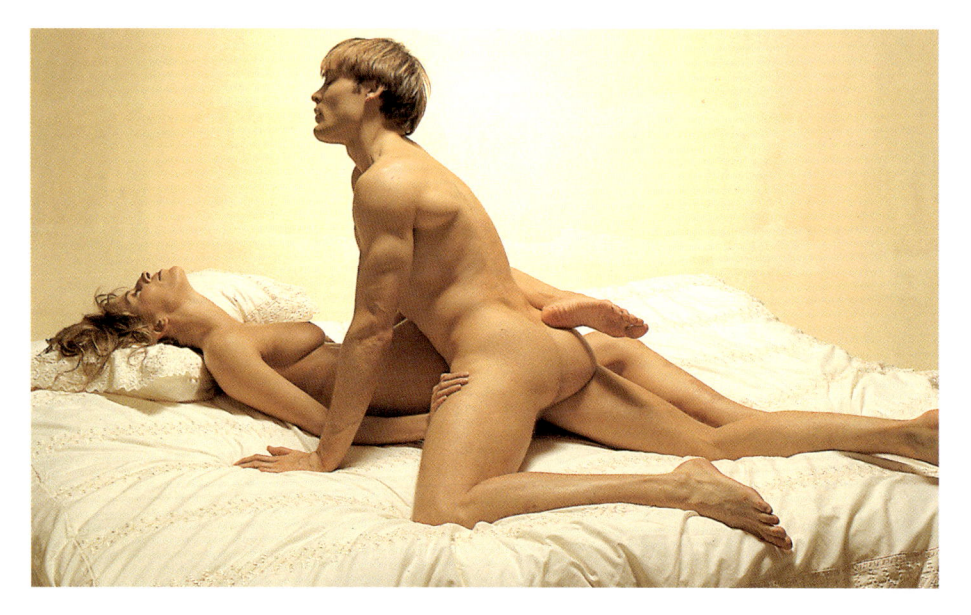

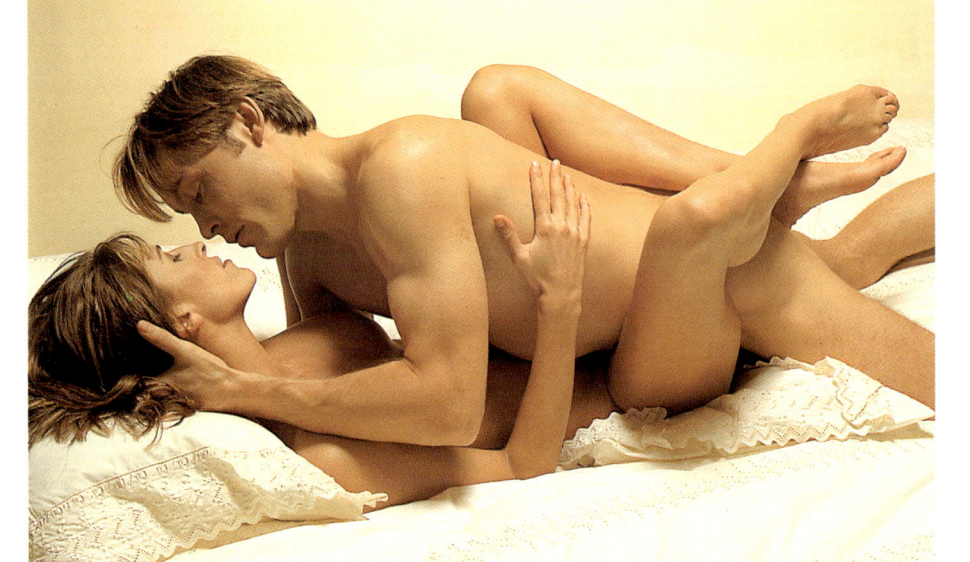

Pulling Close

◀ *While beneath her man, a woman may want to become more involved in the action. One way is for her to wrap her legs around the man's back, pulling him close in to her. This will bring their genitals in very close contact, creating a pleasurable friction on the clitoris, especially when the pelvic motions are circular or rocking from side to side. It is not a position that can be prolonged, however, as the man's movements are somewhat restricted, and it may become tiring for the woman.*

The Basic Positions

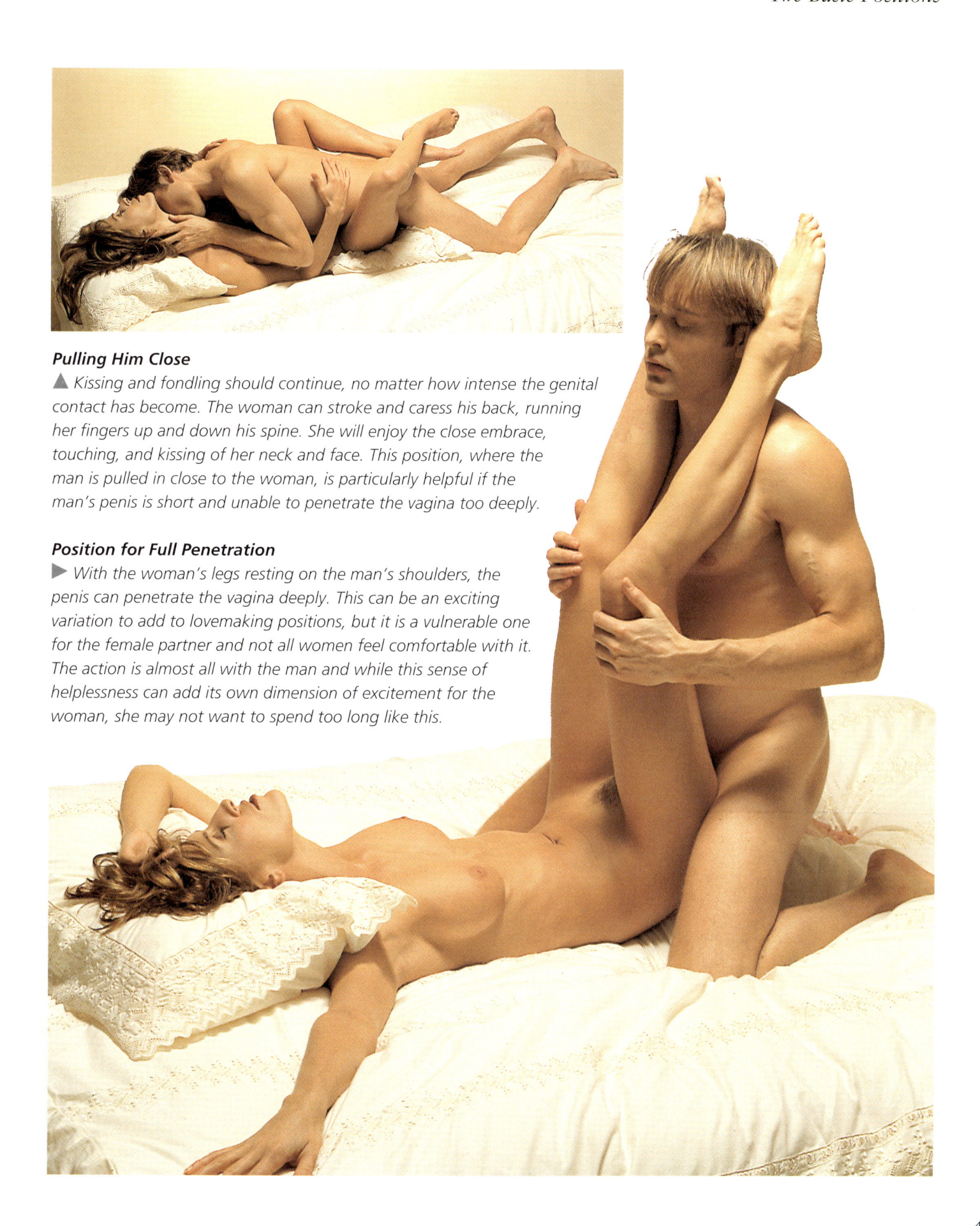

Pulling Him Close
▲ Kissing and fondling should continue, no matter how intense the genital contact has become. The woman can stroke and caress his back, running her fingers up and down his spine. She will enjoy the close embrace, touching, and kissing of her neck and face. This position, where the man is pulled in close to the woman, is particularly helpful if the man's penis is short and unable to penetrate the vagina too deeply.

Position for Full Penetration
▶ With the woman's legs resting on the man's shoulders, the penis can penetrate the vagina deeply. This can be an exciting variation to add to lovemaking positions, but it is a vulnerable one for the female partner and not all women feel comfortable with it. The action is almost all with the man and while this sense of helplessness can add its own dimension of excitement for the woman, she may not want to spend too long like this.

Basic Techniques

Unlike past decades, few women today would put up with a sexual encounter that only lasted a few minutes. On the other hand, anxiety about performance can lead some men to become too controlled, and that can also cause discomfort if the thrusting becomes prolonged and mechanical and out of tune with a woman's wishes.

Greater sexual awareness and openness have changed some basic patterns of male sexual behaviour. Only three decades ago, the famous American sex researcher Alfred Kinsey stated that, according to his studies, the majority of men interviewed considered it perfectly normal to ejaculate within the first two minutes of intercourse. Nowadays, most men are much better informed about a woman's sexual responses and her orgasmic capacity and it is quite standard for a man to ask his partner how he can give her the most pleasure.

What is more important is that both people continue to explore their potential for pleasure, allowing themselves to be more spontaneous yet constantly sensitive to each other's feelings, sensations and responses.

While the man remains on top of the women, he should ensure that she is able to adjust her movements to increase her pleasure and that both her clitoris and vagina are receiving stimulation. This can be achieved by allowing continuing contact between his pubic bone and her clitoris, or he can add gentle pressure to her vulva with his hand, or stroke her clitoris sensitively with his fingers.

Lifting One Leg

▼ *A more comfortable variation of the legs-raised position is for the man to lift one of his partner's legs over his shoulder. He is then able to thrust and move his body more easily, while also increasing the pressure on her thigh and vulva. The woman needs to be supple enough to stay relaxed, and as deep penetration is also possible, the position should only be adopted when she is fully aroused.*

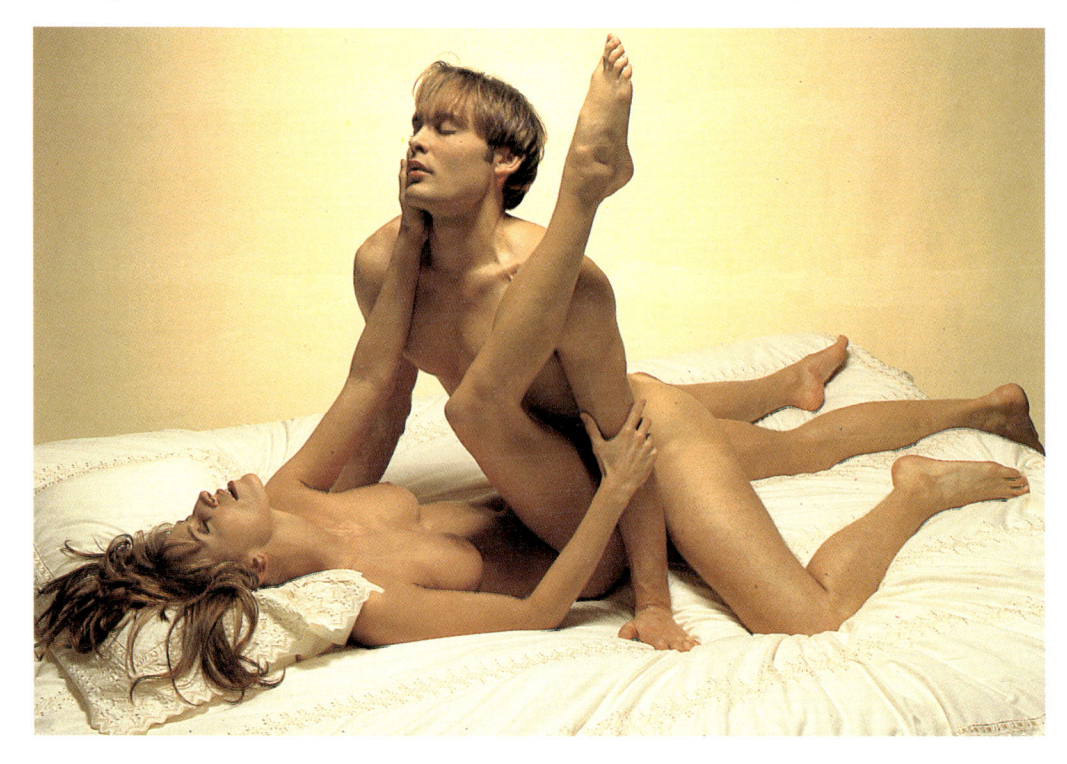

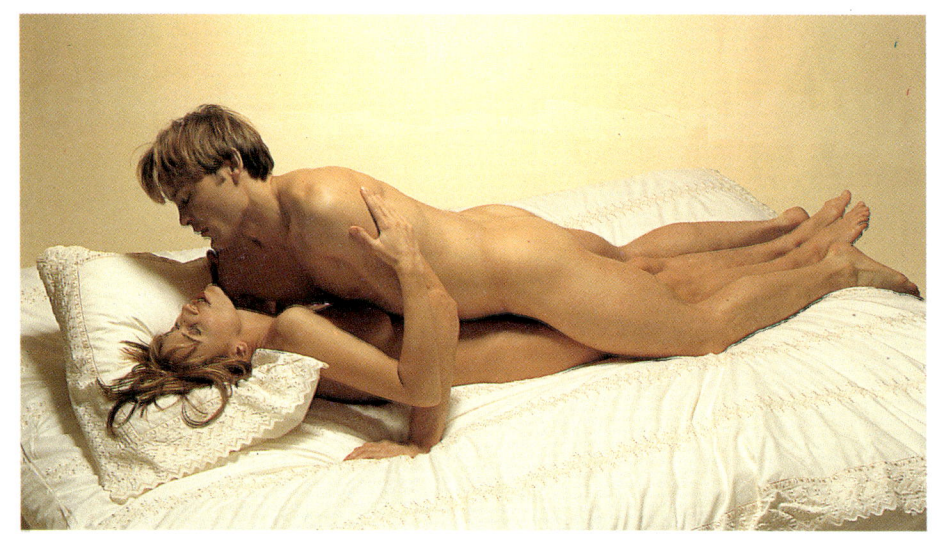

Increasing Pressure

◀ *Here the woman's legs are between the man's as he squeezes her thighs with his. Although she has very little movement in this position, the extra pressure on her vulva is very arousing, while his penis fits tightly into her vagina. To increase stimulation, she can wiggle around a little, or contract her pelvic floor and vaginal muscles to exert extra pressure on his penis.*

The Basic Positions

Opening Wide
▼ If the woman's legs are straight and spread out wide, then her clitoris is in a good position to receive strong stimulation from the man's thrusting movements. He will need to support his own weight with his arms as he rocks his pelvis back and forth. A teasing side-to-side motion will rub and stimulate her whole vulva for even greater arousal.

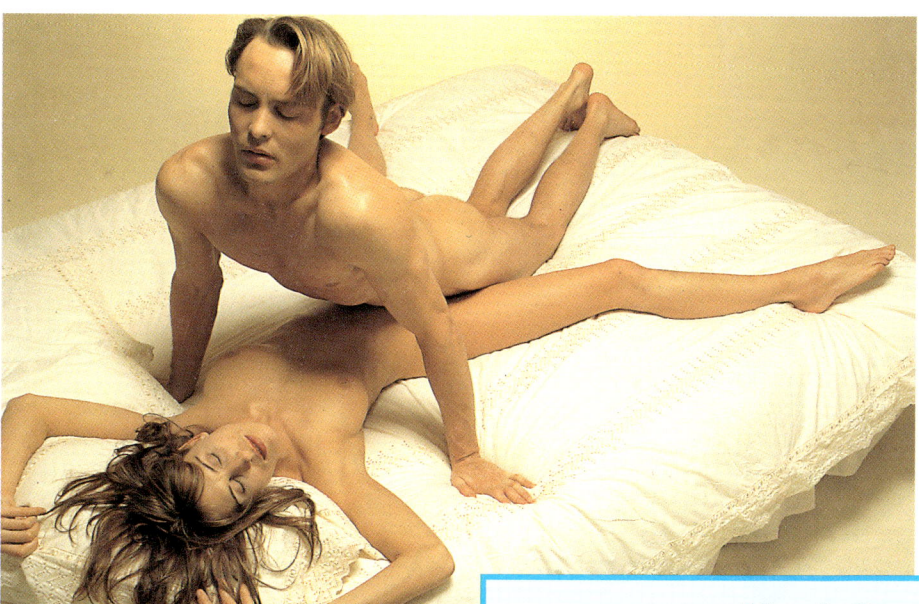

Holding Tight
▼ Although this position does not allow the woman much pelvic movement, she can reach out to hold him tightly around the neck and shoulders and draw him closer to her. Some women like to scratch their partner's back as they become excited – he will enjoy this too, if it is not too rough.

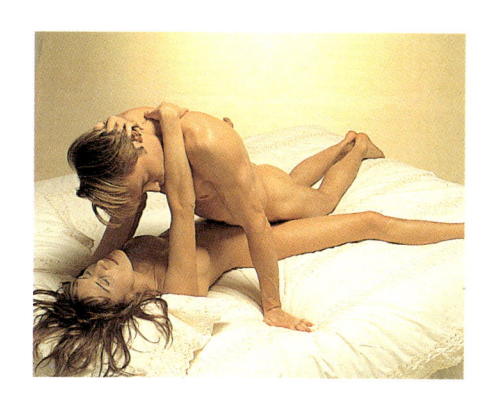

Close Body Contact
▼ While the man is in the more active and dominating position when he is on top of his partner, she can exert her power too by pulling him towards her and enfolding him in her arms so that he surrenders to her embrace. Throughout their lovemaking, there should always be moments of close, intimate and passionate body-to-body contact.

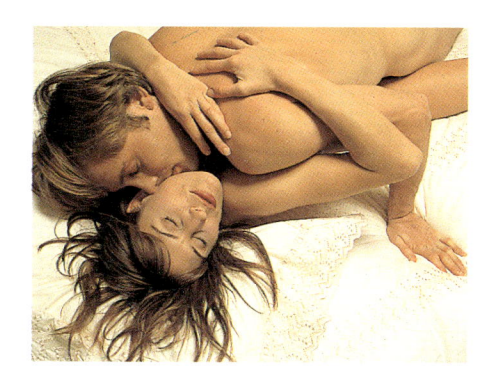

Men's Sexual Attitudes

Simon, 57, divorced, father of three, a teacher: What turns you on most about a woman? *"The eyes and the voice."* What do you enjoy most about lovemaking? *"The sense of merging with another person."* When do you experience your most powerful orgasms? *"When I'm not too tired. It depends on how close and secure I feel with my partner."*

Dean, aged 23, a student, single: What turns you on most about a woman? *"Beauty and a feeling of warmth between me and the woman I'm attracted to."* What do you enjoy most about lovemaking? *"The closeness."* When do you experience your most powerful orgasms? *"When I'm in love. If it's a one-night stand it's more like a release."*

Terry, 42, a postal worker, divorced: What turns you on the most about a woman? *"The eyes, the smell, the breasts, her femininity."* What do you enjoy most about lovemaking? *"The closeness; the bonding, expressing our love."* When do you experience your most powerful orgasms? *"In a good relationship, sex is just more intense; or if I haven't had sex for a while. It's also a special mood, all openness, it is not something that can be planned."*

Paul, 30, a decorator, single: What turns you on most about a woman? *"Everything, and all kinds of women!"* What do you enjoy most about lovemaking? *"The intimacy, the closeness, giving and receiving pleasure."* When do you experience your most powerful orgasms? *"With my current girlfriend."*

Expressing Our Sexuality

The bedroom, of all places, should never be a battleground for power. So the question of who takes the dominant and submissive positions, or the active and passive sexual roles, should be a matter for lovers to decide after they have conducted a shared and joyful exploration into what feels natural, pleasurable, satisfying and sexually creative to them both. These days, most couples like to swap sexual positions and roles because it allows them to experience all the nuances of their sexual nature, which will have both feminine and masculine qualities, regardless of gender. This is how it should be because men and women today are breaking away from gender conditioning in every other aspect of their lives too.

Men do not always want to be "macho", and sometimes need to express the more sensitive side of their nature, while women are no longer content to be typecast purely in the "gentler sex" role. Since our sexuality is a profound expression of who we are, there should be enough scope within any sexual relationship for it to reflect the whole diversity of our inner selves.

Over the last three decades, women have enjoyed more sexual freedom than ever before. This may partly be due to the availability of efficient contraception, which has reduced their anxieties about unwanted pregnancy, and liberated them from the constraints of their biology to enjoy sex for reasons of pure intimacy and pleasure. In addition, women now know that they have an equal, if not greater orgasmic capacity than their male partners. Gone are the days when a sexually ecstatic woman was considered to be an aberration of her sex.

Women want and expect to have a satisfying sex life, and to take charge of their bodies in order to do so.

While it is largely true that for a woman the emotional, sensual and nurturing aspects of a relationship remain integral to her sexual happiness, she may also desire to reach the heights of sheer physical pleasure during lovemaking for which her body is uniquely designed.

The Woman-on-Top Position

A woman is able to express her innate sensuality and eroticism to a greater degree in the woman-on-top sexual positions than when the man

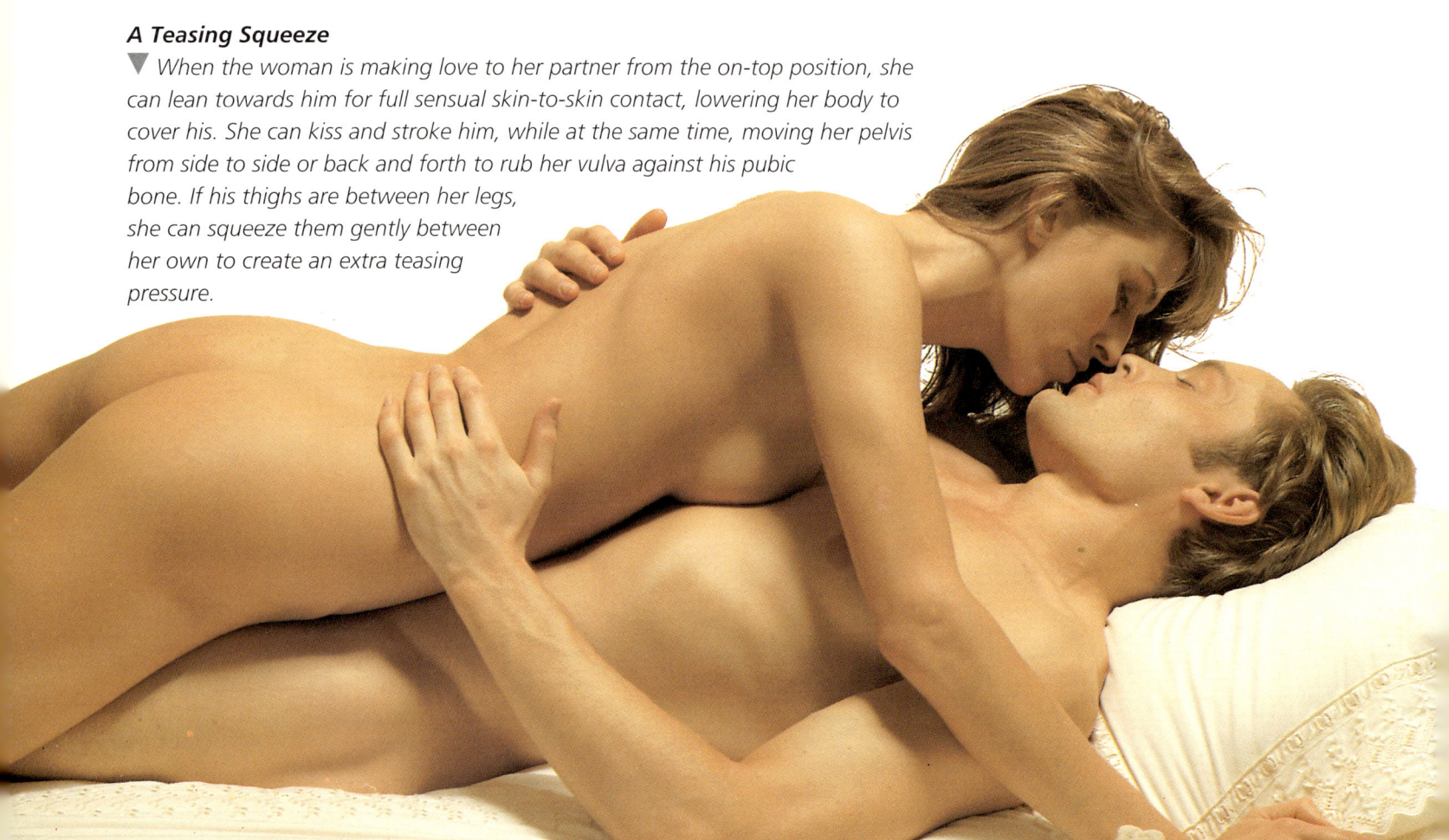

A Teasing Squeeze

▼ *When the woman is making love to her partner from the on-top position, she can lean towards him for full sensual skin-to-skin contact, lowering her body to cover his. She can kiss and stroke him, while at the same time, moving her pelvis from side to side or back and forth to rub her vulva against his pubic bone. If his thighs are between her legs, she can squeeze them gently between her own to create an extra teasing pressure.*

Expressing Our Sexuality

Relaxing Change of Role
◀ If the man is lying beneath the woman, he no longer has to worry about his weight on her body or about maintaining a sexual performance. It can be a relief to a man to be able to surrender himself into the more passive role, and totally relax while he receives her tender and nourishing caresses. She can kiss him gently all over his face, and tenderly stroke his head, while rotating her pelvis to maintain genital stimulation at the same time so that his whole body begins to melt into hers.

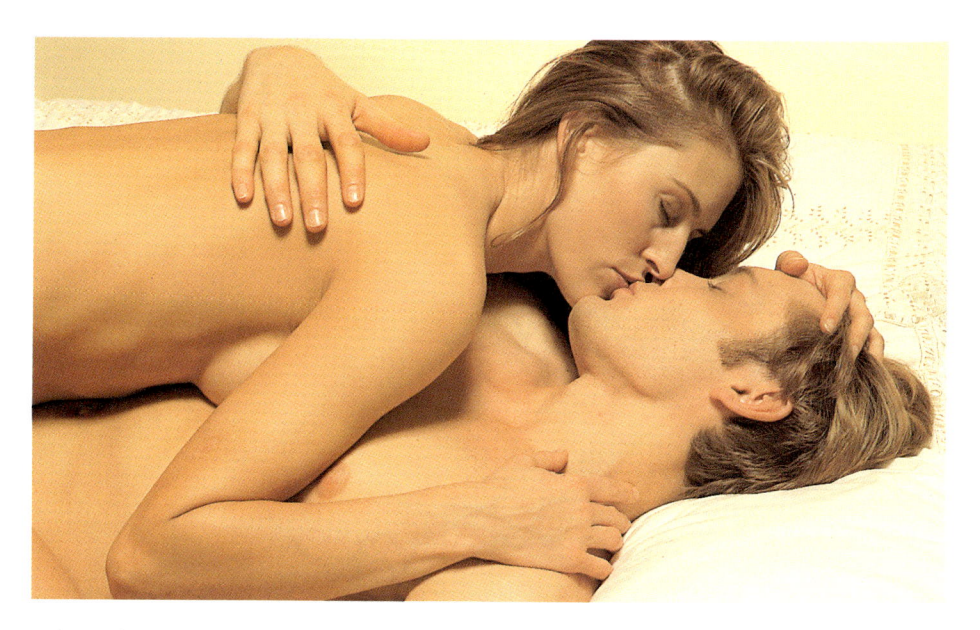

takes the active role. She has more freedom of movement, is less burdened by weight, and can gain the maximum stimulation for orgasmic excitation.

Most of the positions illustrated in this section not only allow a woman to enjoy the pleasure of taking her lover's penis inside her vagina, but also the choice of movements whereby her vulva and clitoris receive adequate friction too. Deep penetration is possible with many of these positions, particularly when she is squatting over her man, yet at the same time, she is better able to control the depth according to what feels comfortable.

For the man, having a partner on top and in charge of the movements can come as a great relief, especially if he is fatigued or would like some respite from the role of main performer. Not only is it erotically and visually arousing for him to watch his woman express her sexuality so powerfully, he can enjoy relaxing into the more passive side of his own sexual nature.

Couples can use the woman-on-top position for the whole duration of a lovemaking episode, or incorporate it into any number of other exciting sexual manoeuvres. A change of positions should be made gracefully, slowing down the pace of

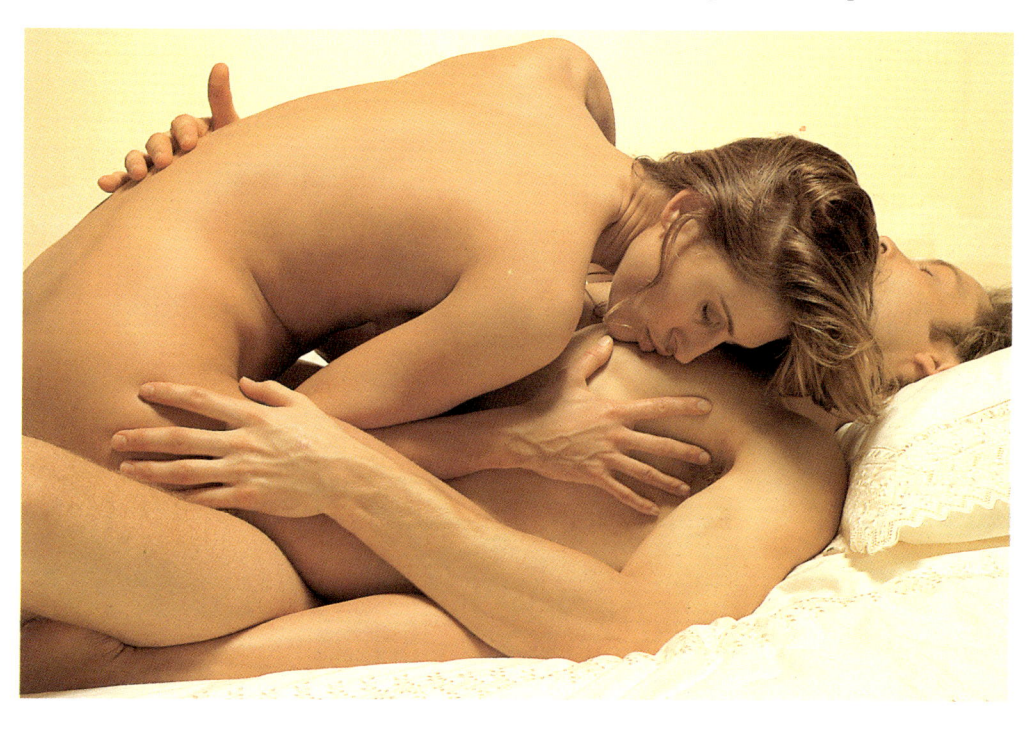

Sensual Stimulation
▶ Many women enjoy the possibility of extending sensual play into lovemaking, and this position allows them to continue giving erotic stimulation to different parts of the man's body. Even while they are making love, she can kiss and lick her way down his body, turning him on to even greater heights of arousal. Flicking her tongue across his nipples and then blowing gently on them with her warm breath will drive him wild. If she is only moving her pelvis slightly at this point, she can contract her vaginal muscles around his penis to exert an extremely pleasurable pressure on it, as well as increasing her own genital sensations.

Basic Techniques

action if necessary so that both partners can adjust their limbs and posture to become comfortable. When the rhythm and motion of lovemaking is harmonious and fluid, a couple can constantly change positions without interrupting their intercourse. Sometimes, however, it may be necessary for the man to withdraw his penis from the vagina for some moments in order to avoid clumsy movements.

The woman-on-top position requires some caution from the woman as she lowers herself onto her lover's penis. Sudden, abrupt or speedy movements from her before he has found a comfortable fit can injure him by bending his penis at an acute angle. She needs to remain aware of his comfort too if she is abandoning herself to uninhibited movement.

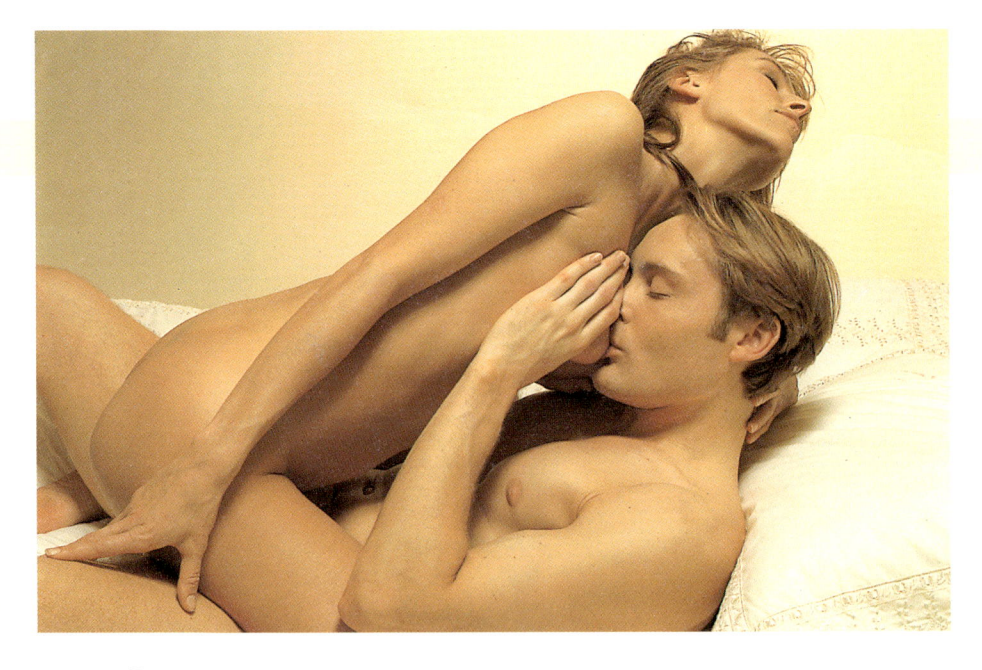

Controlling Penetration
▲ *While the woman is moving up and down on the man's penis, she is able to control the depth of its penetration into her vagina. She can tantalizingly raise herself upwards so that the tip of the penis is gripped by the lower end of her vagina only, though she should take care that it does not slip out. Then she can make subtle up and down movements, to intensify stimulation to these mutually nerve-packed genital zones. Or she can lower herself so that the penis satisfyingly fills her whole vagina. Even more pleasure is generated if she plays between the deeper and more shallow levels of penetration, constantly surprising him with her changes of motion. If, at this point, he lifts up to lick, kiss or suck her nipples, he can take her to the edge of orgasmic ecstasy.*

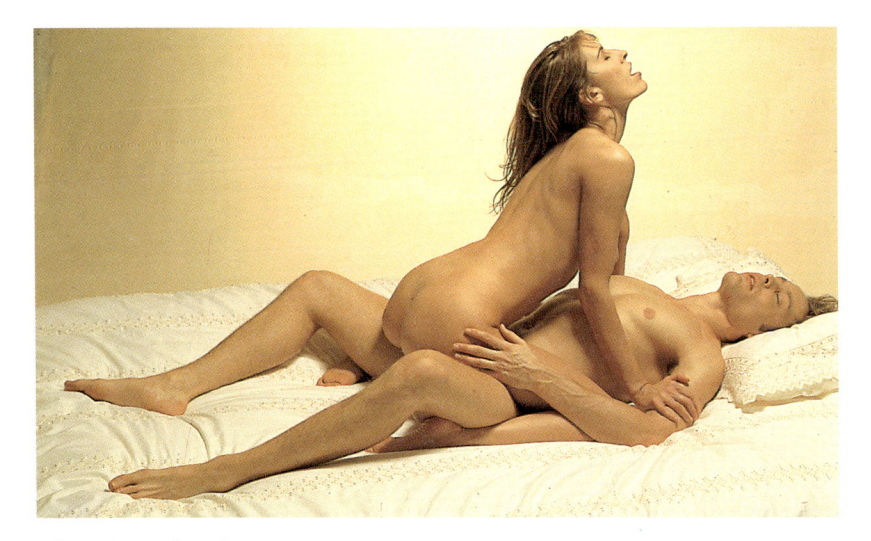

Pelvic Gyrations
◀ *Intense genital stimulation can be achieved once the woman lifts her body away from her partner and begins to gyrate her pelvis in varying motions to gain maximum vaginal and clitoral stimulation. While the contact between the lovers' bodies becomes less intimate, the arousal grows stronger as they both let go into their own waves of pleasure and movement. She can sway her body from side to side so that his erect penis strokes every part of her vaginal wall, and she can rub her vulva against his pubic bone for extra pressure on her clitoris. While the man's movements are more restricted in this position, he can wiggle his pelvis to increase the effect, or use his feet to lever his lower body up and down to add some deep thrusting motions. He should also use his hands to stroke and caress her.*

Clitoral Stimulation

Many women complain that men either ignore the clitoris, concentrating too much on vaginal thrusting, or they zone in too much on the clitoris, to the exclusion of the rest of the body. This looks like a no-win situation for the man. Happily, there is a way he can give her the clitoral stimulation she needs, and without her feeling she is being tuned up like a car before a motor race.

It is important for the woman to continue receiving clitoral stimulation throughout intercourse and during orgasm. This can be achieved by positions, which either partner can take, that give the woman freedom of movement and allow her vulva to press against the man's

Expressing Our Sexuality

pubic bone. During penetrative sex, the man or the woman can also press on, or sensually stimulate, her clitoris manually. Stroking of the vaginal lips and over the mons pubis will also stimulate the clitoris, and may be more arousing and enjoyable than pressure placed directly onto it. Remember, though, that the clitoris is a delicate organ with a high density of sensitive nerves, so frantic rubbing or excessive pressure can be irritating and even painful.

While a woman may desire and need clitoral stimulation to reach the peak of sexual arousal, she may not want to receive it to the exclusion of loving, tender touches and kisses bestowed on the rest of her body. This also applies to her breasts, which when stroked, kissed and licked during intercourse can take her into sexual bliss, yet she does not want them to be the sole centre of attention while the rest of her is ignored. Every part of a woman's body is erogenous, and she can be greatly turned on by the emotional depth of the lovemaking too.

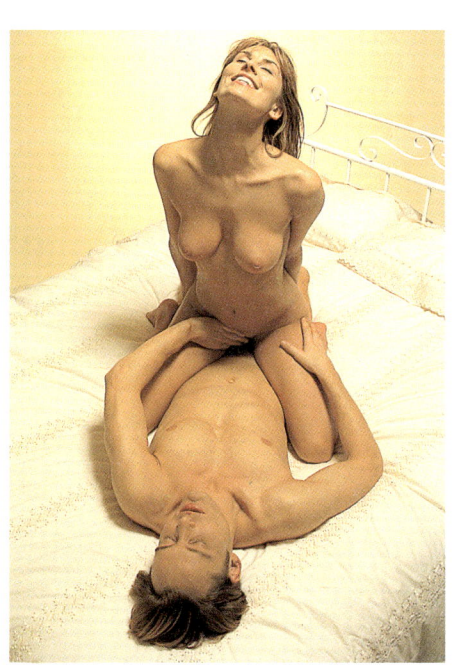

Boosting the Sexual Charge
▼ To keep a sustained and arousing pressure on her clitoris, the woman can raise her back and push her vulva towards the man's pelvic bone, leaning into it without motion for several moments. She can heighten her pleasure by tightening her buttocks and thigh muscles, thereby constricting her vaginal muscles in order to hug the penis, and this will increase the sexual charge in her genitals. Creating this kind of voluntary tension in the muscles of the genital area can bring some women to orgasm.

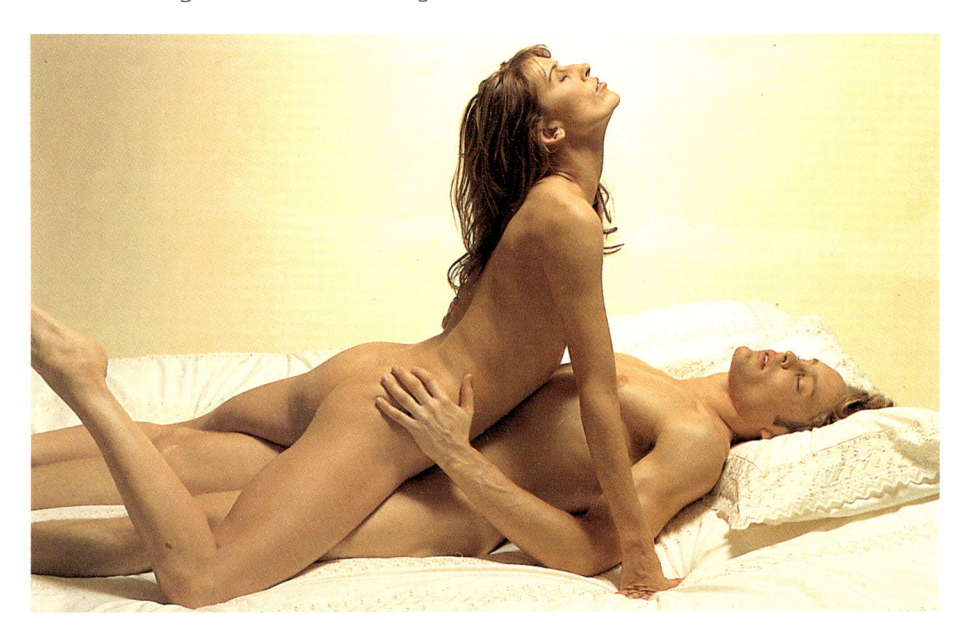

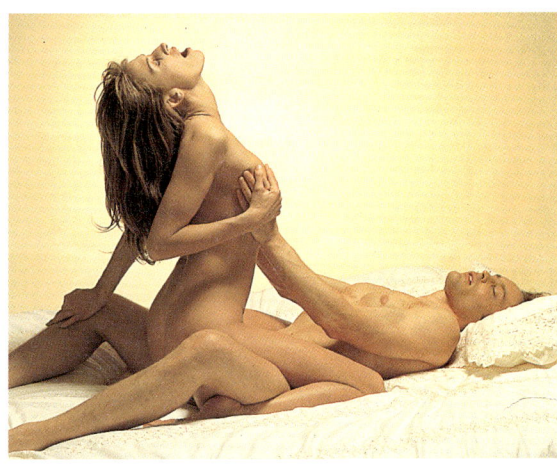

Freedom of Expression
◀ A woman has a tremendous capacity for experiencing ecstatic sexual joy, and in this position, where she rides her man, she is free to move and express herself fully without inhibition or restriction of movement. She is able to raise and lower herself on the penis, bringing intense pleasure to the man, and enabling him to penetrate her deeply. She can also grind her vulva against his pubic bone to provide extra stimulation to her clitoris. As she abandons herself to her rapture, the man can touch her breasts and nipples.

Arousing Caresses
◀ As the man lies back in this position, he can use his hands to stroke and caress his partner's whole body. He can also increase her arousal by stroking her vulva or rubbing her clitoris while she moves on top of him. At the same time, she is able to reach back with her hands to gently fondle his scrotum, which will certainly add to his pleasure.

49

Basic Techniques

Most women would probably say that they want all the tender, erotic touching and caressing of sensual play to continue after penetration, plus the right amount of clitoral stimulation – and they want their lovemaking to be exciting, yet relaxed and spontaneous too.

They do not want to feel that they are being programmed for an orgasm by excessive mechanical stimulation, or that their total sensuality is being neglected.

Ecstatic Moments

When a woman feels confident enough to take the more active sexual role, she can really let go into her orgasmic sexual energy. Suddenly her whole body is free, and she can move, turn and sway so that the waves of pleasure can rush through every part of her. If she has a partner who relishes her ecstatic expression, the experience can be intensely erotic for them both.

If she is truly uninhibited, she may even shout and scream, moan, or even cry and laugh in turns, and all of this can be very exciting to a man who is not afraid to see powerful female sexual energy unleashed. Or she may want to move in a very soft and sensual way, stroking and kissing her man, teasing him with playful and arousing movements, and touching his heart deeply with her gentle and nurturing femininity.

Taking Charge

One of the advantages for the woman when she assumes the on-top position is that she can take control of the movements to satisfy her needs in all the previously mentioned ways. Also, when a man is in the passive role, he is likely to be more attentive to her whole body, reaching out to touch and caress her because he is able to relinquish the tension of being the main performer. Yet at the same time, a woman needs to carry the same awareness that she expects from her man when he is the dominant sexual partner. Just like a woman, a man does not want to feel that his body is being used purely for sexual gratification, as if it is somehow separate from his whole person.

If both want to enjoy a prolonged session of lovemaking, she needs to be in tune with his sexual responses, so that the stimulation he is receiving does not propel him too quickly to his orgasm threshold. For a man, there is a certain point of no return, when he no longer has control over the process of ejaculation. The woman should remain alert to his signals, slowing down the pace of her movements, or even staying still, until the excitement level has subsided sufficiently to allow sexual activity to continue.

However, men who are prone to premature or early ejaculation can benefit from having their partner take the top position since it is likely to create less intense stimulation to the penis and can slow down the ejaculatory process.

Sensate Exercise

As the woman rides her man, she can begin to move slowly up and down on his penis, lowering herself so it penetrates deep into her vagina, and then raising herself so she is barely containing its tip. Closing her eyes, she should then try to merge herself entirely into each sensation, letting

Slow the Pace

▼ Even at the height of ecstasy, it is wonderful to slow down the pace of action to simply feel the sensations which are arising like pulsing waves in the body. The woman can brace her back, clasping the man's legs behind her and then breathe deeply together with her lover. In this position, the penis will be exerting its pressure onto the front wall of her vagina to add increased stimulation to her G-spot.

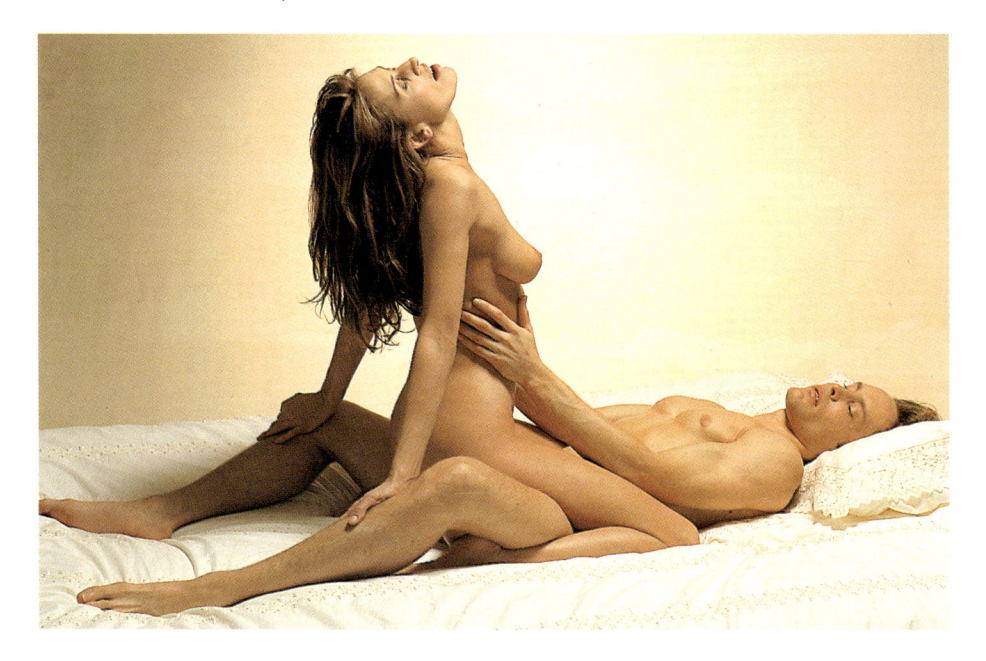

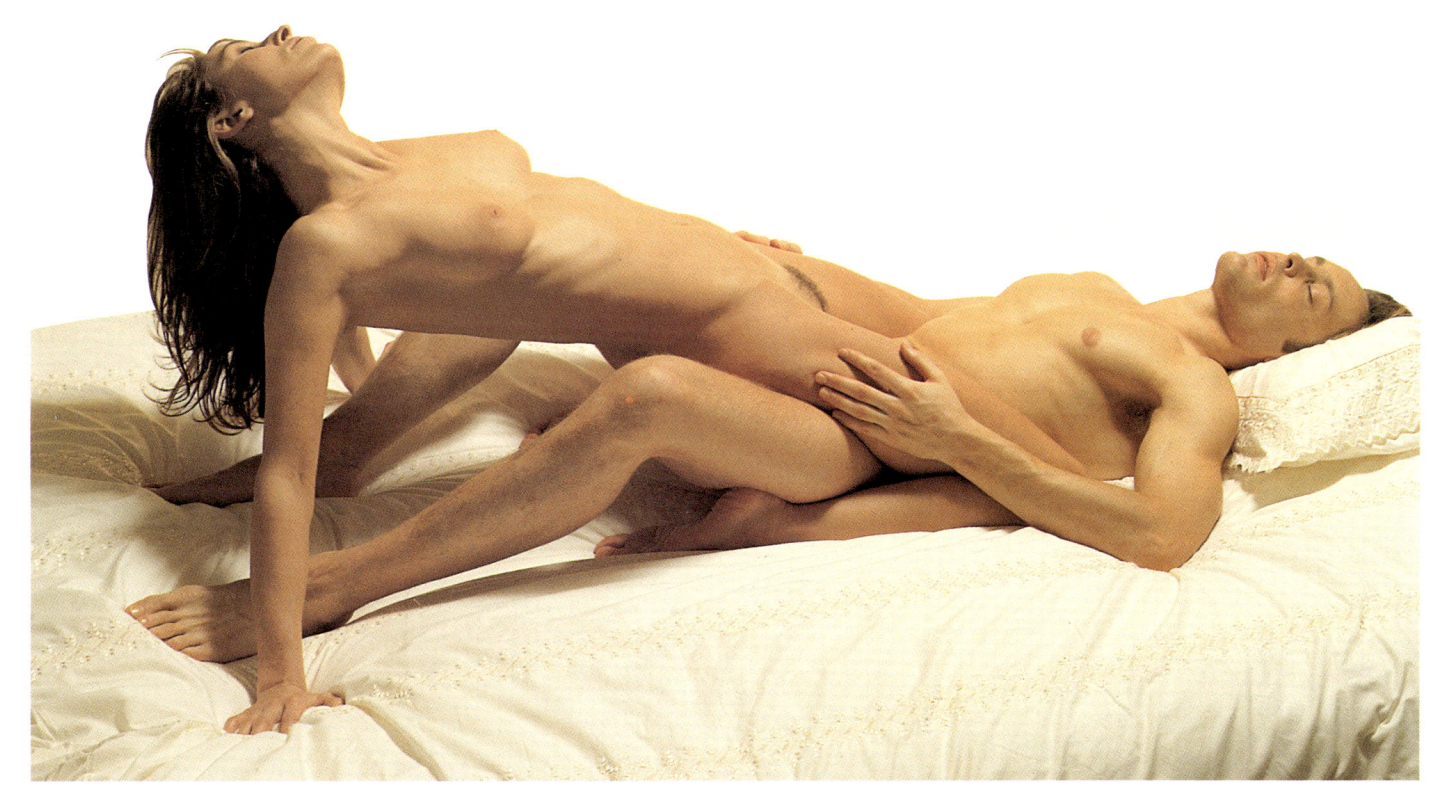

Vary the Movements
▲ Lowering herself back gently, the woman can arch and extend the whole trunk of her body as she leans against the support of her partner's raised thighs, and takes her own weight into her arms. With the pressure of his penis against the front wall of her vagina, she can rock back and forth with tiny movements to stimulate this highly erogenous zone. She is now exposing her vulva to her lover, and he can lovingly caress this intimate area, and her thighs.

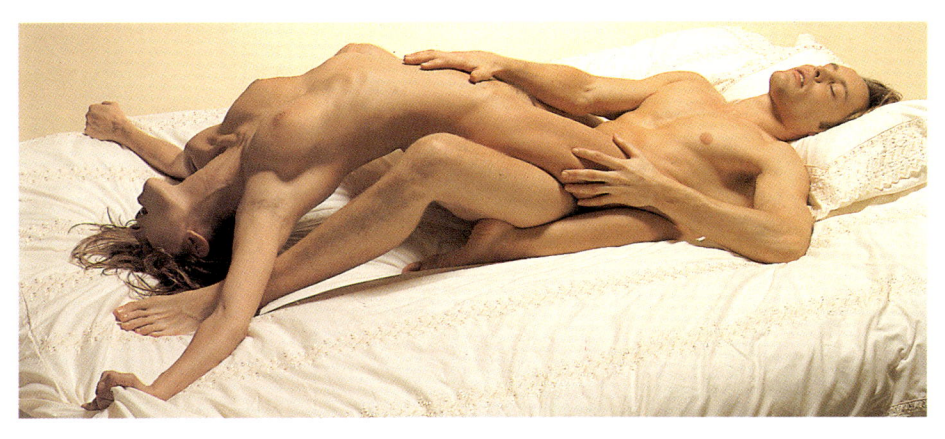

Opening Up to the Pleasure
▲ If she is supple enough she can lean right back into this almost yogic posture where her head rests on the mattress by her lover's feet, and her arms are spread-eagled so that the front of her body is completely open and extended. This will enable her to breathe very deeply so her whole body becomes infused with vitality. She is now in a perfect position for her lover to touch and caress her belly and thighs, before stroking and rubbing her clitoris and labia to give her immense delight and possibly bring her to orgasm.

Moments of Merging
◀ Between the waves of high energy activity and rapturous movement, it is always wonderful to rest awhile in a position that brings you both back to a sense of merging and melting with each other. The man will be happy to enfold his partner again in his arms, drawing the softness of her body close to his. These are the precious moments of stillness and silence in lovemaking, where both people can breathe together in harmony, connecting deeply through their love and intimacy for each other.

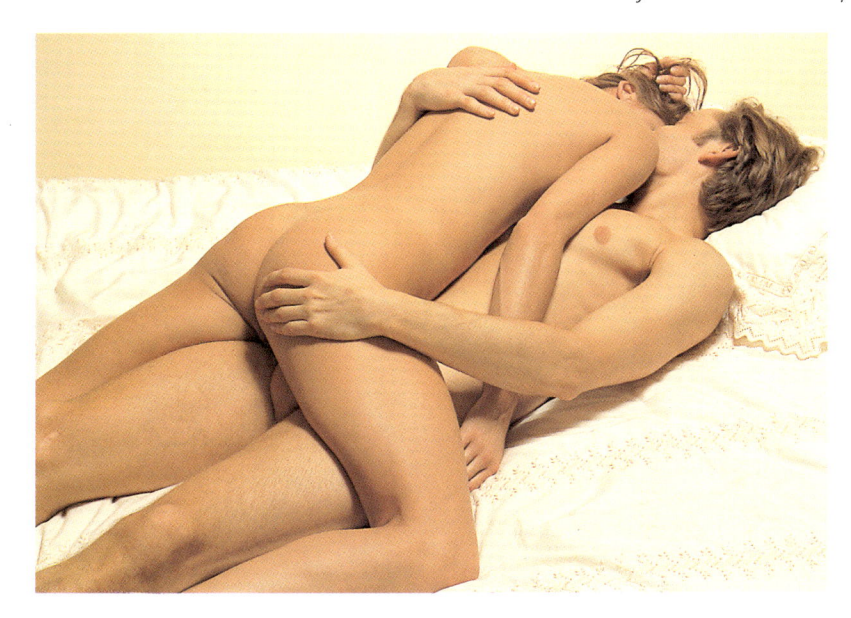

Basic Techniques

herself imagine what each subtle change of depth and movement must feel like for her partner. She can also ask him to describe those feelings to her. Gradually, those sensations will transfer themselves into her sexual consciousness.

If the woman becomes extremely sensitive to her man, she may actually begin to feel what he is experiencing, as if the sensations his penis are receiving are also occurring within her own body. It is an experiment certainly worth trying, for it can lead to a deepening of mutual sexual joy and understanding.

Feeling Confident

There are some women who simply do not feel comfortable about taking the sexual initiative or adopting the superior position while making love. There can be all kinds of reasons for this and no one should feel forced into doing something which makes them feel ill at ease.

If it is simply embarrassment, it is worth gathering the confidence to give it a try, and almost certainly the male partner will love the new variation and the chance to lie back and enjoy. If, however, the man insists on always taking the dominant sexual role, this may be a symptom of a deeper problem within the relationship. No woman should allow herself to feel sexually repressed, and if she feels that she is, the couple may benefit from talking the issues over carefully, or seeking advice from a relationship counsellor.

A woman may be reluctant to assume the on-top position because of a sense of low self-esteem regarding her body. Perhaps she is shy to expose it so boldly to her partner, or maybe she feels overweight and too heavy to climb on top of her man. Most women make critical judgements about their bodies, but more often than not these views are not shared by their partners.

Feeling good about your body is more to do with your self-regard than your actual weight. You can be big and beautiful or thin and beautiful, if you are truly in touch with your inner beauty. However, if your concerns about your body image are actually interfering with your sexual relationship, and stopping you from expressing yourself to your full potential, then it is worth doing something about it.

New Angles of Pleasure

▼ *In this position, the woman squats or kneels with her back to her partner. Although there is less intimacy, because they are not able to see each other's faces, it can be an exciting variation to add to the sexual repertoire. The woman should lower herself carefully onto the penis so that it enters her vagina at a comfortable angle. Penetration can be very deep with any of the woman-on-top squatting positions, so care should be taken to avoid thrusting movements which may cause the penis to jar the cervix. To maintain the squatting position, the woman will need to be quite supple in her hips and legs; kneeling astride the partner may be easier for her. The advantage of this position is that the woman is free to stimulate her own clitoris, while the man surrenders to the pleasurable sensations of her movements.*

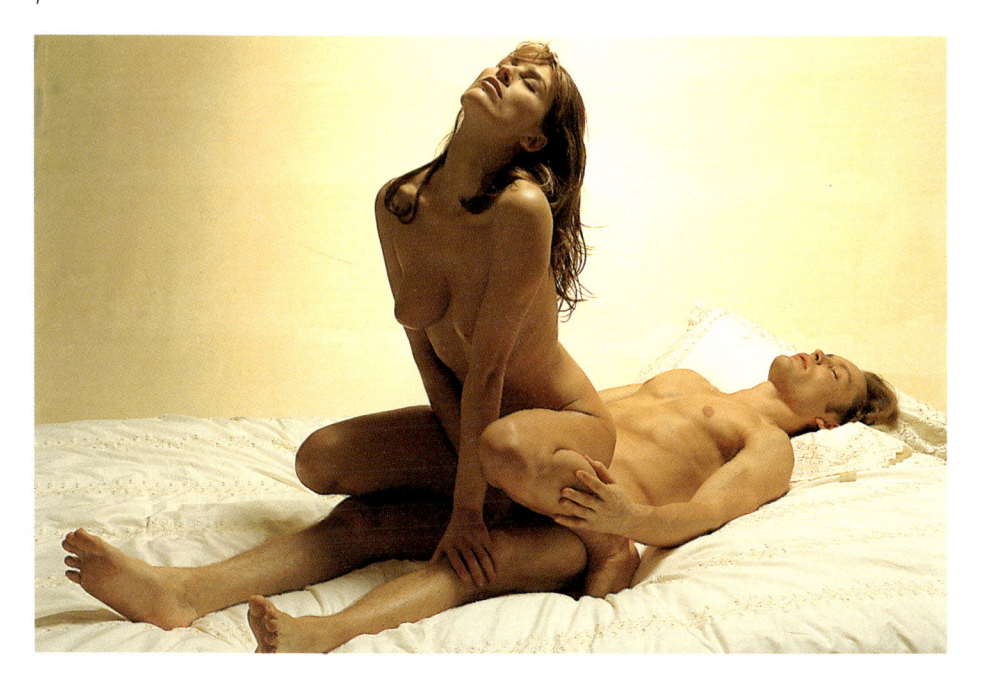

A balanced diet, containing lots of fruit, vegetables and grains will give you vitality and energy and help you to stabilize your weight. Exercise will strengthen your muscles, giving you extra power for some of the more exciting sexual manoeuvres. Toning up your abdomen, buttocks and thighs will not only make you feel good, but add to your agility and suppleness and ability to accomplish an exciting range of sexual positions. Working on your pelvic floor exercises will benefit your vaginal muscle control to the delight of you and your man, and may increase the intensity of your orgasm.

Expressing Our Sexuality

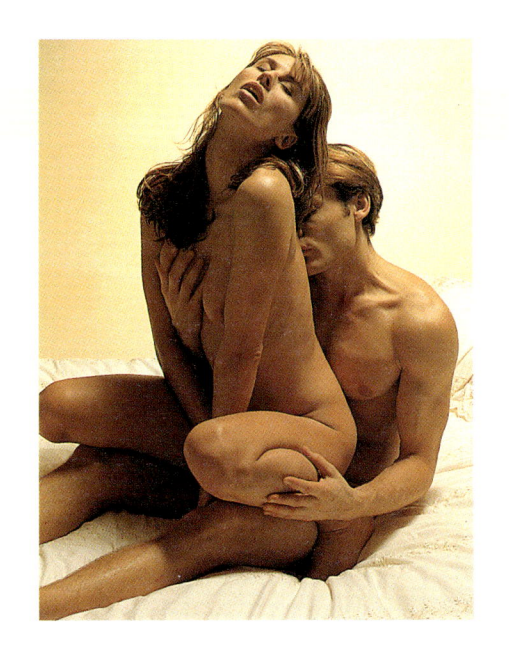

Sensuously Slow Motions
◀ If the man is sitting up when the woman kneels or squats with her back to him, then much greater physical contact and intimacy can ensue. Her back and buttocks will be moving against and stroking the front of his body, and he will be able to kiss and caress her. Intimate contact on the back of her body will be especially pleasant for her as this area is largely neglected during more traditional sexual postures. He can also reach around to stroke her breasts, belly and thighs. Using her feet and legs for leverage in her movements up and down on the penis, she may particularly enjoy savouring the sensual feeling and the slow motions of this position. In addition, she can continue to stimulate her own clitoris, or lovingly stroke her partner's scrotum.

Visual Variations
▶ While many women may be shy of exposing their buttocks and thighs so prominently to their partners, both sexes can find this variation of the woman-on-top position with her back towards the man a very exciting part of their love play. A man, in particular may be very visually stimulated by looking at his partner's buttocks, especially if she is kneeling and leaning forward so it is on display. Gentle stimulation on her anal area with his fingers can also increase her sexual arousal, though for hygiene reasons the fingers should not then be transferred to her vagina until the hands are washed. The woman's movements can become quite active in this position, as she lifts and lowers herself on the penis, or she can tantalizingly raise herself so the lower end of her vagina clasps just the tip of the man's penis, to make small but deliciously sensual and erotically exciting motions.

Heightened Bodily Contact
▶ If the woman is light and supple enough, she can follow on from the previous position, to lean her body back to lie flat against her partner's trunk. This will bring them both back into a very intimate contact as the length of her upper body sinks into the front of his. In this position, the couple should take time to relax deeply and breathe together, allowing a sense of physical and emotional merging. The pressure of his penis inside her vagina will rest against its front wall, supplying an intense stimulation to her G-spot area. While there is little movement in this position, the woman can tighten her vaginal muscles around the penis to exert pleasurable contractions onto it. The open and exposed position of the woman's body means that both of them can touch and caress her breasts and vulva at the same time.

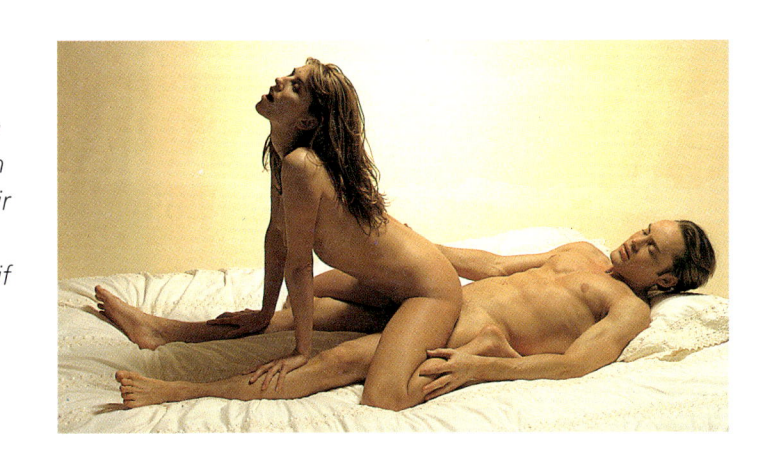

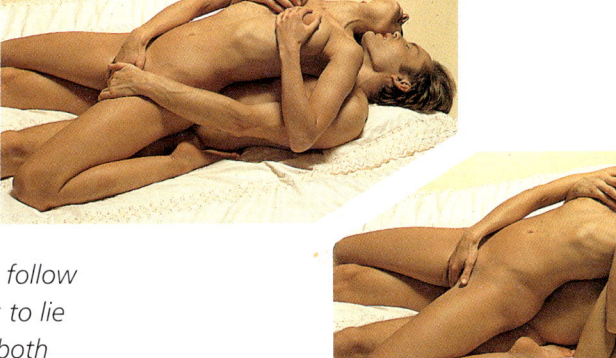

Stimulating Strokes
▲ When the woman has lowered the back of her body against her partner's chest and belly, as in the previously described position, she can also easily masturbate herself to reach a peak of arousal or orgasm while the man strokes and palpates her breasts and nipples. This can be tremendously exciting for the man as he feels the waves of pleasure running through her body vibrate against his skin, and as she surrenders to her involuntary contractions against the safe support of his body.

53

Basic Techniques

Sitting Positions

Sitting positions allow the man and the woman to feel equally involved in their lovemaking, and can add a completely different emotional and physical dimension to their sexual life. The position itself does not allow for a great deal of movement, and is more often used in between other manoeuvres, or when the couple needs to find a more restful connection during intercourse. Yet it can create a very profound feeling of intimacy and bonding between both people, allowing them to have close eye and body contact. Holding each other, and breathing together, can be emotionally fulfilling. It can also transform the excitement and passion of lovemaking into something transcendental: a shared experience with a more meditative quality of deep merging and union of mind, body and spirit.

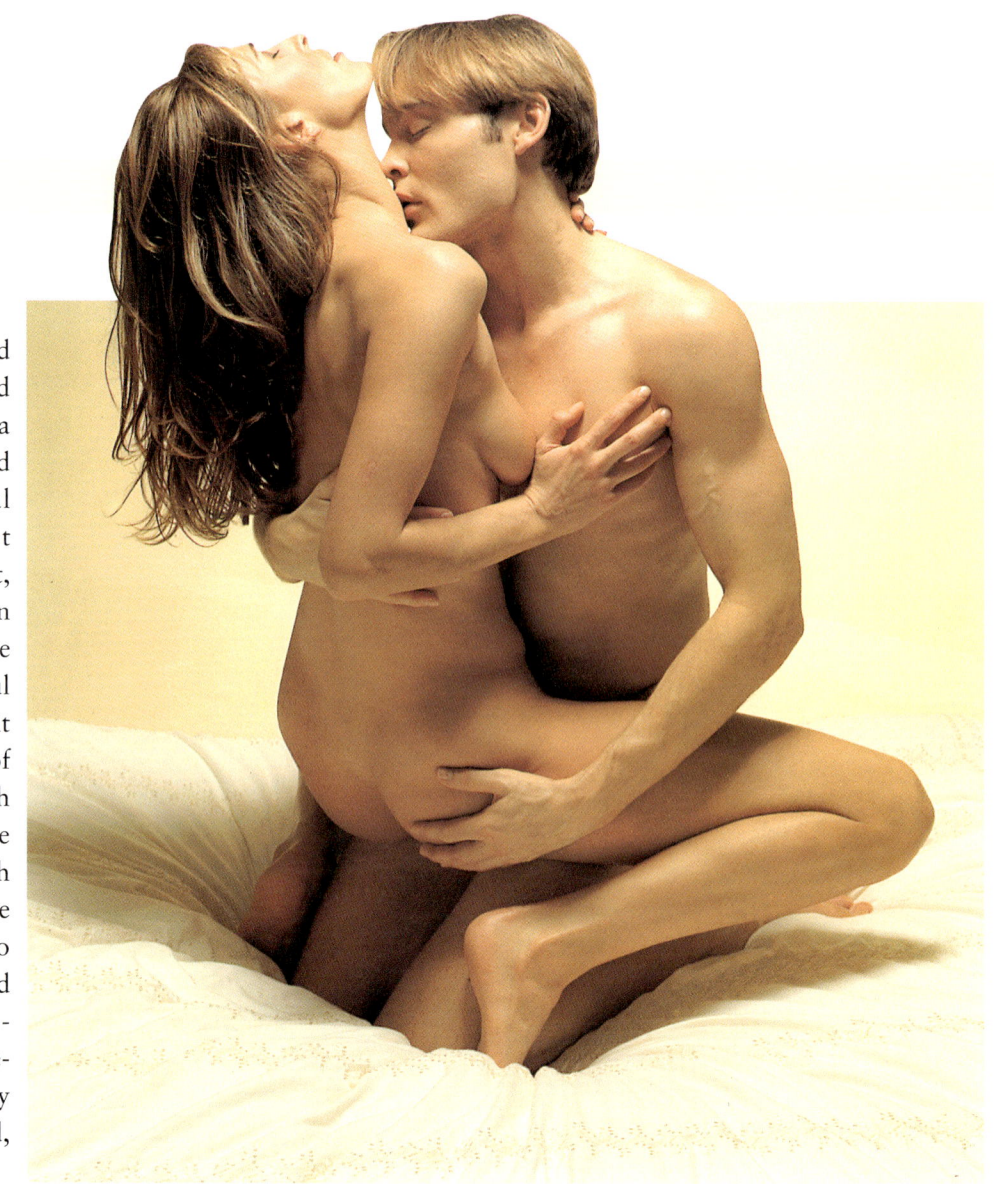

Women's Sexual Attitudes

Vanessa, 27, graphic artist and single. What turns you on most about a man? *"His humour, his eyes, his sensuality."* What do you enjoy most about lovemaking? *"The tenderness and intimacy, lots of cuddling and kissing."* When do you experience your strongest orgasms? *"When I trust my lover completely with my vulnerability."*

Renuka, 31, a personal assistant and married. What turns you on most about a man? *"I was attracted to my husband because he was good looking and kind."* What do you enjoy most about lovemaking? *"When he takes control and is powerful and strong. It makes me feel very feminine."* When do you experience your strongest orgasms? *"When we are relaxed and I am not worrying about the children."*

Deidre, 42, psychologist and divorced. What turns you on most about a man? *"His charisma, his looks, and his self-confidence."* What do you enjoy most about lovemaking? *"I enjoy mostly everything, especially if we can laugh and have fun."* When do you experience your strongest orgasms? *"When I am in love."*

Carolyn, 22, married with one baby. What turns you on most about a man? *"Physically, I would have to say his height, his build and his buttocks. Emotionally, I would pick his ability to communicate and love me."* What do you enjoy most about lovemaking? *"When it is slow and gentle yet very erotic."* When do you experience your strongest orgasms? *"When we are making love at the same rhythm and pace, and when we feel especially close with each other."*

Freda, 35, artist and divorced. What turns you on most about a man? *"Everything, I love them all."* What do you enjoy most about lovemaking? *"When it is hot, passionate and lusty."* When do you experience your strongest orgasms? *"When I feel free enough to scream and shout and generally let go."*

Expressing Our Sexuality

Intimate Exchange

◀ *The closeness of the bodies, and the feeling of freedom and ease in the back and spine, can make the sitting position in lovemaking one of great intimacy and pleasure. It is a sexual posture which can feel erotically different from most others, and is best used in moments of deep emotional and sensual exchange. Neither partner is playing a dominant role, as both people are assuming a vertical posture. The woman kneels or squats astride her partner's thighs, and therefore, penetration can become very deep.*

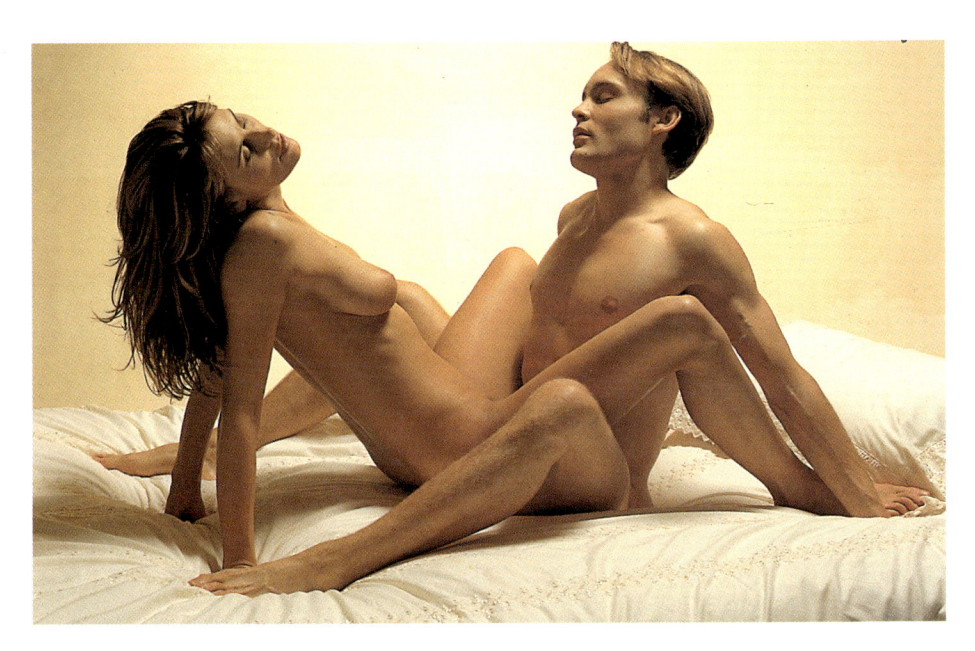

Synchronized Sexuality

◀ *While making love in the sitting position, more movement can be attained if the couple separate their bodies, leaning back and supporting their own weight on their arms and hands. The woman can use the strength in her leg muscles to lever herself up and down on the shaft of the penis, and the man can thrust into her. Movements should synchronize, or be made by one or the other partner. The more separated position of the bodies also enables the man to stimulate the woman's clitoris with his fingers.*

Resolving Harmoniously

▶ *The intimacy and equality of the sitting positions make them some of the most satisfying and pleasurable in the repertoire. Such harmonious lovemaking can draw the man and woman into a deep sense of joyful union, which can be beautifully resolved and reinforced by sinking back gently into each other's arms and lying quietly together in blissful repose.*

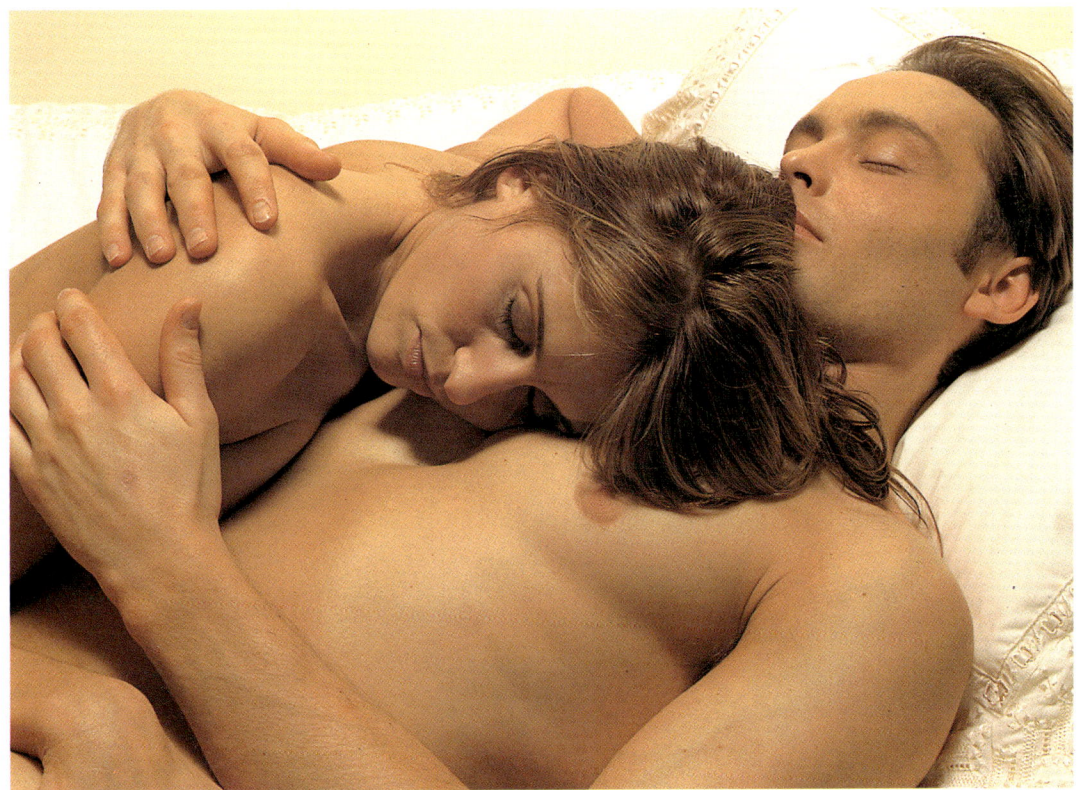

Orgasm

Orgasm is the culmination of lovemaking – the sweet release of powerful sensations which are discharged when sexual arousal has reached its peak. For both the man and the woman, it can be a most exquisite and joyful physical experience. Orgasm need not be just a genital affair – a pleasurable release of pent-up sexual tension from the pelvic region. It is possible for the whole body to surrender to the pulsating waves of orgasmic energy.

Orgasm is not just a physical process – it is a holistic experience. It can encompass the whole spectrum of what it means to be a human being – involving also our love, our emotions and our spiritual nature.

It would be wrong, however, to assume that every orgasm should leave you feeling as if "the earth shook". There will be many occasions when the moments of climax and ejaculation will feel more like tender seconds of release, or gentle vibrations in the sexual organs. For the orgasm will largely reflect your mood at the time, whether you are tired, or under stress, or in tune with your partner. Sometimes it can even be a real source of disappointment, a feeling of being a bit let down. Honesty, exploration and experimentation will help most couples to improve their orgasmic ability and to find a greater compatibility in their lovemaking.

Most of all, do not let orgasm become an obsession in your lovemaking. Setting it as the goal of intercourse can create tensions in body and mind, detracting from the joy of the moment and actually interfering with the orgasmic process. Orgasm can be the cherry on the cake, but the

A Melting Moment
▶ *Both the man and the woman can feel as if they are melting and merging and letting go into something that is greater than themselves. For some moments the individual ego is dissolved, and for this reason orgasm has often been described as a potentially transforming experience.*

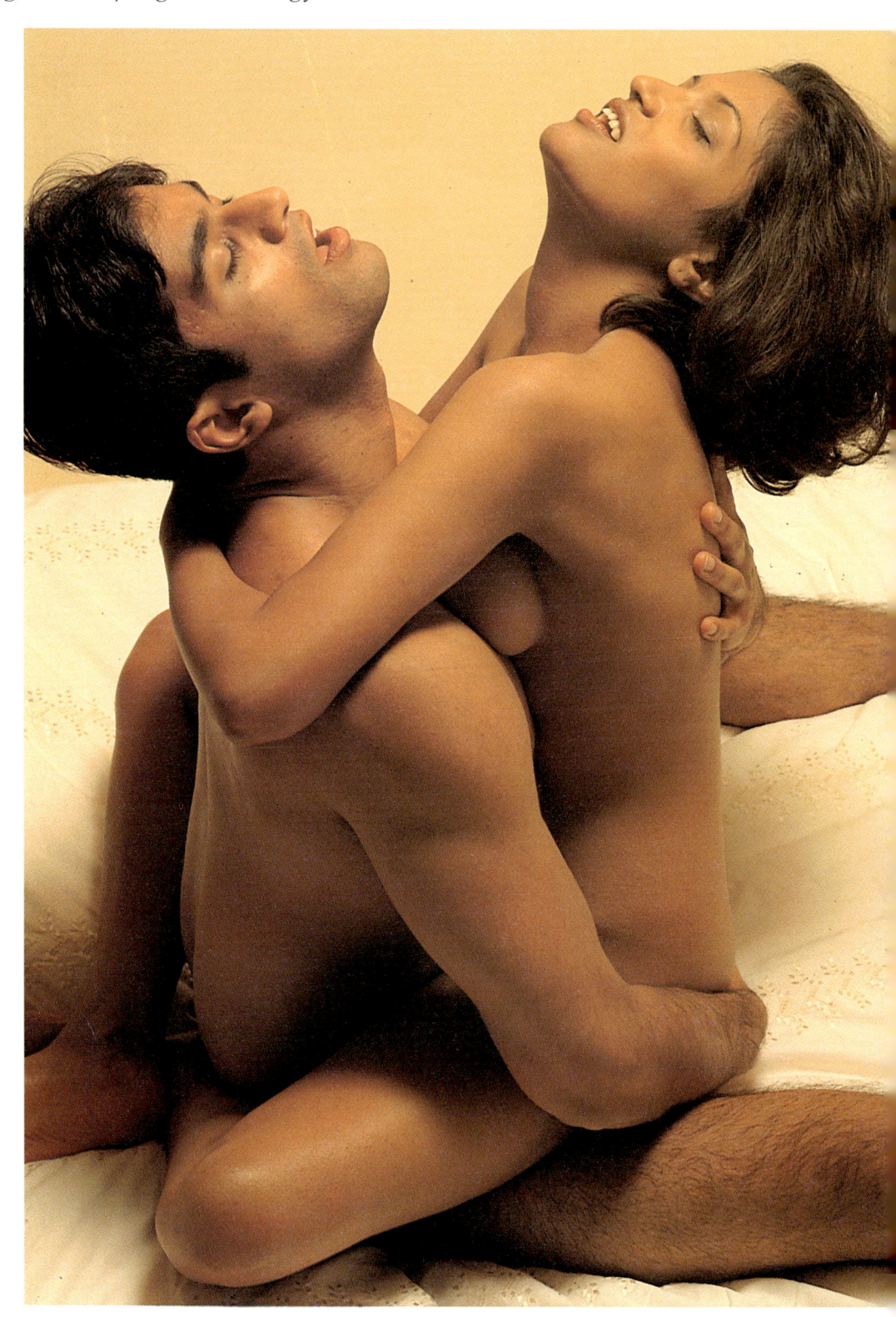

Orgasmic Variety

cake itself is also delicious and should be enjoyed for its own sake!

It is not necessary to have penetrative sex in order to have an orgasm. It can be attained from self-masturbation, mutual masturbation, and oral sex. Sometimes, during intercourse, a couple may choose to switch to oral sex to complete the orgasmic experience. A man who is concerned that he might not sustain his erection, or that he might ejaculate too soon, may even perform cunnilingus so that his partner has an orgasm before he enters her. So orgasm is very versatile and can be adapted to the mood of the individual or the lovers concerned.

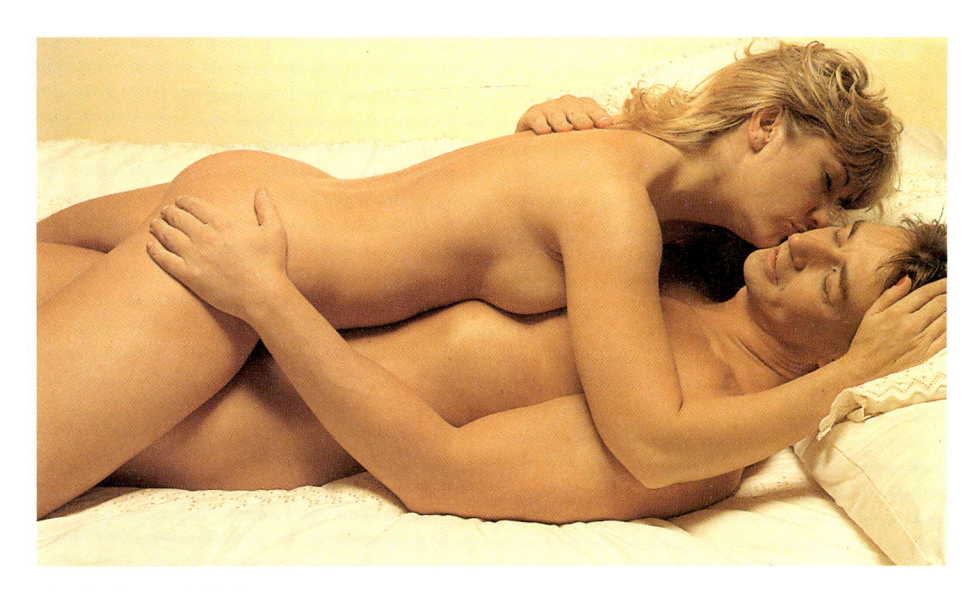

Seek New Heights
▲ Become more sensual and relaxed with each other so your bodies begin to resonate together. Try different positions for making love to see which ones can bring you to greater heights of arousal.

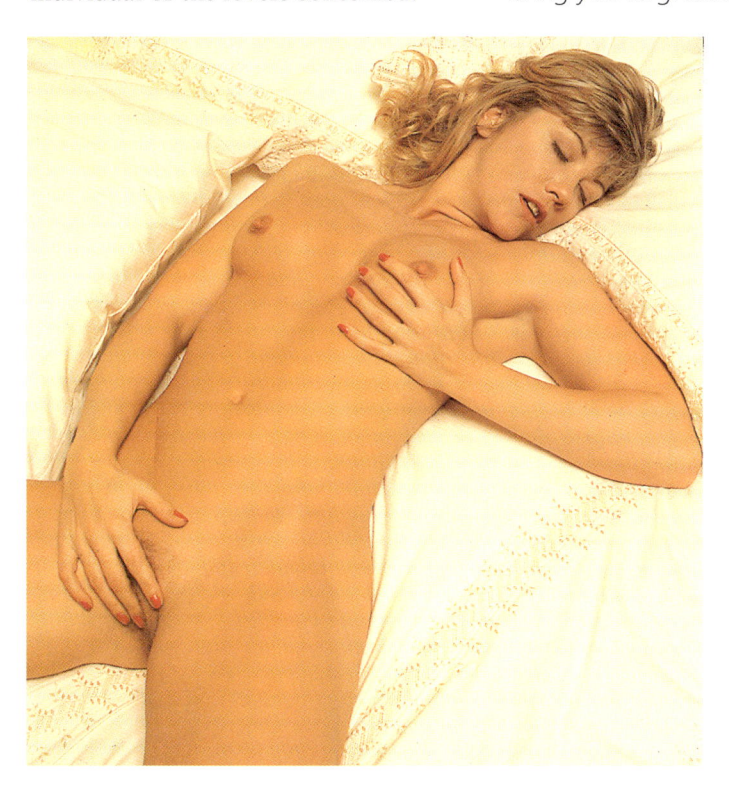

Self-Discovery
▲ Quite often, self-masturbation is recommended as an exercise for people who are experiencing difficulty in obtaining an orgasm with a sexual partner. By bringing yourself to orgasm, you can learn exactly what kind of stimulation you enjoy and also become more relaxed with your own sexual organs and bodily responses.

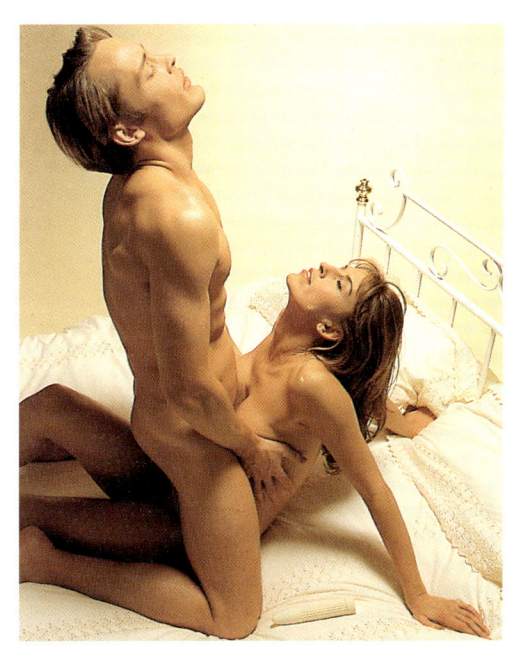

Varying Orgasm
▲ There are times when a man may choose not to ejaculate into his partner's vagina. Maybe penetrative sex is unwise because of a current infection, or there is a risk of pregnancy, or perhaps the couple want to add a little variety to their repertoire. In such cases the man can reach his orgasm threshold and then ejaculate onto his partner's belly, or even between the warm soft mounds of her breasts. (It goes without saying that he should only do this with her consent.)

Basic Techniques

The Body's Response in Orgasm

Studies conducted into human sexual behaviour by American researchers William Masters and Virginia Johnson in the 1950s revealed for the first time that men and women follow a very similar physiological pattern before, during, and after orgasm. They discovered that the sexual response of men and women is divided into four phases: the arousal or excitement phase, the plateau phase, orgasm or climax, and the resolution or recovery phase.

However, they also discovered that the sexes differ in many respects. For example, the plateau phase in males can be much shorter than in females, with the result that the man may ejaculate before the woman has had an orgasm, unless he makes an effort to prolong this phase. In contrast, the resolution phase can be much shorter in females compared with men, enabling many women to achieve several orgasms during a single lovemaking session.

In addition, Masters and Johnson showed that the woman's clitoris is as erogenic as the man's penis, and its sustained stimulation during intercourse may be necessary if she is to achieve orgasm. They also noted other distinct parallels between the male and female physiological responses, such as the buildup of neuro-muscular tension, the increase in heart rate and blood pressure, the quickening of breathing, and, if it occurs, a reddening or flushing that can spread over the skin.

Male Physical Response

Orgasm is triggered in the man when the muscular tension in his body and nerve stimulation of the sex organs

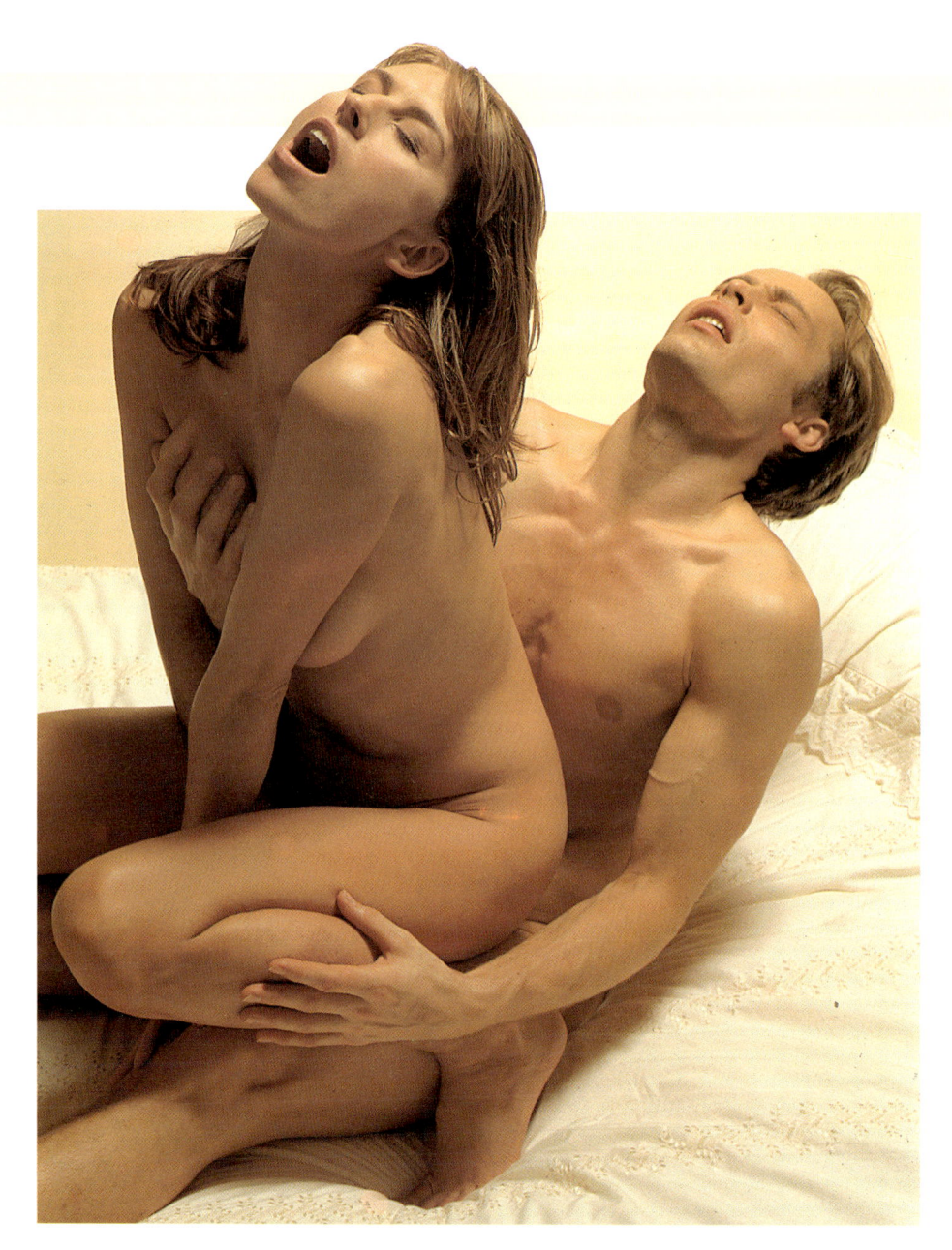

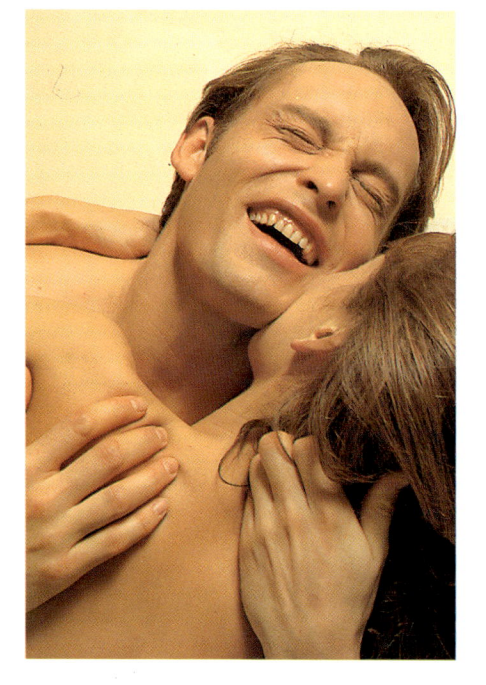

The Pleasure Surge
▲ *During orgasm, both sexes experience rhythmic contractions in the sex organs and pelvic floor muscles, followed by a release of tension which creates a surge of pleasurable sensations spreading through the body.*

Spasms of Ecstasy
◀ *Some men seem to experience sexual contractions only in their genital area, while others feel them throughout the body. During these moments of orgasm, a man may shout or cry out, and his face may contort for a few ecstatic moments as a result of muscular spasms.*

Orgasm

has reached the orgasm peak in what has been termed "the point of no return". Just before ejaculation, rhythmic contractions of muscles around the prostate gland, the seminal vesicles, and the epididymides, push seminal fluids and sperm into the base of the urethra – the urethral bulb – where they mix together. At this stage, the man's testicles are fully elevated and the opening between his urethra and bladder closes.

Extra Stimulation
▼ *If a man ejaculates prior to the woman's climax, and so loses his erection, she cannot reach orgasm unless additional stimulation is provided, either by him or by herself. This can be achieved by the man performing cunnilingus, or manual stimulation of her clitoris. Alternatively, he can kiss, stroke and lick her body and breasts, while she masturbates herself to orgasm.*

At ejaculation, intense rhythmic contractions of the urethral bulb and spasms of the pelvic floor muscles pump the semen through the penis, where it spurts out at the tip. These ejaculatory contractions follow each other in rapid succession. Initially they can be very powerful, though they progressively decrease in strength. At the same time the man experiences the intensely pleasurable sensations of orgasm.

Female Physical Response

Women do not always have an orgasm, even though they may have attained a high level of arousal during the excitement and plateau stage, and there can be a number of reasons for this. Some women may not reach orgasm at all during lovemaking, or during a particular episode of sexual activity, but this does not necessarily detract from the pleasure they have experienced during the other stages of intercourse, and they may feel sexually fulfilled just the same. In addition, a woman can be more easily distracted by her thoughts or concerns at this stage, in which case

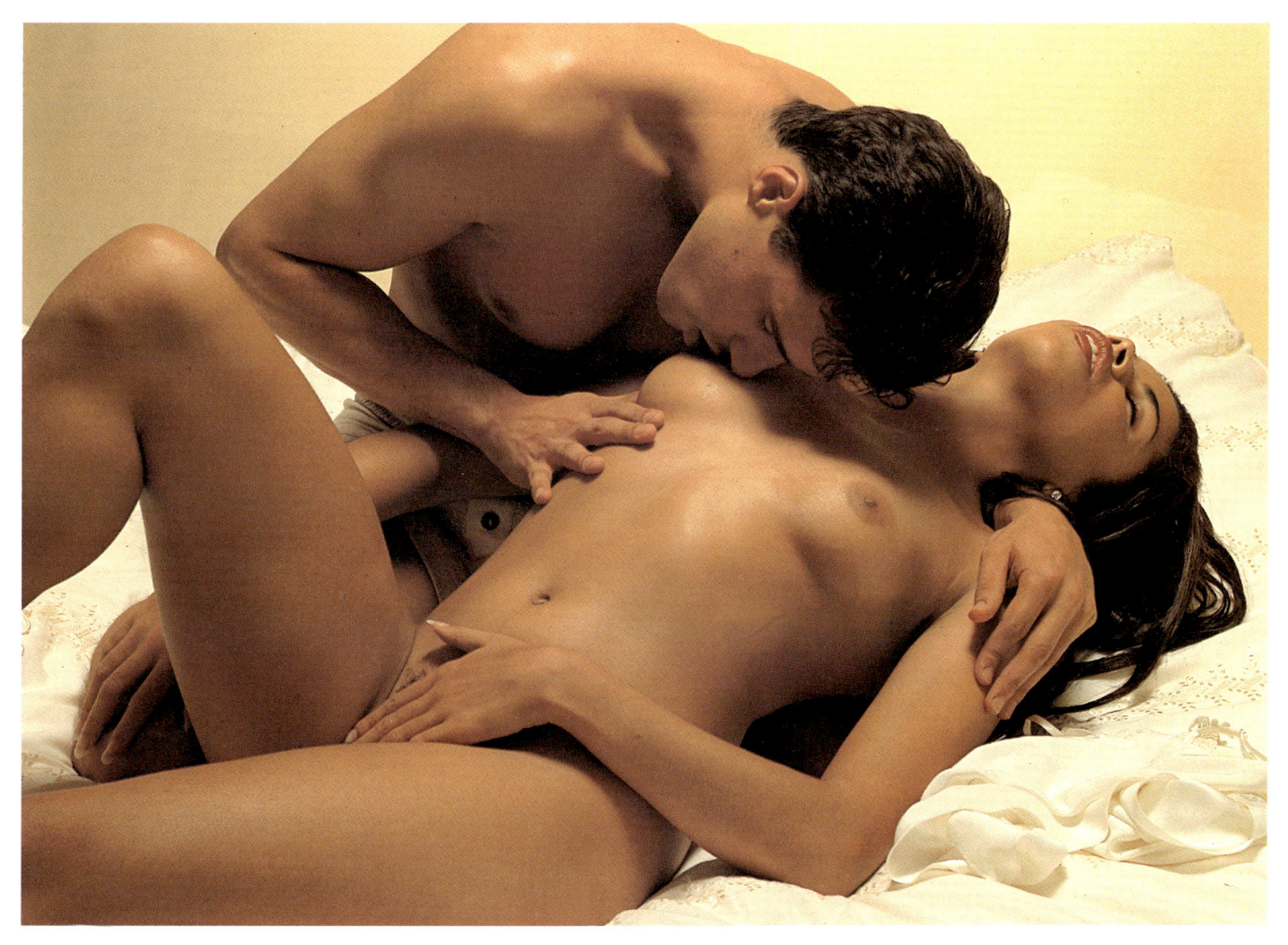

Basic Techniques

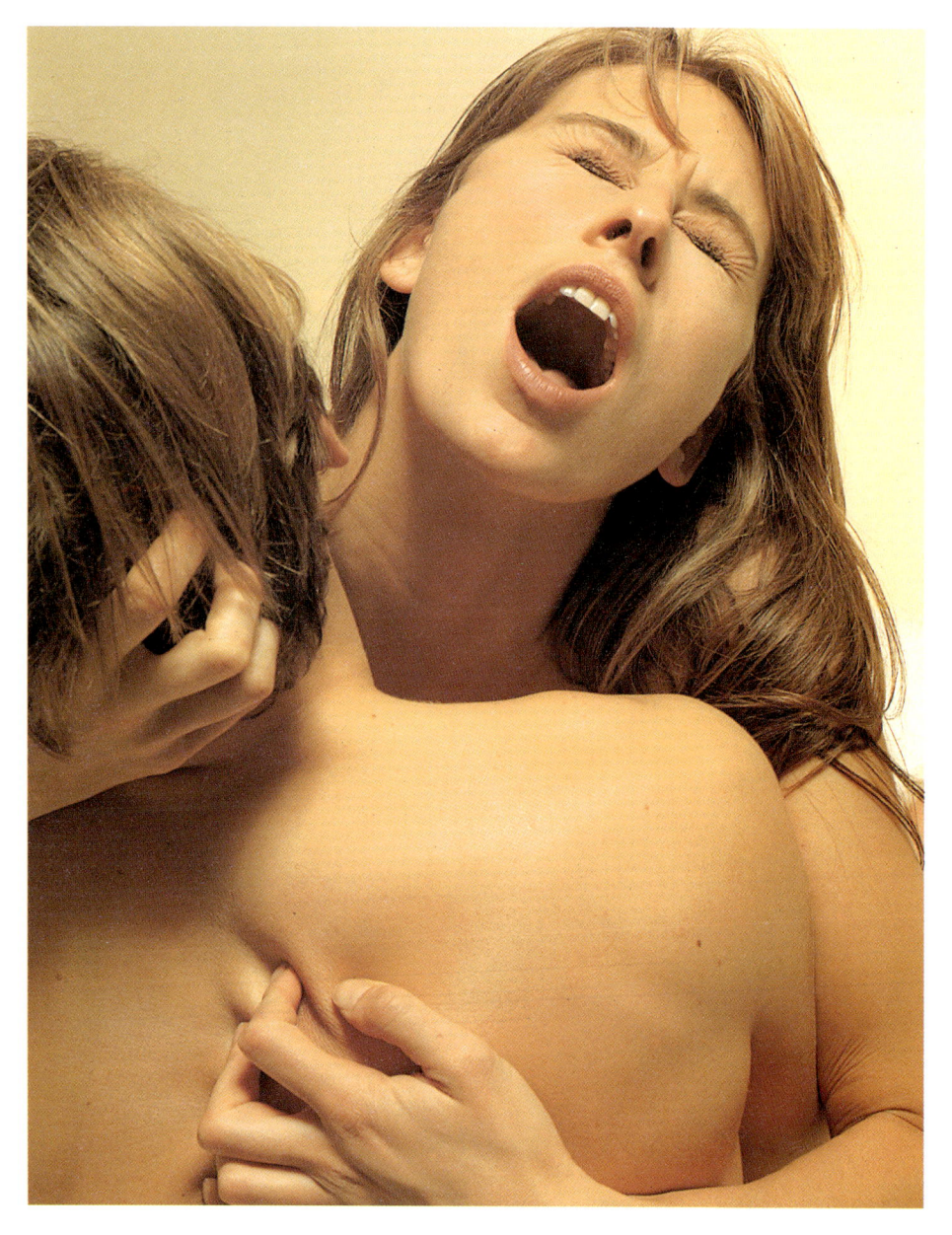

Losing Control
◀ *During this time, the woman loses voluntary control over her muscles, so her face may spasm, and even her fingers and toes can curl. Often in the moments of climax, a woman will cry out or scream, and even dig her fingernails into her partner's back.*

These involuntary contractions work as a pump to release the vaso-congested genital area, so if a woman has almost reached the point of climax, but orgasm is interrupted, for whatever reason, this pent-up feeling of tension in her genitals can make her feel physically very uncomfortable and emotionally let down. She must either wait for this physiological feeling to subside by itself, or for her partner to bring her to orgasm – by oral or manual stimulation if he has already ejaculated. Alternatively, she can masturbate herself to reach her climax.

Faking Orgasms

It is worth mentioning here that many women feel obliged to fake orgasms, leading their partner to mistakenly believe they have reached a climax. Sometimes a woman will do this to finish a lovemaking session because she is bored or tired and her partner's efforts to please her are putting her under an unnecessary pressure. Perhaps her arousal level has dipped, and her vaginal juices have dried, so the prolonged intercourse is making her sore. For whatever reason, a woman may then fake an orgasm to please her partner and to soothe his sexual ego.

Many women, for all sorts of reasons, find it very difficult to be truthful in these sensitive moments. In such situations, the faked orgasm

even the effort of trying to reach an orgasm can be counter-productive.

Most women do not reach orgasm through vaginal friction alone, and need more direct clitoral stimulation during intercourse, either by skilfully applied pressure from the man's pubic bone, by her own movements, or by additional oral or manual stimulation.

When the conditions are right for the woman to have an orgasm, she may begin to feel it as an intense sensation of warmth spreading from her clitoris throughout her body, and a throbbing sensation in her vagina and the muscles in her pelvic region.

When this tension reaches its peak, it gives way to powerful rhythmic contractions which can occur in the lower portion of the vagina, the uterus, and around the anus. For many women, these waves of sensation can pulsate through their whole body. The first contractions are the strongest, but they may be followed by a series of milder pulsations – rather like the aftershocks that often follow an earthquake.

Orgasm

is something akin to a "little white lie". Problems arise if faking an orgasm is a constant pattern of behaviour in a couple's sex life. In this case, it is better if the woman can reveal to her partner that she is unable to climax while making love. Together they can then explore all kinds of sensual ways of bringing her greater pleasure. Perhaps they need to spend more time on foreplay, so the woman is more fully aroused. Or they could experiment with different lovemaking positions so that she can receive the right kind of clitoral stimulation – the woman-on-top positions may help. The issues involved may be even deeper, possibly relating to a sexual anxiety, and it would be beneficial for the woman, and even her partner, to seek professional help from a sex counsellor.

Multiple Orgasms

As the resolution, or recovery, phase in females can be very short – just a few seconds in some cases – some women are capable of attaining multiple orgasms one after another during sex. This is not possible for men because the male recovery phase takes anything from several minutes to many hours. However, there are many women who feel satiated after reaching one orgasm and, like men, will temporarily lose interest in continuing intercourse, although their arousal may return sooner.

There has been a considerable amount of discussion in the media about a woman's multi-orgasmic capacity. In one way this is useful information, for it alerts both men and women to the fact that female sexuality is powerful and profound. It is worth bearing in mind that it has only been in the last 50 years that a woman's orgasmic nature has been fully acknowledged by Western scientists and doctors.

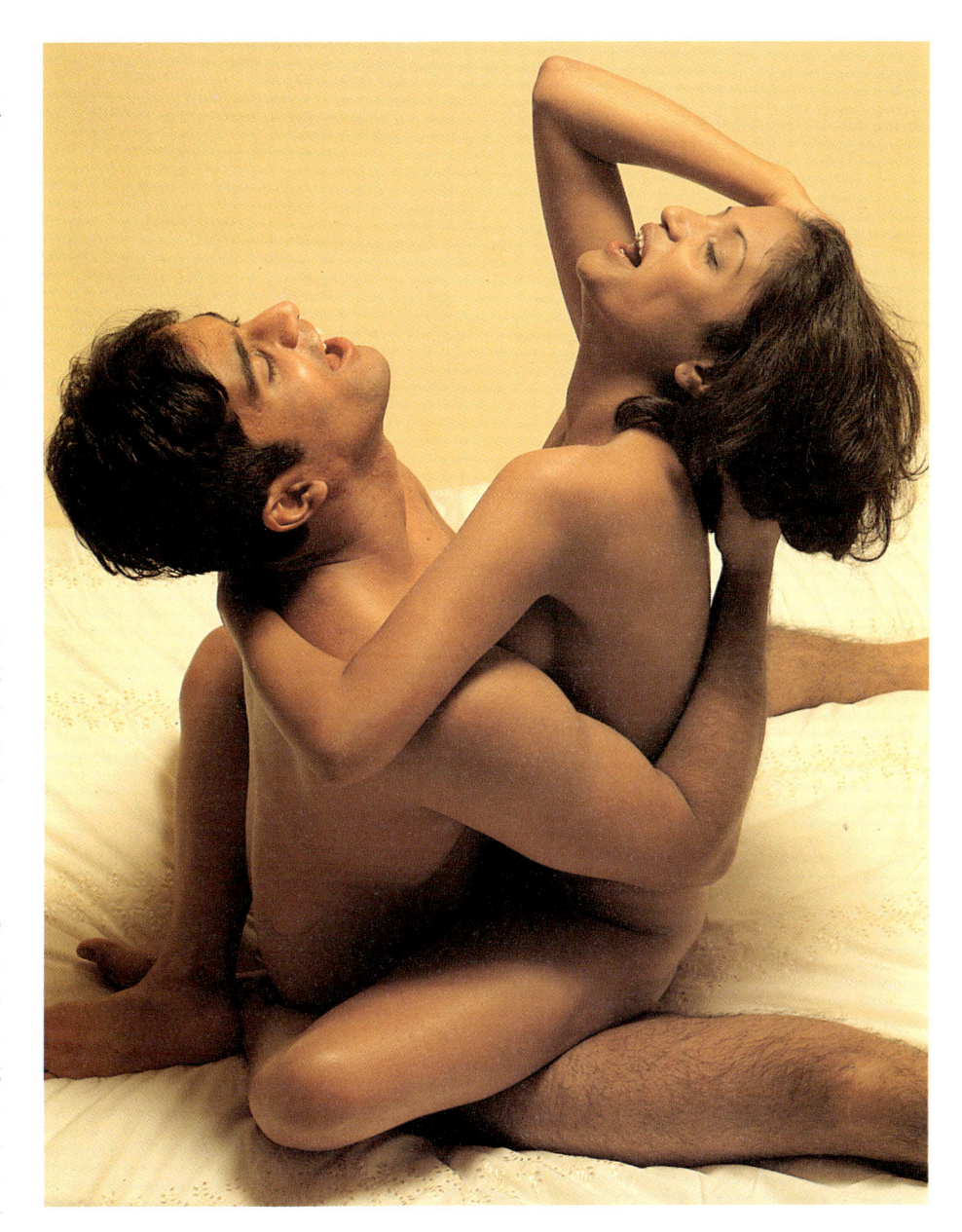

However, the hype over multiple orgasms can cause problems by creating tensions for men and women. A man may feel he is a failure as a sexual performer if his partner fails to achieve a certain quota of orgasms, while the woman may believe there is something lacking in her for being unable to climax over and over again. Every loving couple can benefit from exploring their full sexual potential, but ultimately their orgasmic capacity should be measured in terms of quality rather than quantity, just like every other aspect of lovemaking.

Prolonging the Plateau
▲ *If the man is able to prolong the plateau phase of lovemaking – delaying or abstaining from his own orgasm – the woman may be able to have one climax after another. This capacity for multiple orgasms differs from one woman to the next.*

Basic Techniques

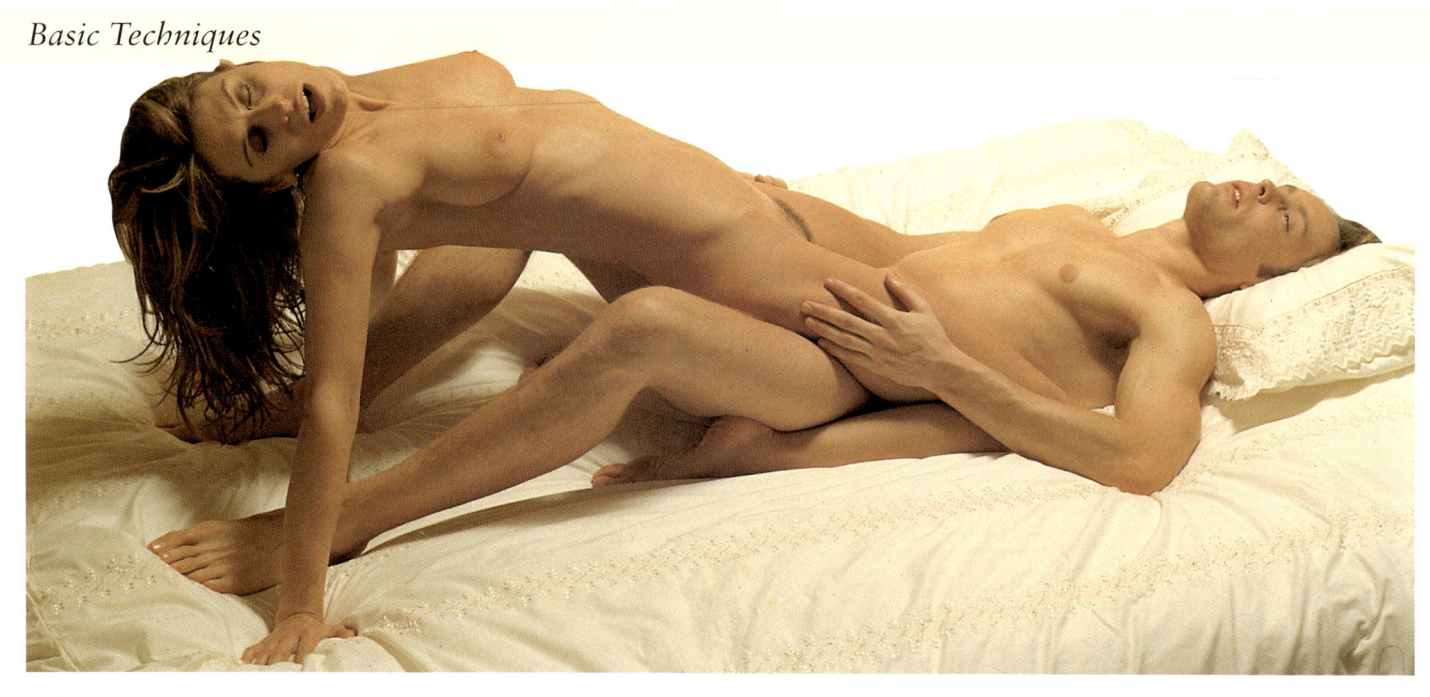

The G-Spot

We now know that the clitoris is the most erotically sensitive part of a woman's body and that it plays a fundamental part in her orgasmic process. However, in recent years there has been much debate about the woman's G-spot, so called after its discovery by the German gynaecologist Ernst Gräfenberg. Pressure on the G-spot, which is a complex of nerve endings located on the front wall of the vagina, is said to induce a particularly intense form of vaginal orgasm. Gräfenberg's studies went even further, stating that when the G-spot is adequately stimulated the urethra ejaculates a clear fluid which has "no urinary character". This exciting discovery has been refuted by other doctors and scientists, who continue to believe that the fluid is indistinguishable from urine. Many doctors also deny the existence of the woman's G-spot. However, there is evidence to suggest that, in some women at least, this orgasm-triggering nerve bundle really does exist. It is definitely worth exploring.

Locating the G-spot
▶ You can gently probe your own vagina, to see if your finger pressure can find the magic spot, or you can ask your partner to do it for you. The G-spot is said to be located on the front wall of the vagina 5–7.5cm/ 2–3in from the vaginal entrance.

Stimulating the G-spot
▲ The G-spot can be stimulated by lovemaking positions in which the man's penis rubs against the front wall of the vagina, provided he can maintain this action for some time. In the position shown here, the woman leans back to allow the penis to press firmly against her G-spot.

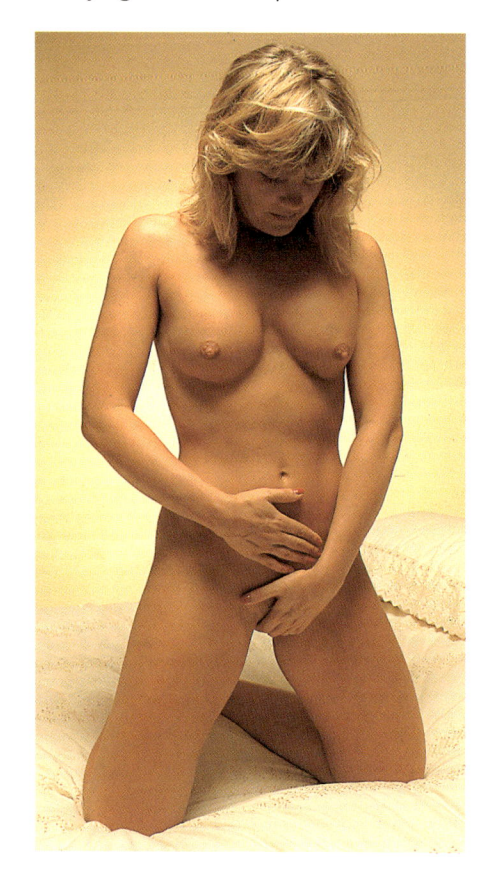

Simultaneous Orgasms

When a man and a woman have orgasms simultaneously it can be a peak experience in making love, but it is not absolutely necessary for a satisfying sexual life. Most couples can have an extremely happy sexual relationship without ever achieving simultaneous orgasms.

If the man should happen to ejaculate first, he can continue to stimulate his partner to reach her climax with oral or manual techniques. Alternatively, if the woman orgasms before the man, she is usually physically able to continue intercourse and can then devote herself to his pleasure. She may even climax again if she is multi-orgasmic.

Simultaneous orgasms can happen when the couple are in harmony with each other's arousal signals. They may intuitively know when to hold back and when to go forward, slowing down if one or the other is

62

Orgasm

dangerously close to the orgasm threshold. Talking to each other while making love can add an exciting dimension of shared intimacy, so do not be shy to tell your partner you need to take it easy, or that you need more stimulation, or request that he or she "hold on a second". Say these things seductively; you do not want to make them sound like an order. After a while, these verbal signals will become part of your love-play.

Resolution

Resolution is the final phase of the sexual cycle of response, as defined by Masters and Johnson. Here, for both the man and the woman, the body now returns to its normal pre-arousal state. In a man, the immediate stage after ejaculation is termed the refractory period, and it is impossible for him to resume sexual activity at this time. The length of time the phase lasts varies greatly from one man to another, but in most cases it increases with age.

Most men feel depleted after orgasm and need a period of time to recover, often wanting to withdraw into themselves, or go to sleep. However, a post-orgasmic woman can often remain in a state of sexual excitement after climaxing and may want the lovemaking to continue. As explained, a woman is often capable of going on to achieve more orgasms.

The main difference between the sexes immediately after orgasm is that the man is more likely to require peace and quiet, while his partner needs intimacy to continue, if only in the form of cuddling, touching, and talking. This fundamental difference in the male and female response in the moments immediately after making love can create real problems in a relationship. Quite clearly, both have needs which must be met.

If a man consistently "turns off" after orgasm, his partner is likely to construe his actions as a sign that he does not care about her. His behaviour may render the whole sexual experience null and void for her and she may feel bitterly rejected. For the man, his need to rest may be paramount, and in fearing that he cannot meet his partner's demands he may cut off from her even more.

If after-sex behaviour is disrupting the harmony of your love life, it is really worthwhile talking about the issue with each other. It is best to try to understand your partner's needs and point of view, rather than becoming angry or defensive.

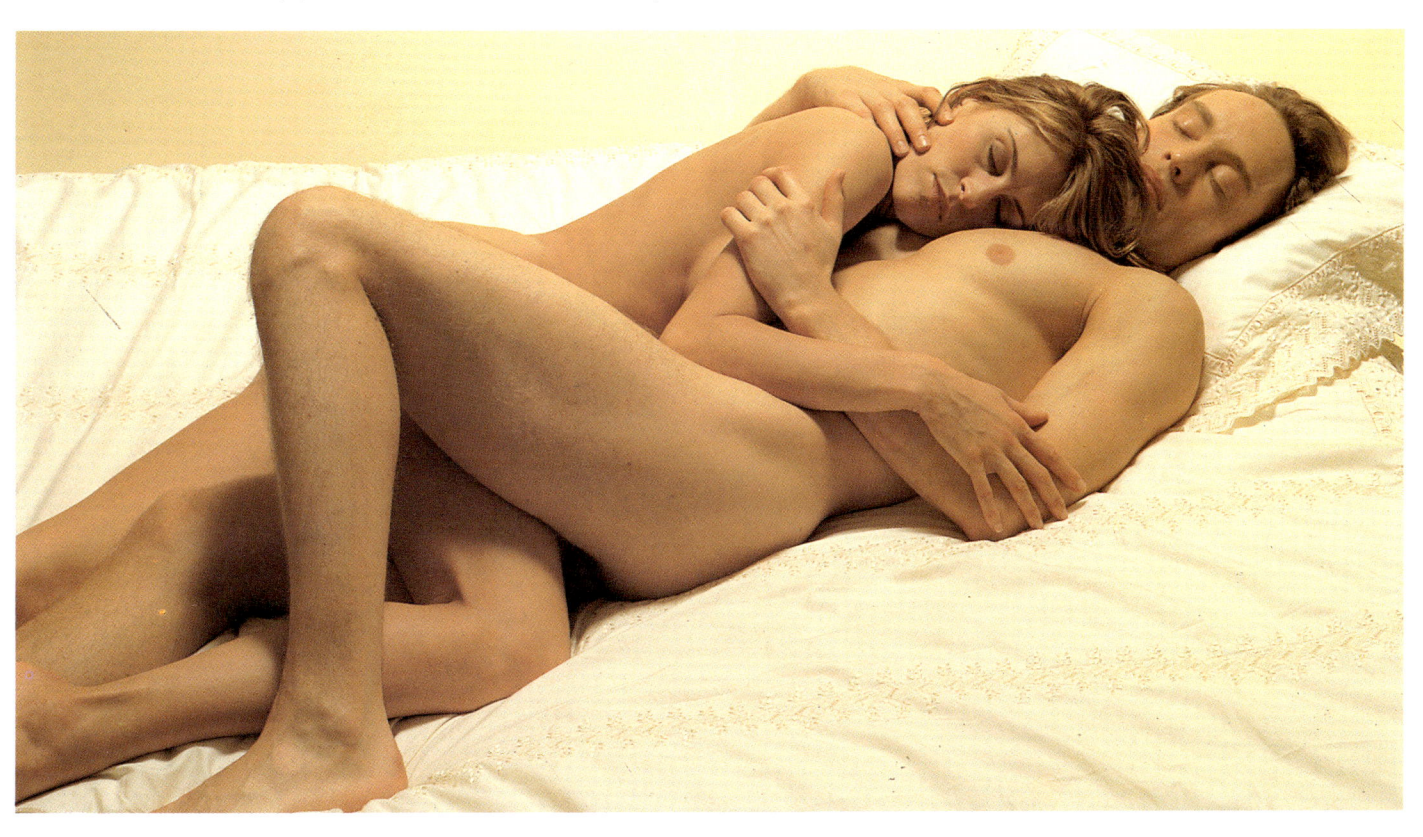

Enjoy the Intimacy
▼ *During the resolution phase after orgasm, a couple can lie together in each other's arms, simply enjoying their close physical presence and the intimacy of the moment, allowing themselves to relax deeply.*

Adventurous Lovemaking

There is nothing new about adventurous sexual positions, despite the plethora of advice that is currently in vogue. Detailed texts and manuscripts on the best ways to achieve sexual happiness, and explicit descriptions of sexual positions and practices, have appeared in many ancient cultures, including India, China and the Middle East. Some of these texts dealt with the pursuit of sensual and erotic pleasure, others were medically informed scripts to help couples achieve sexual health and happiness, and some referred to sexo-yogic practices through which men and women could attain a higher spiritual state of consciousness.

The Kama Sutra of Vatsyayana, which was written in India in about the fourth century AD, is one of the most famous of the texts giving frank and exact advice on how to achieve sexual fulfilment. The first English version of *The Kama Sutra* was translated from Sanskrit by the great Victorian explorer Sir Richard Burton in 1883, and privately printed for The Kama Sastra Society of London and Benares. At that time, this organization was devoted to the acquisition and translation of important and historical texts dedicated to the subject of erotic love.

It was not until 1964, however, that the text was widely published in the West, when its forthright descriptions of the sexual behaviour of the Indian bourgeoisie of an earlier era caused a considerable stir among the public. In particular, its ample detail of a variety of erotic practices and sexual positions really excited the readers' imaginations. The publication of *The Kama Sutra* during the 1960s was one of the many events of that decade that heralded a more open attitude to sexuality.

The Kama Sutra does not, in fact, concern itself solely with sexual issues, but also extols the merits of perfecting a life filled with art, pleasure and recreational activities which would have been deemed appropriate to the wealthy and privileged classes of fourth-century India. It is based on the principle of kama, or desire, which is the celebration of the physical senses and the longing for love. In a spiritual context, this can be perceived as the human yearning to be united with the Divine.

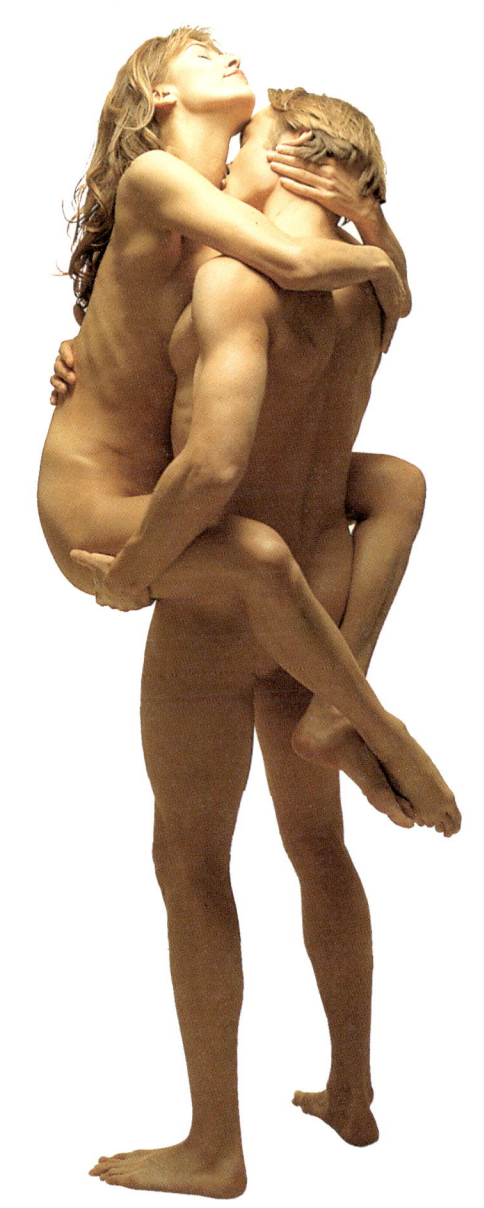

It is the section on sexual union, however, which has spanned the divide of culture and history to become meaningful and relevant to modern readers. *The Kama Sutra* does not shrink from an explicit discussion on sexuality, even though it embraces the social mores of its time, some of which may seem alien to the contemporary reader.

It talks candidly about every aspect of erotic behaviour, including how to touch and caress, the art of kissing, biting and scratching, varying sexual positions, themes of domination and submission, and oral and even anal sex. This is not a text book

The Standing Position
◀ *Among the many positions of intercourse suggested by* The Kama Sutra *is the one it calls the "supported congress". This is a standing position in which the lovers support themselves, either against each other, or propped up against a wall. If you choose to try the standing position, use it to add variation and adventure to your other lovemaking manoeuvres, rather than as the sole position for intercourse, because, while it is fun and sensual, it can also become awkward and tiring, especially for the man. The woman will need to be lighter than her partner if he is to pick her up and hold her securely. She can swing her legs up around his waist and clasp him around the shoulders and neck, while he supports her buttocks and back with his hands.*

Adventurous Lovemaking

Advanced Standing Position
▶ *To make the standing lovemaking position a little more acrobatic and adventurous, the woman can lower herself slowly down towards the floor, supporting her upper body with her hands against the ground, while her partner secures her lower back and waist with a firm and secure hold. He can then move her pelvis gently to and fro to create the thrusting sensations. This is an exciting and unusual sexual position but should only be attempted by those lovers who are supple and fit. It cannot be maintained for too long before either partner becomes tired. The man should then carefully assist the woman in raising herself upwards, taking care she does not strain her back, or, alternatively, he can slowly and gently sink down on his knees until it is possible to lay her whole back safely against the floor.*

for the inhibited, or for puritans, or those who are content with the missionary position for sex.

It encourages its readers to explore every aspect of their sexuality, from their bestial instincts to their more sensitive and tender expressions of sexual love. It impresses upon men the importance of satisfying a woman sexually, speaks of woman-on-top positions, and comments that the use of certain types of sexual behaviour should "...generate love, friendship, and respect in the hearts of women".

Exploring Variety
To describe lovemaking positions with the kind of practical detail that appears in this section of the book necessitates adopting a somewhat clinical approach to the subject, and this has the unfortunate tendency of divorcing sexual activity from its wider context of affection, intimacy, tenderness and passion. By discussing movements, angles of penetration and the various techniques of arousal for either partner, it inevitably risks reducing the wonder of making love to that of a how-to guide perhaps more in keeping with a gymnastics or a keep-fit manual.

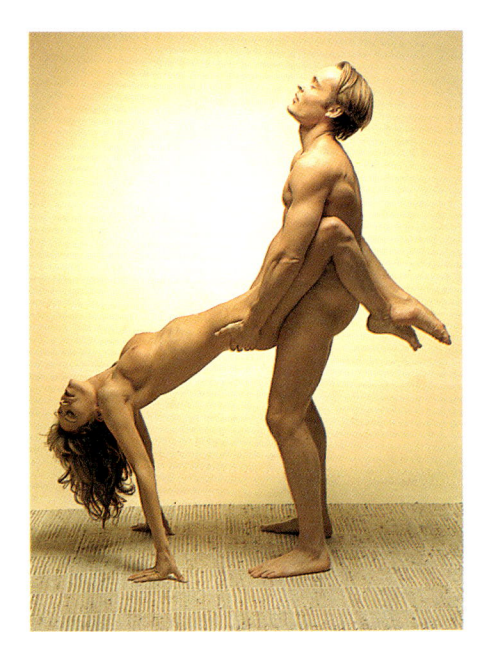

No one can tell two people what is the correct way for them to have intercourse – lovemaking is their own personal act of creativity and an expression of their emotional, psychological and physical make-up. How a couple want to make love, or what they require from a sexual relationship, depends on the needs of the individual or the relationship. Those needs can change from day to day, year to year or from one partnership to another. Telling someone how best to achieve an orgasm cannot possibly address the complex emotions which are also integral to every person's sexuality, or even touch on the shared vulnerability and love which is surely the essence of a truly fulfilling sexual relationship.

Yet in even the most loving partnerships, certain patterns can set in which make the sexual relationship repetitive and eventually boring. Exploration and variety can be as much an enhancement to a sexual relationship as any other aspect of a creative life. Then there are simple physical facts about sexuality that people may simply not know or fully understand because it is often difficult or embarrassing to talk about the nitty-gritty details of sexual performance.

So, for instance, a man could regard himself as an experienced lover, yet despite his Olympian efforts in bed, still fail to satisfy his partner sexually because the positions he favours do not provide the stimulation she needs to achieve an orgasm. The woman, herself, may not understand exactly why she has been unable to reach her peak of arousal, for she may be attracted to her partner and even enjoy those same positions for all the other emotional feelings they provoke.

Examples of this are the various positions shown here where the woman's legs are vertical and resting on the man's shoulders. This position can be exciting for them both, because the man feels powerful and potent, while the woman may enjoy the sensation of surrendering her body to his thrusts. Yet this position precludes the possibility of her receiving direct clitoral stimulation, and is unlikely to lead her to orgasm, so it is not an ideal one to continue for any length of time. Knowing about the subtle variations of position gives partners a greater range of choices and also more understanding of how to fulfil their own and each other's overall sexual and emotional needs.

Adventurous Sex Techniques

Deep Penetration

Some of the more adventurous sexual positions often rely on the man being considerably more active than his female partner, and taking almost complete charge of the movements of intercourse. The positions shown on these pages all require the legs of the passive partner to be held upright or pushed back towards the body, and are mostly variations of the man-on-top position, although the last illustration shown here shows how to

Command the Action

▶ When the woman's legs are raised and leaning against the man's shoulders, he can penetrate her deeply from his kneeling position. She has less movement than him, although her partner can lift and lower her buttocks with his hands. She receives no direct stimulation to her vulva from this position, but her partner can apply some arousing strokes to her clitoral area with his fingers. She may especially enjoy being able to lay back and relax while her partner takes command of the action.

Total Surrender

▶ For deep vaginal penetration, the woman can draw her legs right back into her body, and bend her knees to rest the heels of her feet against his shoulders. The man can then lean into her, pushing her legs even further back, while supporting his weight with his arms and thrusting his pelvis freely. Again, the woman is able to move very little in this position, but can enjoy surrendering to the thrusting sensations. For easier penetration into the vagina, he can raise her hips by placing a pillow beneath her buttocks.

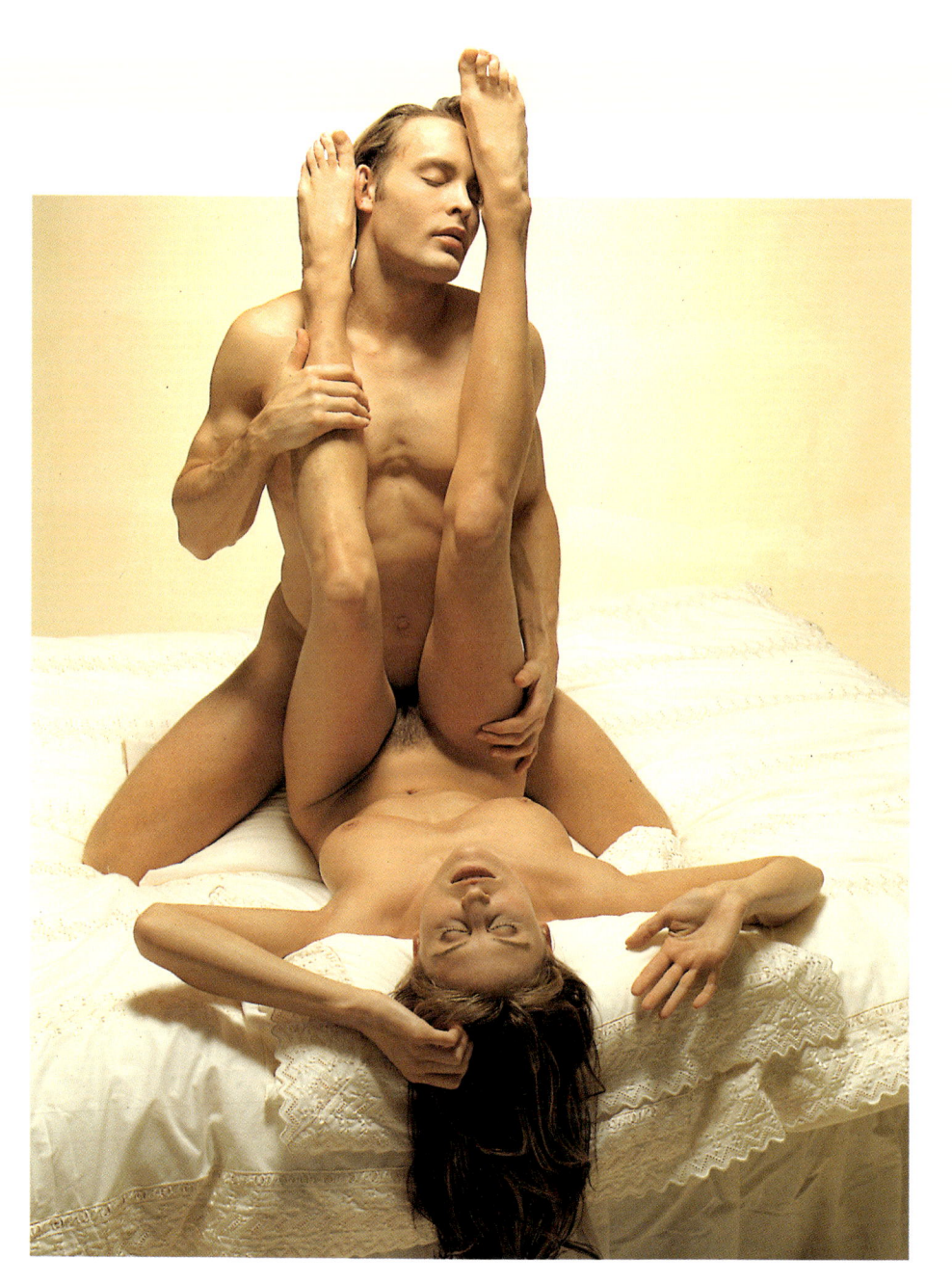

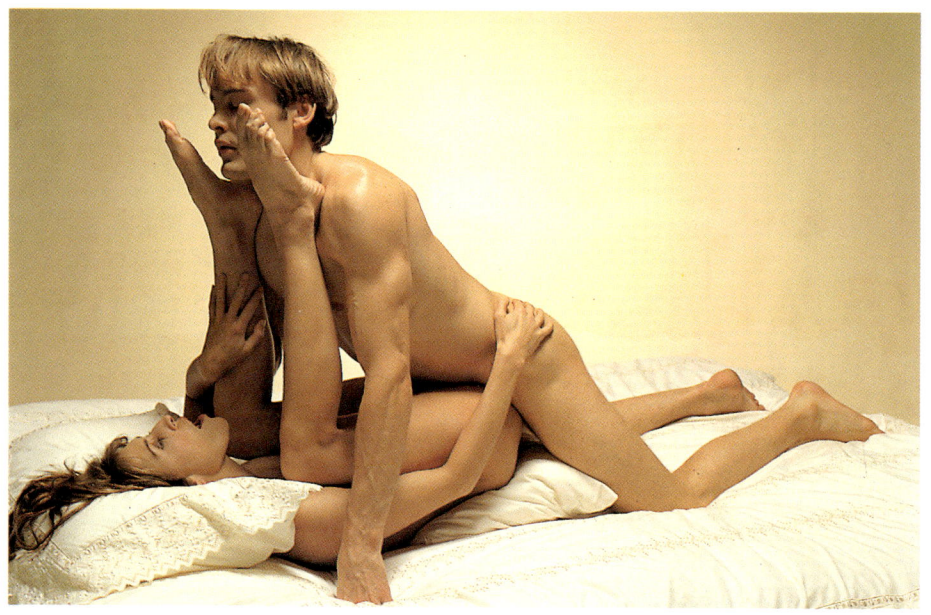

Adventurous Lovemaking

reverse the roles so that the man assumes the more passive and traditionally feminine posture of drawing back the legs.

When the woman takes this passive position, she needs to be supple in her joints and limbs to remain comfortable, and it is advisable for the man not to keep her in this pose for too long. It is best used as an interesting variant to other movements which allow the woman greater flexibility of motion. Also, because her vulva is not in direct contact with his body, the woman is unlikely to gain direct clitoral stimulation from this position and so it is unlikely to lead her to orgasm, which is another good reason for the man not to pursue it for too long.

However, he can stimulate her clitoris with his hand, and caress her body while using this more adventurous lovemaking position, but this should be done only in a loving and sensual way. Most women dislike the feeling of being fiddled with in a mechanical way, and prefer arousal to come from a natural, flowing sequence of movements.

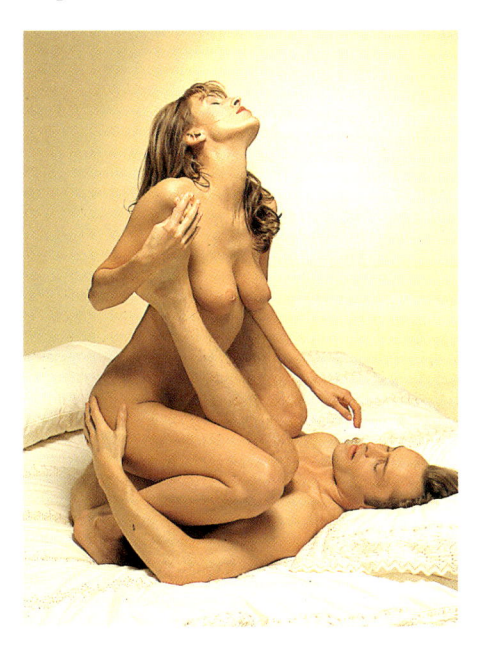

The pleasures to be derived from these positions are that they add variety, they allow deep penetration, which can be very arousing to both partners, and the man is able to express his strength and potency and thrust his pelvis freely. The woman may enjoy the feelings of surrender and "helplessness" that can accompany these positions, and to gain the maximum pleasure from them, she should totally relax her body and yield herself completely to her partner's thrusts.

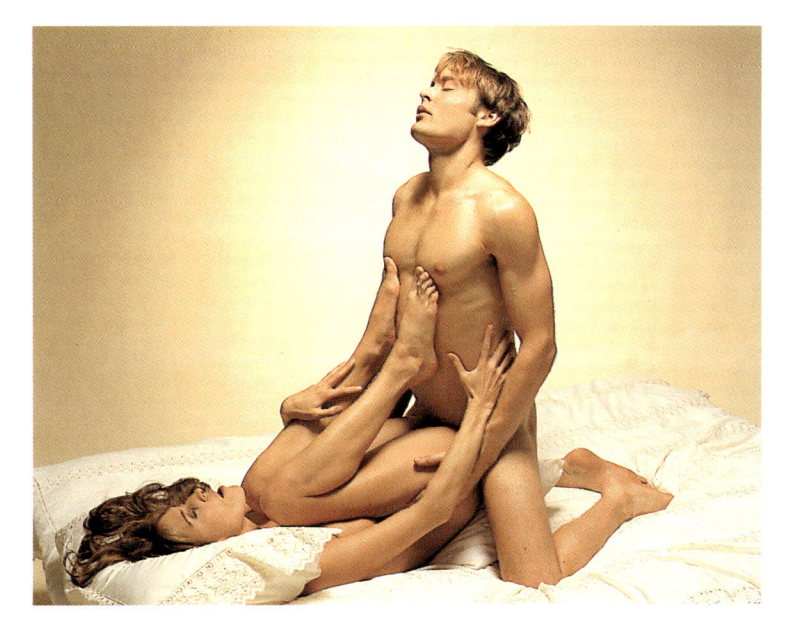

Position of Power
▲ *The woman's body becomes even more compact if she draws her knees towards her breasts and places the soles of her feet comfortably onto the man's chest. This position provides little clitoral stimulation as her vulva is lifted away from her partner and her movements are limited. However, she may find the powerful surge of her partner's thrusts very thrilling and be content to submit to a passive role. While the man can enjoy feelings of power and strength as he makes love to his partner like this, he needs to be careful not to penetrate her so deeply or vigorously that he is hurting her cervix. If, in this position, he stops thrusting for a while and leans his body back a little, he can apply an exciting pressure from his erect penis to the woman's G-spot.*

Role-Reversal
◀ *This position offers a fun and unusual opportunity for role-reversal. Here, the man lies on his back with his knees drawn up and his legs raised so that he is assuming a position viewed more typically as a female one. The woman lowers herself onto his penis carefully, making sure its angle is right and that she does not bend it awkwardly by moving too quickly. She squats, so the backs of her thighs rest against the backs of his, but she supports her weight on her feet, and uses her legs as leverage to move up and down, or she can wiggle her hips from side to side. Only a supple man will be able to maintain this position for long, but it will certainly help him to understand a woman's perspective of the submissive role.*

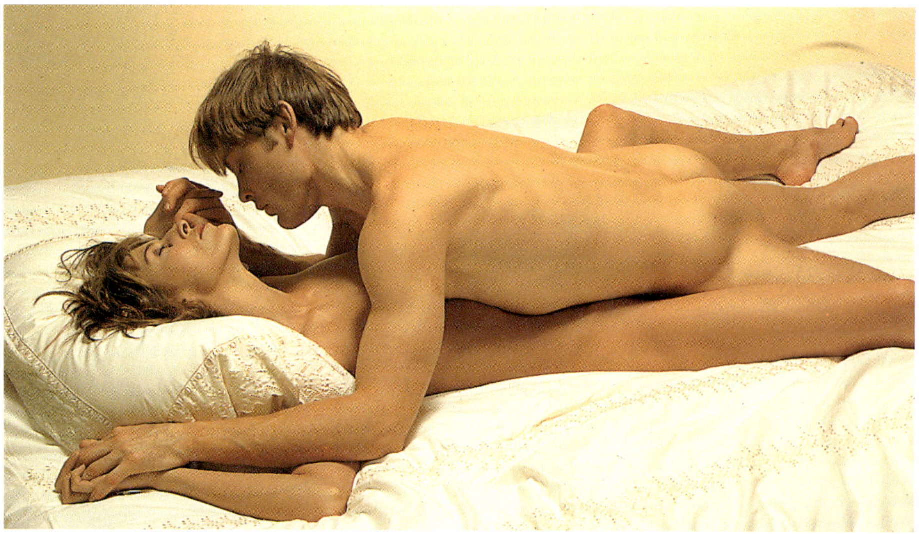

Adventurous Sex Techniques

Restraint in Lovemaking

The themes of domination and submission frequently provide a strong element of pleasure and desire in many sexual relationships. The feeling of "being taken" by a lover can be deliciously arousing and emotionally fulfilling for either sex, although it is usually only one aspect of a more all-rounded sexual relationship, where the active and passive sexual roles are equally shared.

Many couples, however, would not wish to go as far as acting out restraint or bondage practices, but find other ways to express more naturally the fluctuating surges in their need to dominate or submit to their partners. The two illustrations shown here capture the moments when sexual arousal has reached a particular peak, and one partner takes on the more powerful role and temporarily restrains the movements of the passive partner by pinning his or her arms, hands and body while taking command of the sexual activity.

Usually, this is initiated by the body language of the more submissive partner, who splays out the limbs in a position of surrender. Both men and women can enjoy either role, depending on which one of them is taking the on-top or beneath position at the time.

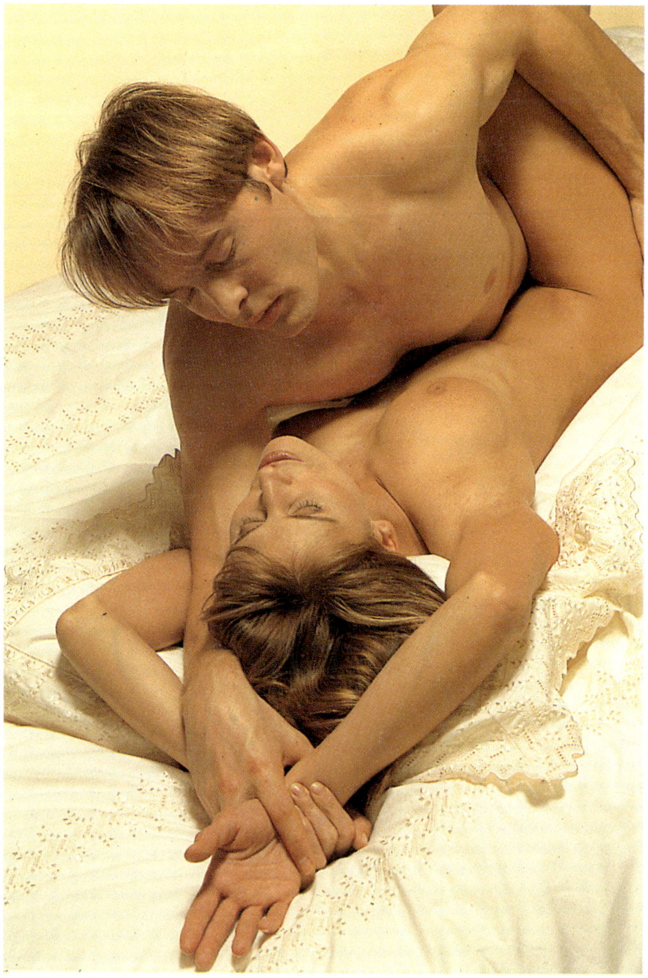

Sexual Surrender
▶ While a woman may like to play an active and equal role in lovemaking, she may also love those moments when her partner takes charge and she can surrender to his masculine power. When her arms have stretched out above her head, he can bind her hands together with one of his own. With the other hand, he can hold her buttocks, or raise one hip towards his body, so he can alter the angle of his thrusts. This allows his penis to also stroke along the sides of the vaginal walls to stimulate them.

Domination and Submission
◀ As the passion rises during lovemaking, a woman may stretch her arms out behind her head, and spread her legs so that she assumes a posture of supine submission. The man can then hold her hands down with his own, and bring his body close on top of hers, so his position is more one of domination. This element of restraint in lovemaking can be very arousing to both partners at certain moments. When the woman's legs are opened out and straight, her vulva is in contact with her partner's pubic bone, and though she can make little movement of her own, she will receive strong clitoral stimulation which may precipitate an orgasm for her.

68

Adventurous Lovemaking

Rear-Entry Lovemaking

Rear-entry lovemaking means the man inserts his penis into the woman's vagina from a position behind his partner's body. It is more commonly known as the "doggie position", so-called because this is the basic sexual position that is common to most animals, including dogs. Some women find the rather

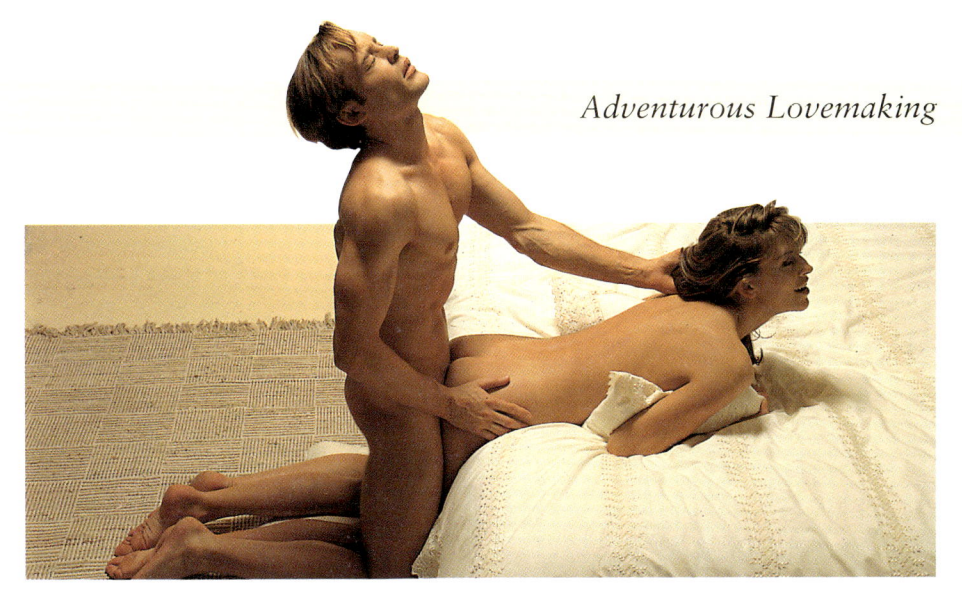

Rear-Entry Sex

▲ If the woman kneels on the floor and lays the upper half of her body across the bed, she can position herself comfortably for rear-entry sex, especially if she pads her chest with a cushion. The man then kneels behind her, so the floor gives him some solid support for his movements. If the woman enjoys making love in the "doggie position", she may be aroused by the slightly dominating aspect of her partner and by her own more submissive stance. Although they are not face to face, the man can be very intimate with her body, and can stroke her hair, back, and buttocks easily. He can also lift her away from the bed slightly to fondle her breasts, caress her belly, or to stimulate her vulva and clitoris with his fingers while making his thrusting movements.

Armchair Sex

◀ An armchair lends itself very well to rear-entry lovemaking, if the furniture is deep enough to take both partners onto its seat. She can lean her body against the padded support of the back of the chair and avoid any feeling of collapsing forward under the pressure of his thrusts. The man can then kneel behind her and, as she leans forward, enter her vagina from the rear position. He can use his hands to stroke and caress her erogenous zones, or to pull her hips closer to him.

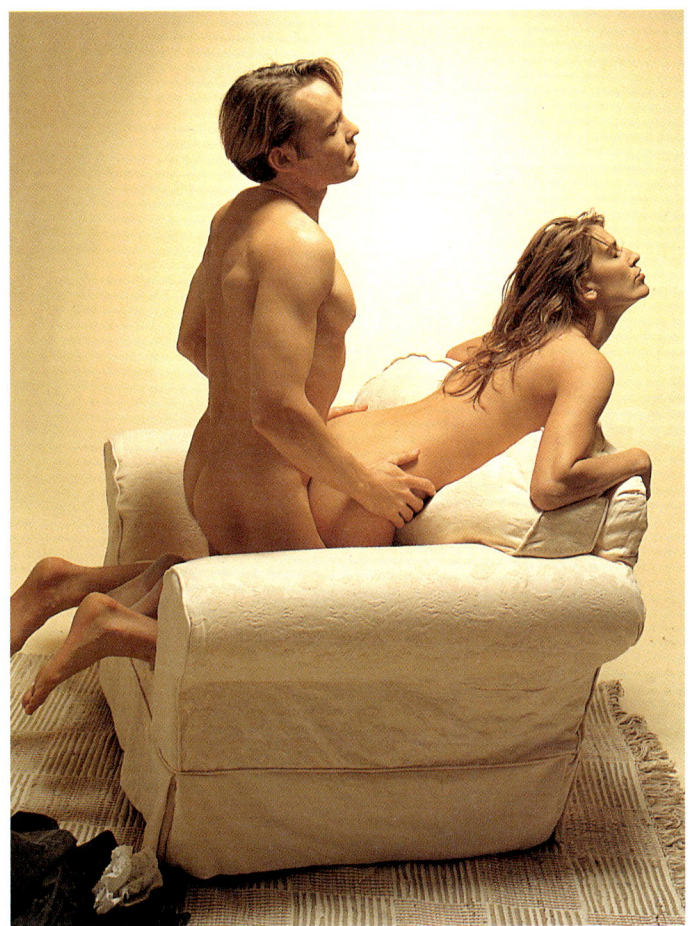

bestial connotations of this posture to be demeaning, and do not enjoy making love with their backs turned to their partners, or to have their buttocks so exposed. Other women find rear-entry intercourse very exciting, and enjoy the rather primitive nature of its stance, and the feeling of surrender that it engenders.

Rear-entry lovemaking can be enjoyed as a variation to other positions, and it is potentially very sexually satisfying to both partners because it allows for deep vaginal penetration. This position has been recommended by some fertility specialists for couples who are trying to conceive a baby because it assists the sperm to pool near the mouth of the cervix. It can also be a comfortable position for a pregnant woman to adopt, although the man must take care not to penetrate her too deeply or vigorously in this situation.

A pregnant woman, or any woman, can make herself more comfortable in this position by kneeling, head-down, on the bed with her back to the man, and padding her belly and chest with pillows.

A bonus for the man is that it provides an ample view of the woman's buttocks, and this can be a

Adventurous Sex Techniques

powerfully arousing visual stimulus for him. For some women, however, the idea of revealing their buttocks so prominently may cause anxiety, especially if they are concerned about their weight or body image.

However, the buttocks are a highly erogenous zone in both sexes, and respond erotically to stroking, squeezing, patting, and even stronger forms of manual stimulation. In this position the woman receives no direct clitoral stimulation, but this can be rectified by the man caressing her vulva while he thrusts, or by her own self-stimulating strokes. If she is thus pleasured, both partners can reach an orgasm in this position.

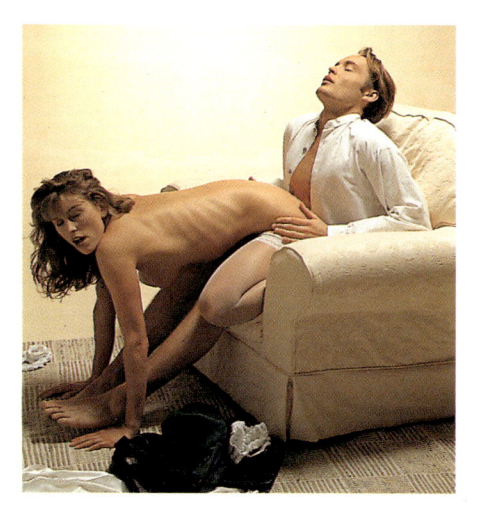

Seat of Pleasure
▲ This is another creative way of enjoying rear-entry sex in the comfort of the armchair. The woman starts by kneeling astride her partner's lap but with her back turned to him, and then carefully guides his penis into her vagina. Once the penis is fully erect, she can then lean forward slowly and support herself by placing her hands on the floor. The man's movements are limited, but he can lift her hips up and down with his hands to create more friction, and the woman can also wiggle sexily from side to side to increase the arousal for them both.

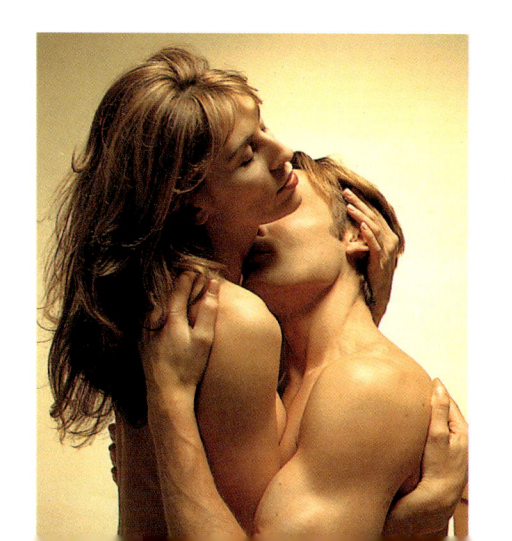

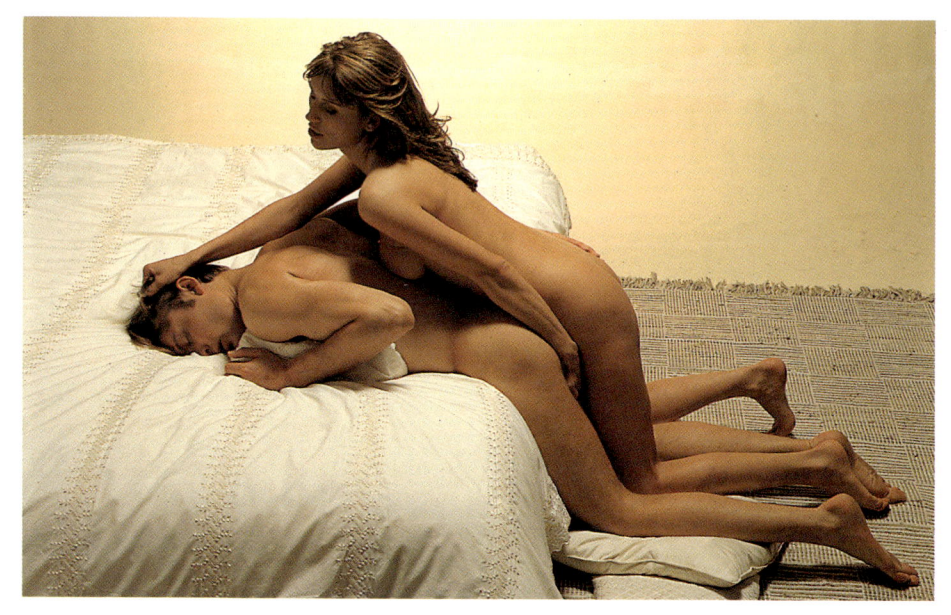

A Fun Variation
▲ Anatomically, it is obviously not possible for the "doggie position" to be reversed for penetrative sex. The couple, however, can enjoy other thrilling sexual sensations by having the man take the usual female position for rear-entry sex. First of all, he can be aroused by assuming the more submissive stance, while experiencing the sensual feel of his partner's breasts and belly moving against his back. He can wiggle his hips to rub himself against the edge of the bed, while the woman can use her hands to squeeze and pat his buttocks, or stroke and fondle his testicles or the erotically sensitive tip of his penis.

Active Sitting Positions
The sitting position for lovemaking is popular for its particular ability to enhance a meditative sexual mood. It can be used while the couple remain on the bed, or chairs or the edge of the bed can be utilized to make it more comfortable for posture and movements. The following examples show the many diverse ways to adapt this particularly sensual and relaxed form of making love.

Slow and Sensual
◀ When making love on a chair, the vertical posture of both partners enables them to relax deeply and bond emotionally and physically. They can embrace each other closely so their bodies are in intimate contact. This position is not chosen for vigorous movement, but more for slow, sensual and tender sex. As the man holds his partner tight to his body, he can lovingly kiss her neck.

Adventurous Lovemaking

Bodies in Harmony
◀ Making love like this can become very still and meditative, and the couple can sometimes just hold each other closely, harmonizing their breathing and even allowing their bodies to rock and sway gently together, but without excitement. During these quieter moments of lovemaking, if the man's penis becomes softer, the woman can tighten her thighs or her vaginal muscles to create just enough pressure and friction to keep it erect. Intimacy here is much more important than excitement.

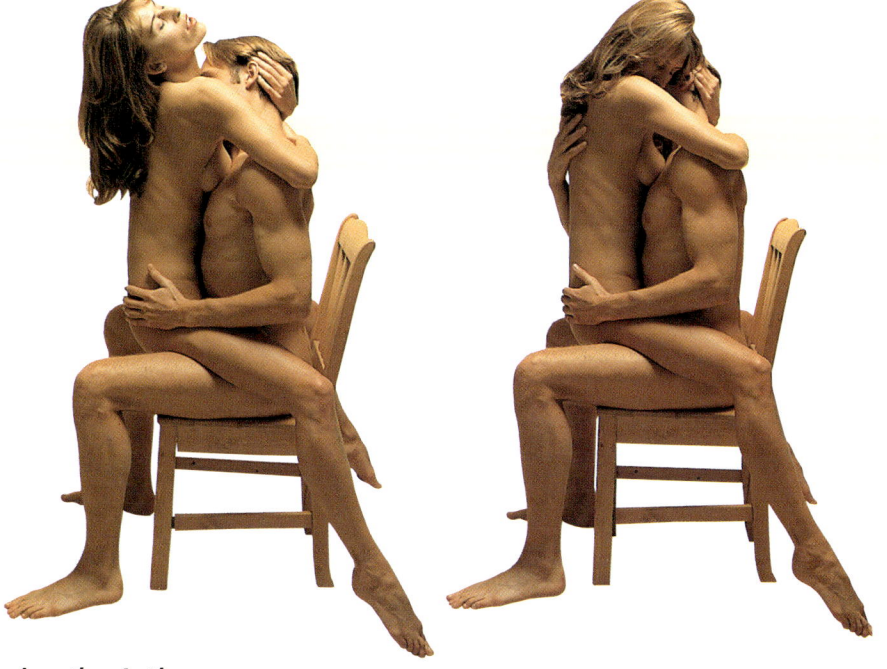

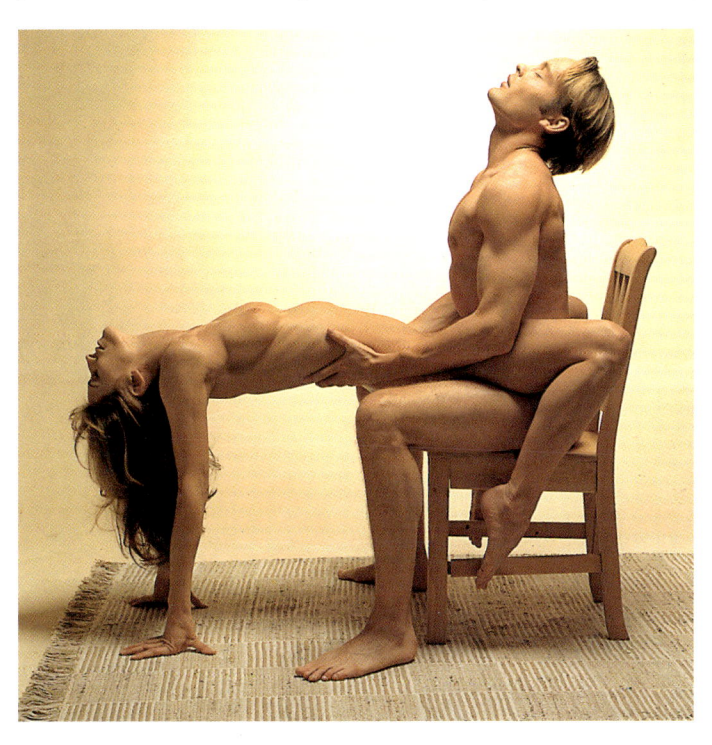

Varying the Action
▲ The woman is the more active partner in this chair-sitting position. She can brace herself against her partner as she hugs him, while rocking her pelvis back and forth. Her motions will arouse and stimulate both of them. He can also place his hands on her hips to raise her up and down to vary the movements.

New Angle of Arousal
▲ If she is supple and confident enough in her body, the woman can slowly lean backwards so that her hands reach to the floor behind her while she is secured by her partner's hold. The angle of her pelvis will enable the erect penis inside her to put sustained pressure on the front wall of her vagina and G-spot, which can be very arousing. The openness and exposure of her body and genitals will be sexually exhilarating to them both. If she allows herself to relax into this position and to breathe deeply, the effort will be worthwhile.

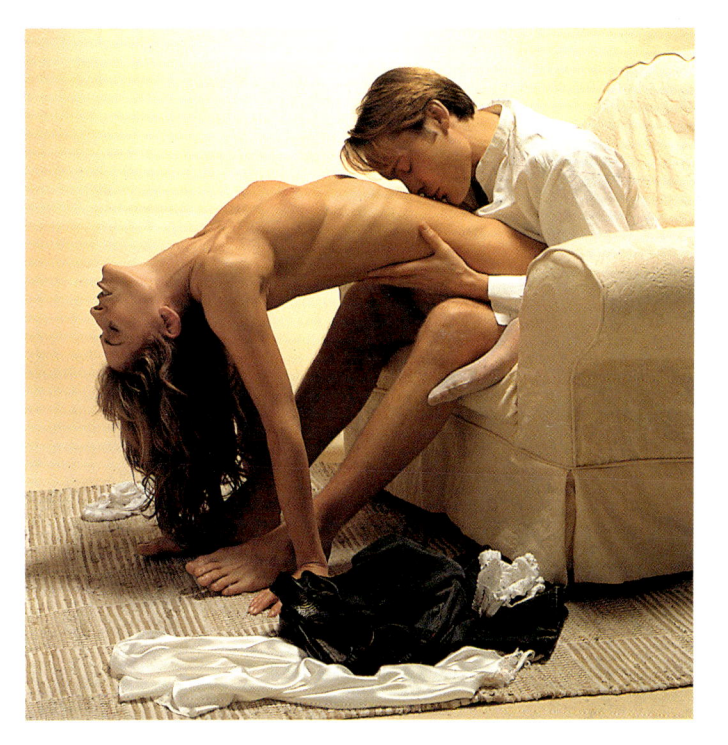

Erotic Charge
▲ The bow-shape of the woman's body as she leans back against the support of her partner's thighs while kneeling astride him in an armchair, will, like the previous position, open and expand her lungs, diaphragm and abdomen so that she can breathe very deeply indeed. This will help her whole body to become charged with vibrant sexual energy. She can also wiggle her hips so that her vulva rubs arousingly against her partner's body. The man can lean forwards to kiss and lick her belly, which will increase the intensity of her sensations.

Adventurous Sex Techniques

Taking It Further

The sitting posture of lovemaking can be one of a whole variety of positions which a couple adopt during a period of coitus to express the wide range of shifting emotional and physical sensations that sweeps through them. By using the edge of the bed for a sexual sitting position, the couple can become more active and passionate than in other sitting situations which are more conducive to meditative lovemaking. Here, the man can balance himself with his feet and hands while the woman is astride his lap, enabling her to move more freely without fear of toppling them both over.

Wild Abandon

▼ Perching on the edge of the bed while making love in the sitting position will enable the man to place his feet firmly on the floor so that the couple have better support and balance if their movements become more abandoned. The woman can grip the man's shoulders firmly, and while leaning her body away from her partner, can gyrate her pelvis vigorously back and forth to create strong sensations of friction.

Synchronized Motion

▼ Pressing one hand against the mattress for additional support, the man can clasp his partner close to him with his other hand, while rocking his hips back and forth. He should co-ordinate his thrusts to move simultaneously with the woman's motions, which are made by her levering herself up and down from flexed knees. When the woman lets go into her sexual energy, she may also begin to toss her head and neck from side to side.

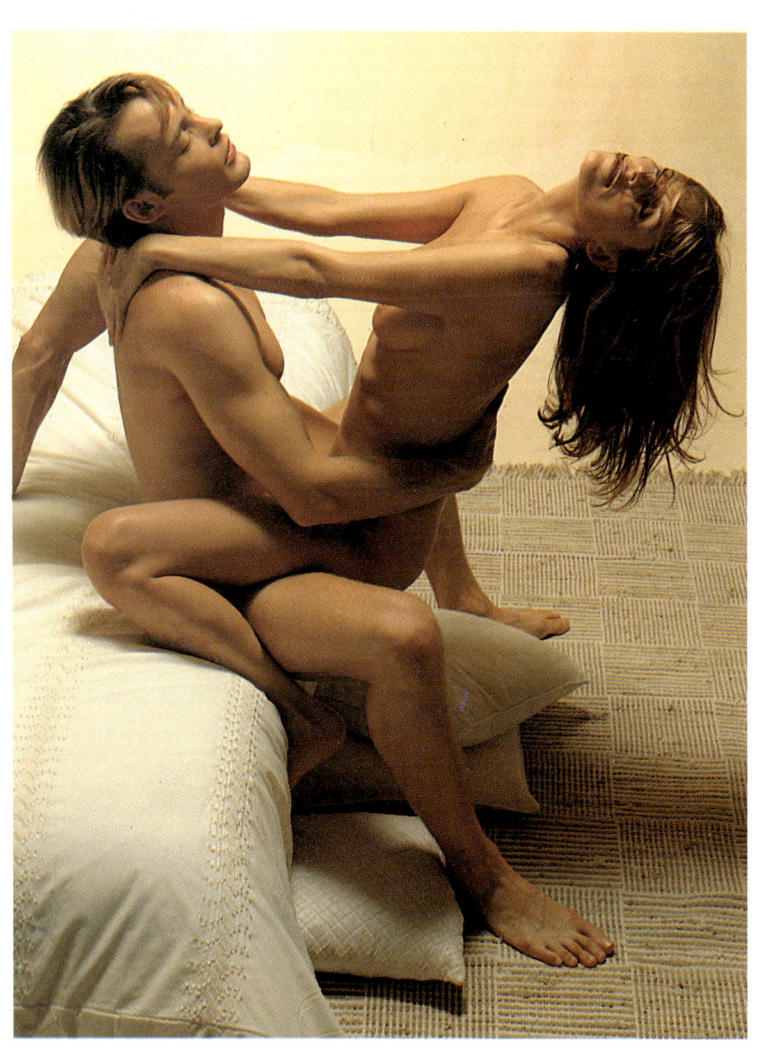

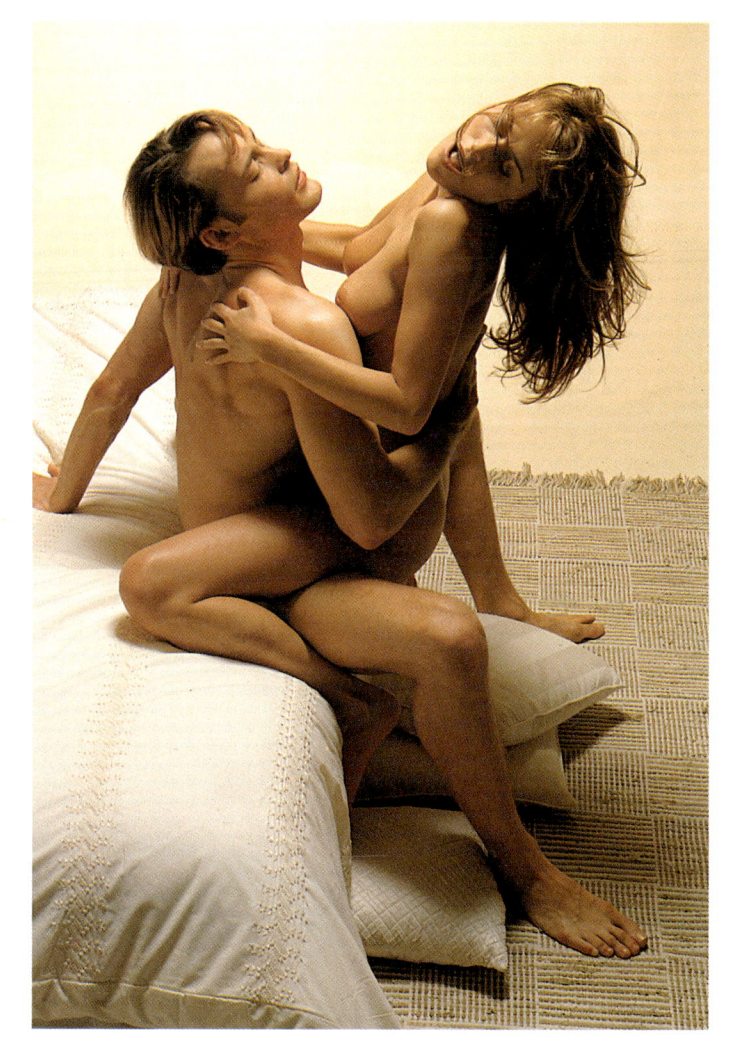

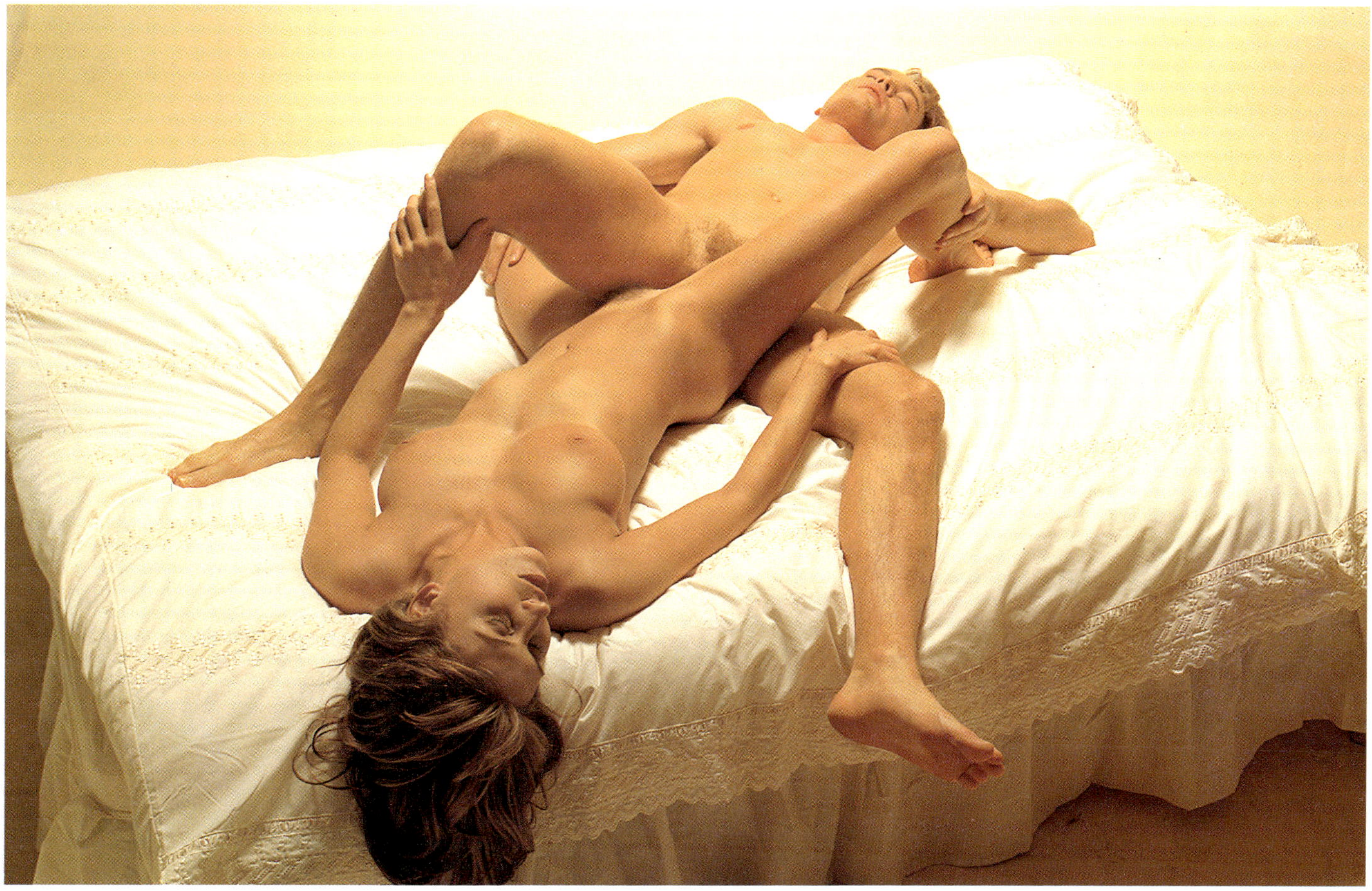

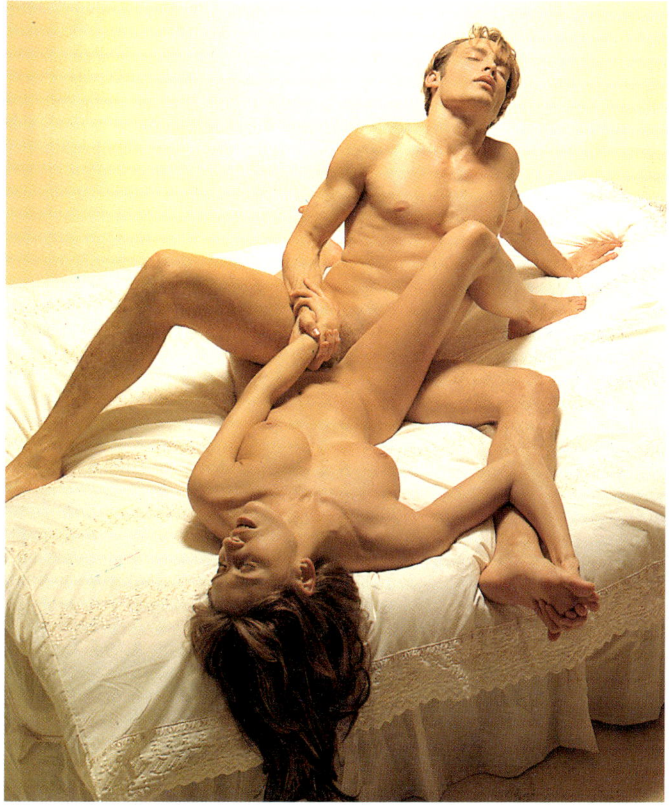

Adventurous Lovemaking

Easing Down
▲ This position follows on naturally and easily from when the woman is sitting astride her partner's lap if they are making love in the sitting position on the bed. She can slowly relax back onto the bed, using her partner's grip to ease herself down gracefully, even while his penis is still erect inside her. Then, with some careful manoeuvring, she can bring the leg that was lying across his thigh to rest beneath it. From this comfortable position she can move her hips from side to side and receive strong clitoral stimulation.

Change of Pace
◄ If the man lies back on the bed after his partner has done so (see illustration above), the couple's position falls into a cross-shape, and they can engage in a very relaxed form of lovemaking which will, at the same time, keep them both in a high state of arousal. By moving their hips around, they will receive adequate friction to keep them both stimulated, but they will be able to rest at the same time. When they are ready to change positions again, the man sits up and then pulls his partner upwards and they can continue with other movements.

Adventurous Sex Techniques

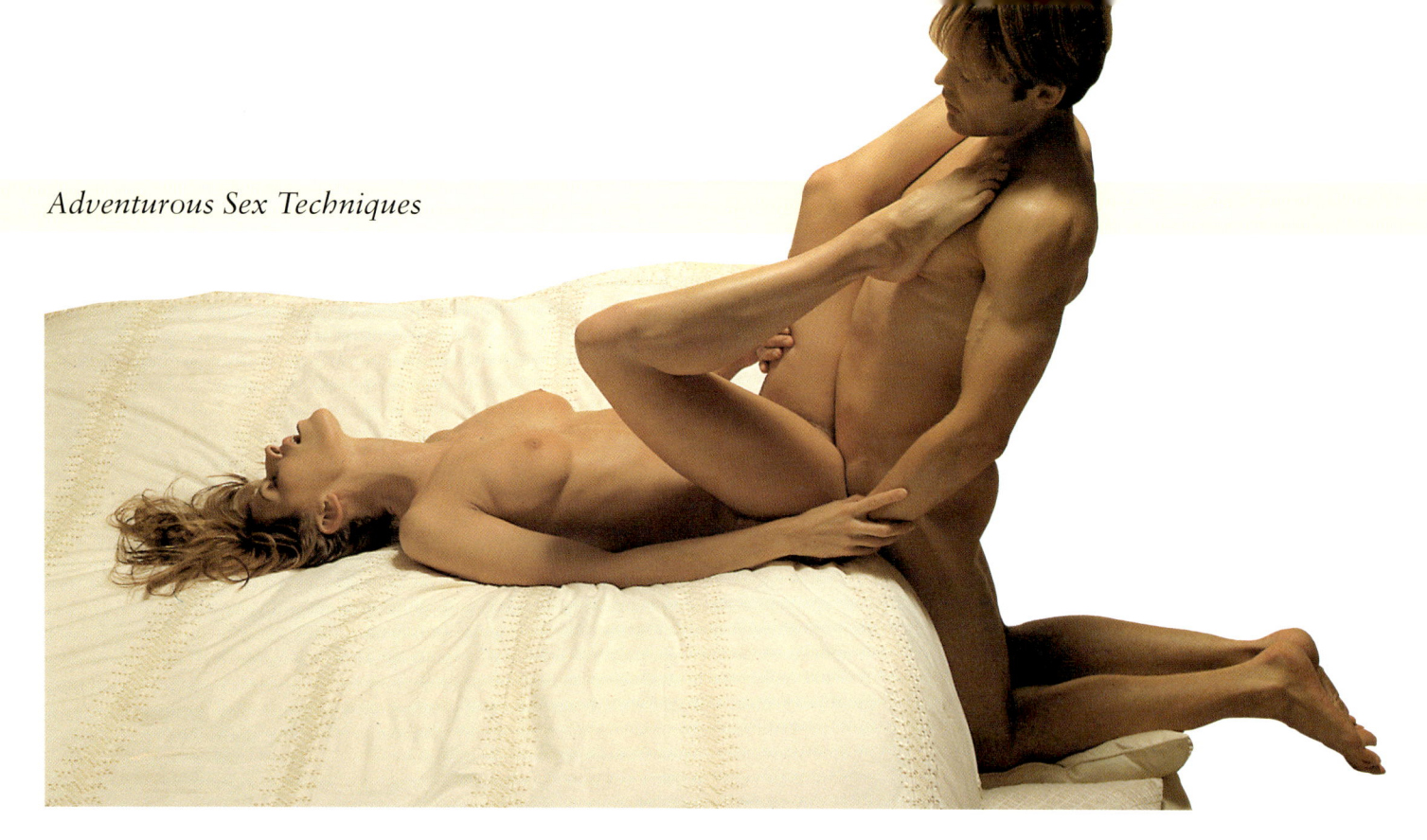

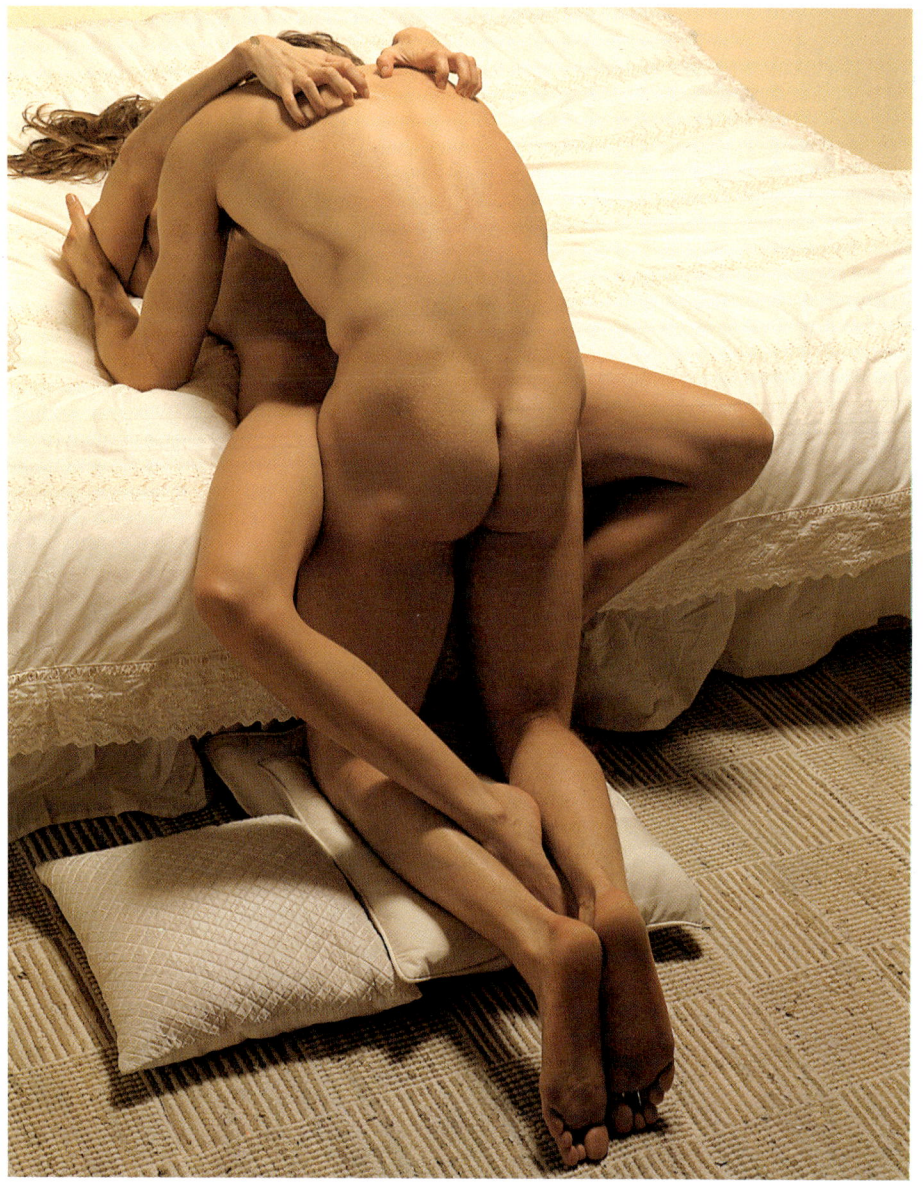

Close to the Edge
▲ If the woman lies on her back, with her buttocks just at the edge of the bed, and the man kneels on the floor in front of her, he can then raise her legs up onto his shoulders so that he can easily insert his penis into her vagina, which in this position will be at the same height. Penetration can be deep and very pleasurable, but he should additionally stimulate her clitoral area with his fingers and caress her body if he makes love to her from this position for long.

Increasing the Stimulation
◀ If the woman lowers her legs and slides her body a little further down over the edge of the bed, the man's thrusting movements are more likely to add a stimulating friction to her vulva, which will increase her sexual arousal. He can also lower his body over hers so that he can kiss her lips and breasts too.

Adventurous Lovemaking

Over the Edge

Sooner or later, if the lovemaking is sufficiently wild and abandoned, the couple will work their way all around the bed. It usually takes some time before two people become so attuned to each other's bodily responses that these movements are compatible and graceful, and do not cause them to interrupt the flow of their intercourse. Winding and unwinding the limbs, rolling over, changing the postures, swapping active and passive roles and positions, all require skilful and nimble movements if they are to be executed with ease and fluidity. However, once a couple are comfortable with each other, they can let themselves go into passionate activity which can take them from one side of the bed to the other, and even over the edge.

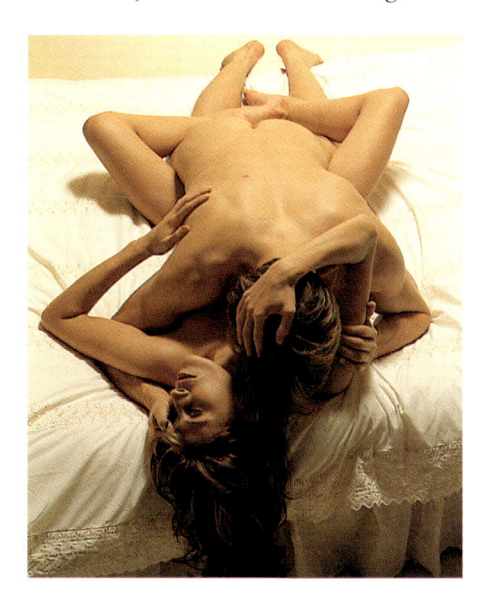

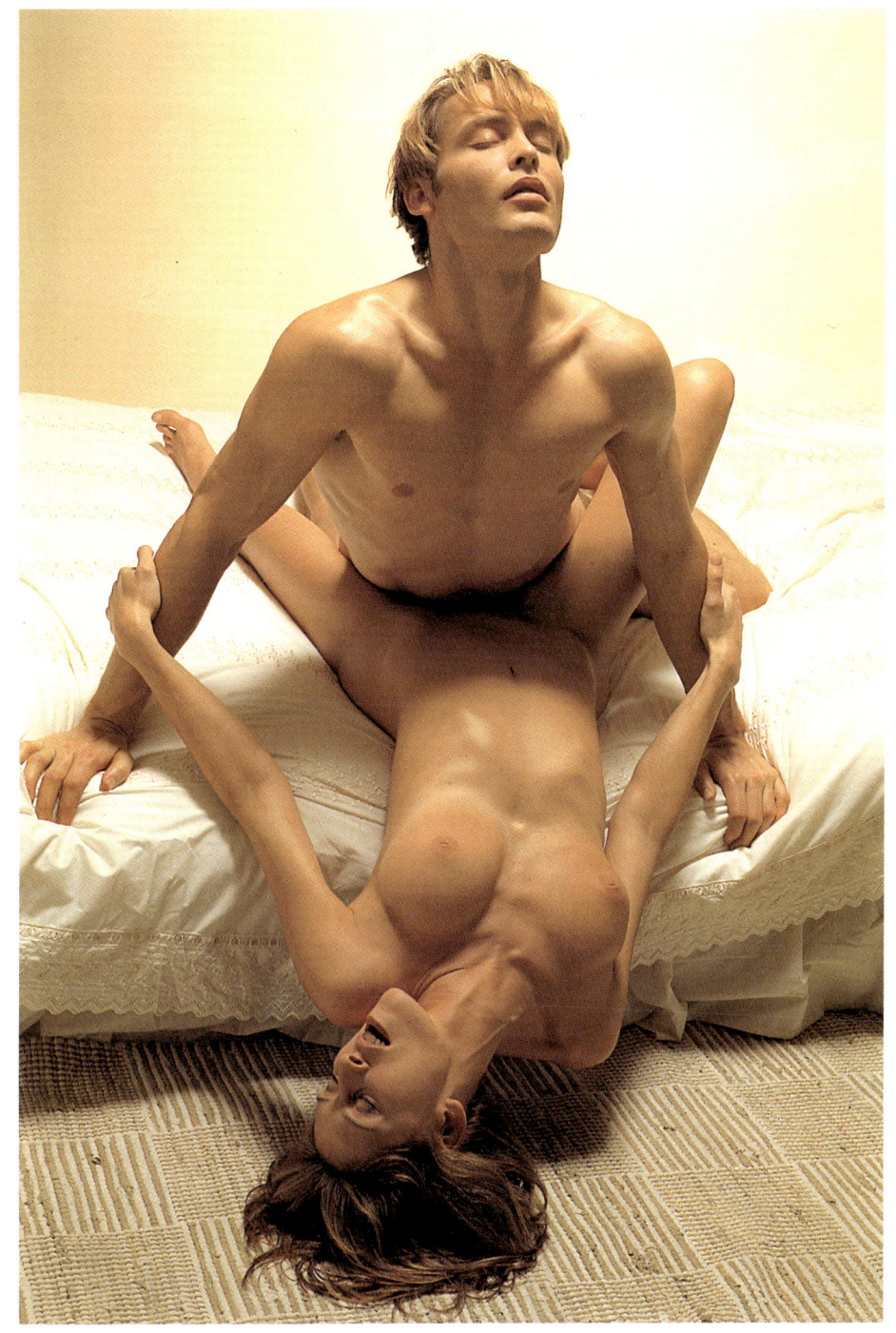

Locked in Congress
▲ Here, the woman is below the man, with her head just slightly off the edge of the mattress. She can hold the man very close to her body while she wraps her feet around his buttocks and locks him into her. This will inhibit his movement a little but the pressure of her feet will add extra pleasurable sensations, and they can just wriggle and rotate their hips for a while to create a whole variety of different stimulating motions.

Exhilarating Sex
▲ The man or woman can end up in a position in which the head is completely off the mattress and is resting against the floor. This can cause an exhilarating rush of blood to the head, but should not be maintained for too long or the pressure can build up too strongly, especially if the person is approaching an orgasm. There is something very liberating, though, about being this abandoned in your lovemaking that you almost topple out of bed.

Masturbating Each Other

Mutual masturbation enhances the sensuality of foreplay by increasing arousal for either partner prior to penetration and intercourse, and it is a sure way to get the love juices flowing. It may also be enjoyed as a complete and totally fulfilling sexual act in itself through which lovers can attain orgasm even without penetrative sex. It is a delightful way to initiate a second round of lovemaking when both people are sufficiently rested from the first bout, and it can be used to lovingly assist a partner to complete sexual satisfaction if the other person has climaxed first or is unable to continue lovemaking.

One of the most important skills in the art of lovemaking is to learn how to masturbate your partner properly. To do it well is to know which touches bring maximum pleasure and to share in your lover's delight. Mastering the skills of masturbation will make you a special and much-appreciated lover.

Many couples, particularly the young, use masturbation as a way of enjoying each other's bodies before committing themselves to a full sexual relationship. It provides a safe means of exploring and becoming familiar with each other's sexual responses as well as enjoying sexual satisfaction without the implications and responsibilities involved in full penetrative intercourse.

Some people find masturbation acceptable but would only allow intercourse within the context of a committed relationship or marriage. Others may wisely consider the consequences of pregnancy or sexually transmitted diseases and prefer to abstain from a full sexual relationship, using masturbation as an alternative until these issues have been safely resolved.

Yet mutual masturbation should remain an integral part of any couple's range of lovemaking techniques, for it continues to provide an erotic enhancement throughout a sexual relationship. Arousing and satisfying your partner by skilful masturbation without asking for anything in return, except the joy gained from his or her pleasure, can be a very erotic experience.

Quick-Release Sex
▼ *Mutual masturbation can provide fast erotic arousal whether it is part of a whole lovemaking session or a separate episode from intercourse. By masturbating each other to orgasm, both of you can receive a satisfying release of sexual tension. Mutual masturbation while still partly clothed can be particularly exciting because it can recall memories of early sexual experimentation, and also because the friction of material against the genitals can be an additional form of stimulation.*

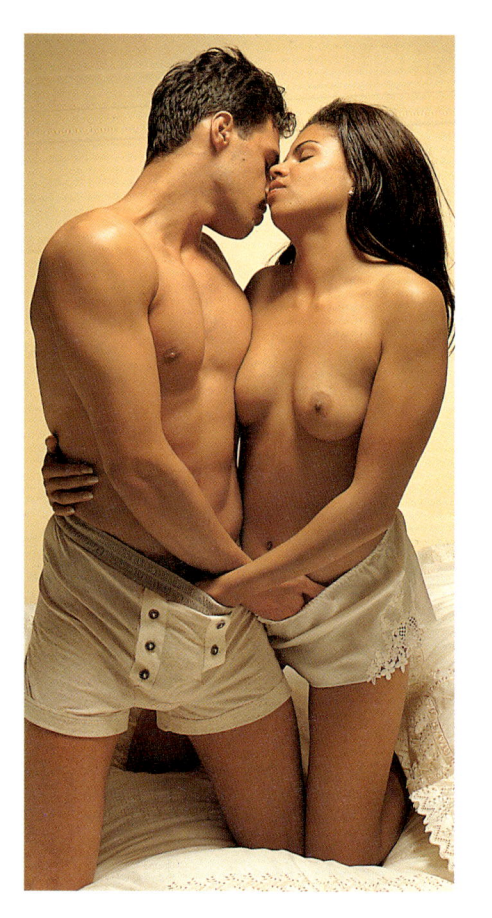

If your libido is at a low ebb, perhaps as a result of tiredness or stress and you are not in the mood for making love, while your partner is, masturbating your lover can be a perfect way to answer both of your needs. If you have a back injury which makes movement difficult, or you are heavily pregnant, then again mutual masturbation can provide an extremely sensual alternative to full sexual intercourse.

In addition to masturbating each other, either of you can indulge in the pleasure of self-masturbation with the other partner closely involved in the process. This can be a very erotic experience, as you watch your partner self-pleasure his or her body next to yours. You participate with touches and caresses to increase the arousal and you can even join in the sighs, moans and changing patterns of breath as if the sensations are being transferred into your body too.

You can take it in turns to masturbate each other, or you may do it simultaneously while standing, kneeling or lying next to your partner so that your bodies begin to vibrate together with the mounting tension of your sexual excitement.

Many lovers feel that the orgasms they experience through masturbation provide a quite different sensation than those resulting from

Masturbating Each Other

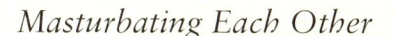

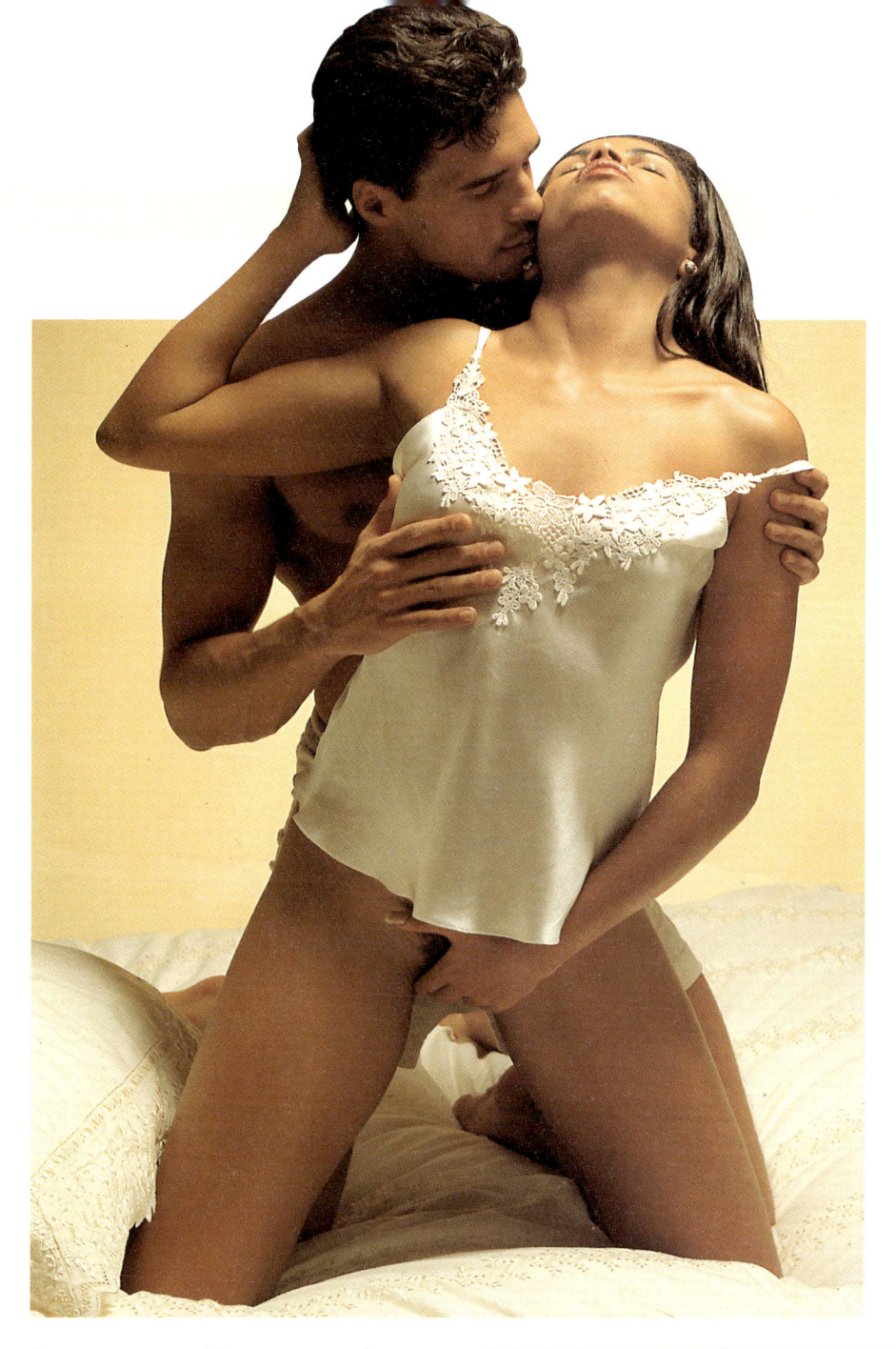

Caresses and Fantasies

◀ You can masturbate yourself to orgasm while your partner holds you close to his body, and touches and caresses your breasts and kisses your face and neck. You can let your own sexual fantasies run free in your mind, or he can even whisper his sexual fantasies to you while you are turning yourself on. Again, this type of masturbation can become even more enticing if you are wearing a silky textured item of clothing, like a camisole, which will rub sensuously against your nipples and skin.

Mutual Pleasuring

▼ You can masturbate each other at the same time. If you are attuned to each other's responses, it may even be possible to reach a simultaneous orgasm, or if not, take it in turns to satisfy one another sexually. Or you may only want to take the arousal level so far with your masturbatory motions before progressing towards other forms of lovemaking. Lie close to each other to have skin-to-skin contact, but position yourselves comfortably so that you can easily touch and stroke each other's genitals.

intercourse. The masturbatory orgasm is sometimes described as being more physically intense than an intercourse orgasm, probably because it ensues from a sustained and specific stimulation applied to the most erotically sensitive areas of the genitals, and possibly because if you are on the receiving end, you can lie back and surrender yourself totally and quite selfishly into its powerful sensations.

For some women, careful and loving masturbation combined with oral stimulation are the only way in which they can achieve orgasmic satisfaction while making love. It may not, however, bring the same deeply

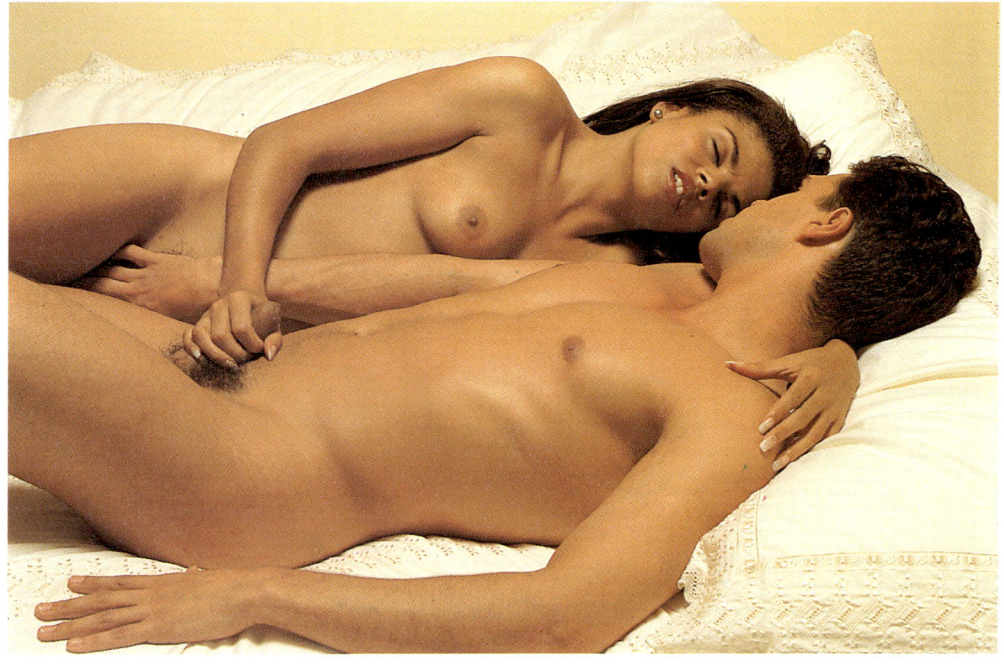

Adventurous Sex Techniques

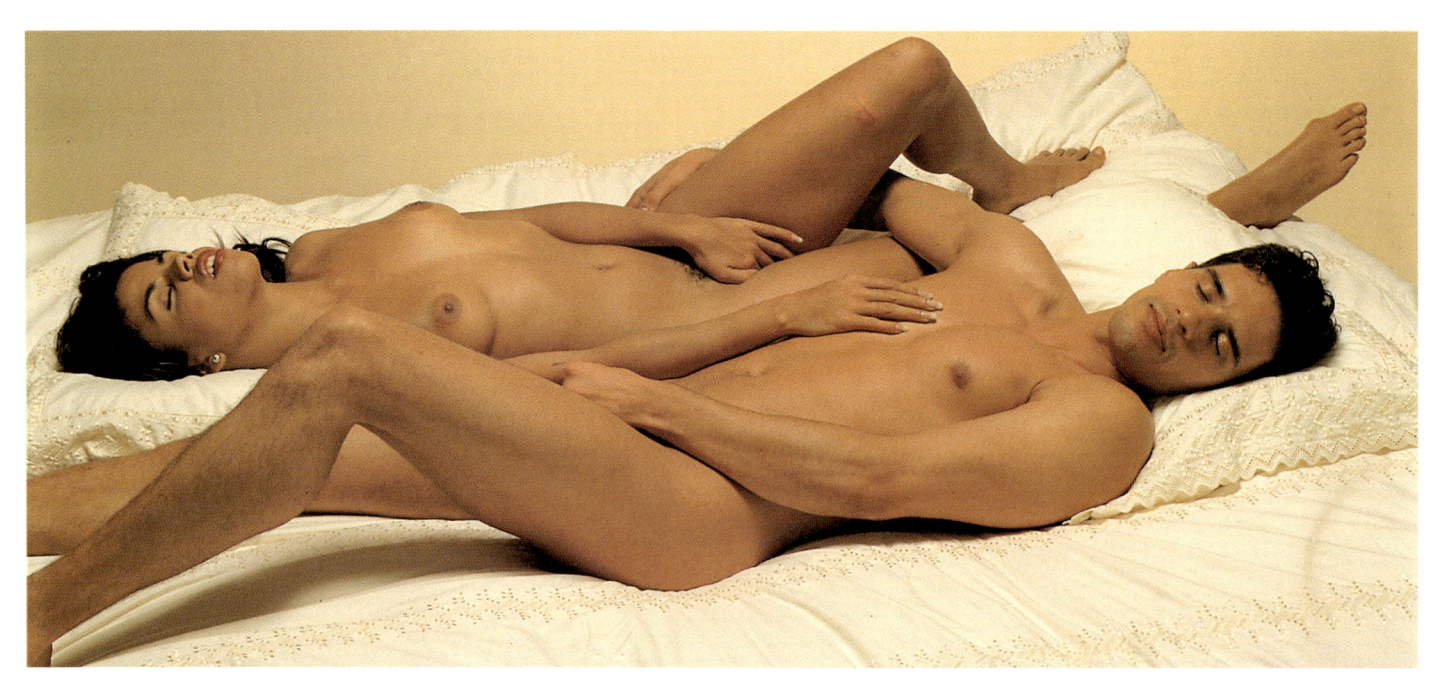

Self-Pleasuring
▲ *Mutual masturbation can be enjoyed when both of you simultaneously pleasure yourselves. One way to do this is to lie comfortably next to each other in a top-to-tail position. Continue tactile contact with each other by resting a hand or arm over the other's body then focus totally into giving yourself pleasure, doing all the things that bring you sexual joy, but at the same time feeling the warmth of your partner close by. Don't be afraid to make sounds, or breathe deeply, because your ecstatic noises will increase your partner's arousal too.*

nourishing sense of emotional bonding and fulfilment which is more likely to occur when a couple climax during the act of penetrative sex. Sexuality, however, is multi-dimensional – a kaleidoscope of physical and emotional experiences – and mutual masturbation is there to be enjoyed as one of its many exquisite hues.

The Right Touch

Most people perfect their masturbation skills on themselves. So it makes sense that the person who can best show you how to apply just the right erotic touch in masturbation is your partner. Only he or she knows the rhythm and pace of the strokes which can be guaranteed to take them to the heights of arousal and on towards a mind-blowing orgasm.

However, that does not exclude the other partner being able to add something entirely new and extremely exciting of their own invention to this type of sexual arousal – so stay open to the possibility of experiencing some hitherto unknown peaks of pleasure.

Men and women, for obvious reasons, masturbate themselves in quite different ways. Generally, a man will focus his attention almost entirely on his penis, though he may possibly include some self-arousing caresses to his scrotum, or finger-pressure on his anus. He is also likely to simulate the action of intercourse by creating the same type of pumping friction on the shaft of his penis, only this time by hand. He almost certainly prefers to use a firm grip of the hand, and may apply increasingly vigorous strokes until the moment of ejaculation.

A woman's way of masturbating herself is likely to be more sensual and slow, and involve more of her body, for she may caress her breasts and rub her nipples, and stroke her belly and thighs as if she is making love to herself. She is unlikely to concentrate her manual stimulation solely on her clitoris, but will move her fingers all around it and over her vaginal lips, separating them carefully to stroke over their folds and occasionally inserting the tips of her fingers to stroke around the lower part of her vagina. She may also rub and vibrate the pubic bone area above her clitoris, and tug gently on her pubic hair to stimulate the highly erotogenic nerve endings at the base of the hair follicles.

A woman is likely to start her self-masturbation in a slow, gentle and languid manner, varying the motions of her strokes, and building up speed

Masturbating Each Other

and pressure only as she approaches her climax. She is more likely to lavish her attentions on her vulva, and less inclined to try to recreate the actions of intercourse, though some women insert a dildo or sex toy into the vagina during self-masturbation to increase the stimulation.

Observing Each Other

Knowing about the different methods employed by men and women during self-pleasuring will help you and your partner to become more sensitive to each other's sexual needs. If you can overcome your shyness, you can watch each other masturbate. If you are observing your partner masturbate, notice everything he or she is doing, which parts of the hands are used, what motions are employed and how the strokes vary at different stages of arousal. Watch your lover's facial expressions and listen to the changing patterns of breath and the sounds he makes, for these will all give you cues to your partner's physical response and arousal patterns during masturbation.

If you are masturbating yourself, tell your partner exactly what you are doing and why a certain stroke or pressure is giving you pleasure. Describe the sensations as well as you can so your partner can begin to absorb all the nuances of those physical feelings into his or her own sexual consciousness. Then, when he or she touches your genitals in a certain way, the physical pleasure you are receiving can also be transmitted to, and consequently experienced by, your partner.

Note, especially, what your partner does as he or she approaches orgasm. Does the friction and stimulation speed up, and does the pressure of palm and fingers increase? What happens on the point of ejaculation and orgasm, and immediately afterwards? In all of these things, your partner is your perfect teacher, but see below for more guidance on masturbation techniques specific to either sex.

Make It Like Music

Mutual masturbation, like oral sex, is a way of getting right down to your partner's genitals. Learn to love them completely so your touches convey your reverence, awe and pleasure for these most intimate parts of your lover's body. Become as familiar with them as you would with any other part of the body. Use your hands and fingers to play on and stroke over your partner's genitals as you would if you were making beautiful music

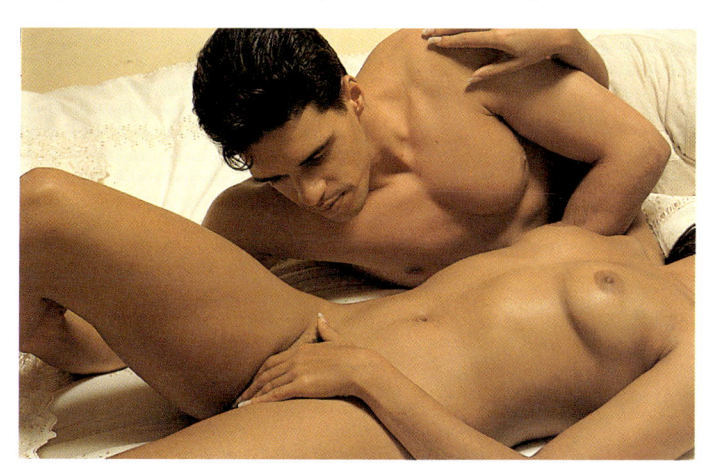

Study Her Style
▲ The best way to learn how she likes to be touched and stimulated in order to attain an orgasm through masturbation is to watch her do it to herself. She can show you exactly what she enjoys, because she has explored the best means of arousal for herself during self-masturbation. Witness carefully how she uses her hand and fingers, what pressure and movements she applies, and what kind of stimulation she gives to her pubic area, her labia and to her clitoris. See how her strokes change from slow to fast, and notice their rhythm and pace.

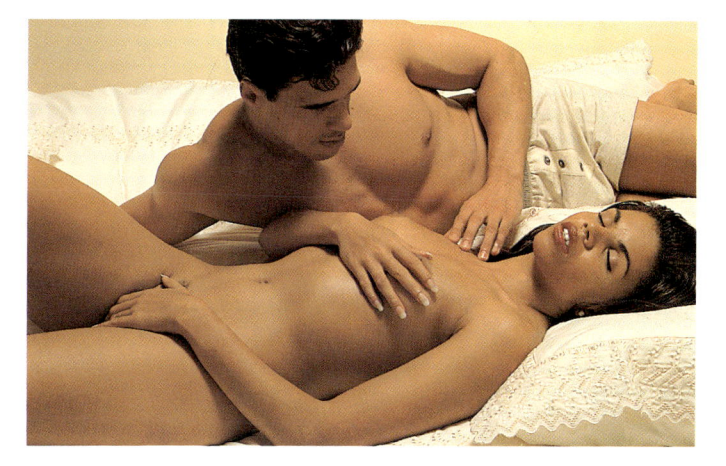

Watch Her Responses
▲ Look also at how her whole body responds to her self-stimulation. Watch how her facial expressions change as she registers the waves of pleasure rising within her. Notice too how she also caresses other parts of her body, not just her genitals, and particularly the way she fondles her breasts and her nipples. You can touch her lightly, but don't interfere with her process right now, because it is important for you to ascertain her full capacity for self-pleasuring and to learn from it so you too can give her equal joy.

Adventurous Sex Techniques

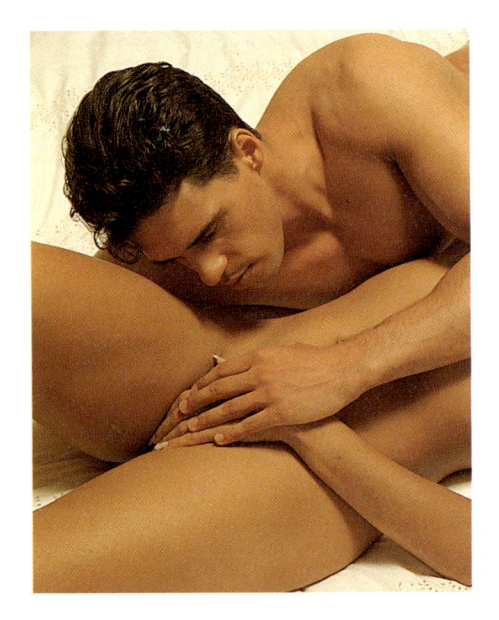

on a classical instrument. Learn to perfect your rhythm and pace, recognize when to be subtle and when to go for the "grande finale".

Masturbating the Male Partner

If you are going to engage yourself fully and wholeheartedly into masturbating your male partner you will want to be comfortable yourself. You can lie beside him, sit or kneel between his legs, or straddle across his body that so you are facing his genitals. Remember that most men prefer the feeling of a firm grip on the shaft of the penis, so it makes sense to use your strongest and most agile hand. You can, however, swap the action over to the other hand if you are going in for a longer bout of masturbation.

You can hold the base of the penis with your more passive hand to keep it steady, and then clasp your active hand around the top end, settling it just below the coronal ridge. (If your partner is uncircumcised, draw the foreskin gently backwards to expose the head of the penis, but do not overstimulate the tip itself as it may

Follow Her Rhythm

◀ Lay your hand gently over hers as she continues to touch, rub and vibrate her fingers against her vulva and clitoris. This is the best way for you to gauge for yourself the manner in which she sexually arouses herself. Try to imagine that your hand is hers, but let hers lead yours in movement and rhythm. Notice how she not only stimulates the clitoris directly, but also strokes her fingers over its surrounding areas and caresses her labia and vagina.

Share His Fantasies

▼ Now it is his turn to tell you exactly how he enjoys to be stimulated during masturbation. Listen and learn carefully from him because he knows best what turns him on. Lay your hand over his to find out how he begins to arouse himself, what strokes he may like to receive on his scrotum, and other parts of his body. If your relationship is open enough, he may like to describe to you the sexual fantasies he uses while masturbating and which help him to achieve an orgasm.

be overly sensitive – unless of course, your partner insists otherwise.)

You can circle the penis with your thumb and index finger to form a ring around it, using this part of your hand as the main tool of stimulation. Alternatively, you can stroke your clasped hand up and down the shaft of the penis from its base to just above the ridge of the glans.

The focal point of stimulation is the erogenously sensitive coronal ridge and the frenulum on the underside, but all-over stroking of the shaft is also pleasurable. You can also roll his penis between your hands, against your thigh and belly, or very erotically between your breasts, although you may need to complete with hand movements to actually bring him to orgasm.

You can start off slowly and sensually, increasing pressure and speed as your strokes progress. Follow what your partner has shown you, varying between short and long, slow and rapid strokes. Build up a rhythm and pace that suits your partner and is in tune with his responses, increasing the tempo as his arousal heightens.

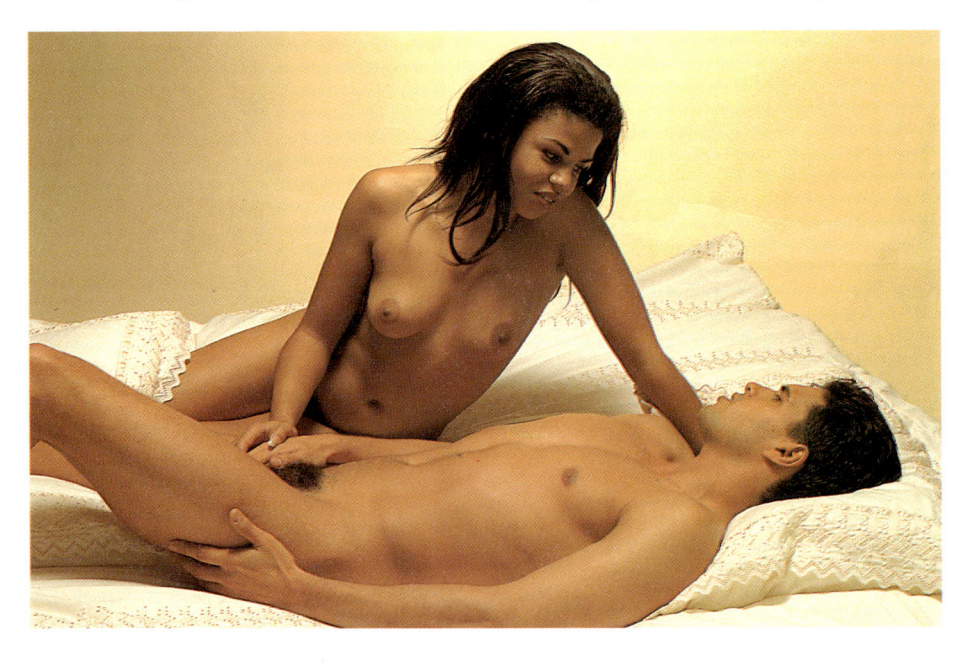

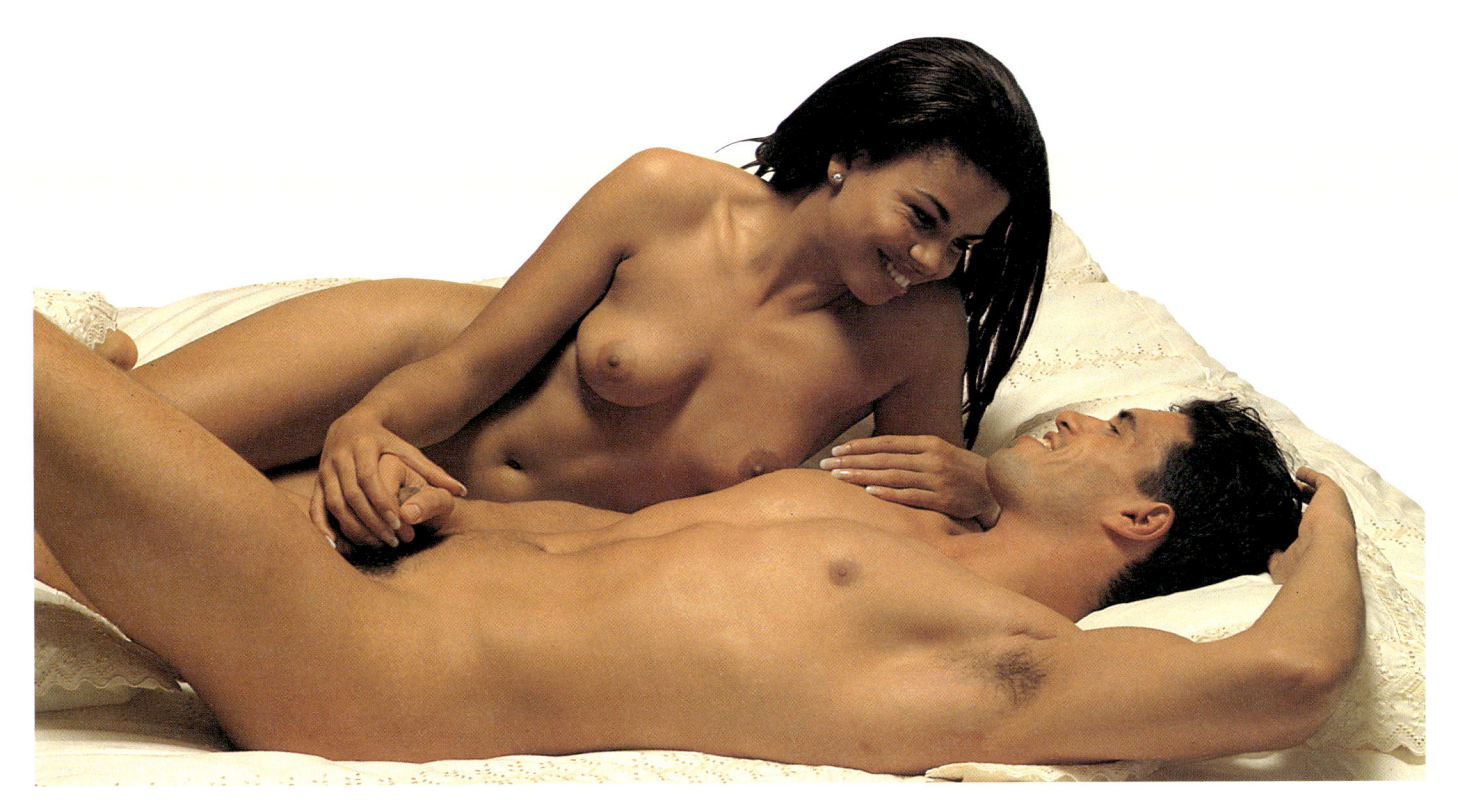

If you both want to prolong the moment of his orgasm, you can slow down teasingly and temporarily just before the ejaculatory process begins, and then start the action all over again. If you do this several times, he may feel as if he is going to burst with increasing sensation and his orgasm, when you allow it to happen, is likely to be very intense.

Learn to recognize the signs that your partner is about to climax so you can speed up your strokes, but stop or slow down once he has started to ejaculate. Continued stimulation at this point may not be welcome as the tip of the penis becomes extremely sensitive and further rubbing can even be painful.

His pleasure may be increased during masturbation if you also caress his thighs and belly, stroke and gently palpate his testicles, apply finger pressure onto his perineum, or press or stroke around his anus. Try it and check out his responses.

Masturbating The Female Partner

Start by stroking, gently rotating and vibrating the flat of one hand over the whole of her vulva, applying some pressure from its heel onto her pubic bone. You should aim to get her love juices to flow, so remember to kiss and caress her whole body, giving loving attention, especially, to her breasts.

Do not zone in right away on her clitoris, and then rub away madly. If you do, you will irritate her, and make this delicate organ feel bruised and sore. Also, remember that she needs to be well lubricated when you are stimulating her clitoral area. Use your finger to gently spread some of her vaginal juices around and over her clitoris. You can also use a little saliva or a drop of KY jelly as a lubricant, but most exciting would be to moisten her with your tongue.

Softly but deftly explore her vulva with your fingers, parting its lips gently and stroking the tip of a finger all around them, and then rub your finger back and forth just above the clitoris. Your middle finger, pointing downwards, is the one long enough to easily stroke over her clitoris, while its tip can gently massage inside her vagina.

Give to her the pleasure she is able to create for herself, applying your strokes with the motions, pressures, and rhythms you have seen her use. Let her guide you with her pelvic movements, and her sighs of delight. Build up your pressure slowly and remember, if she climaxes, to sustain it for the duration of her orgasmic contractions. If the rhythm is wrong or pressure is reduced during these precious moments, you can interrupt the full intensity of her orgasm.

Use Firm Pressure

▲ *A mistake that women often make when masturbating their partner is to use only light pressure because they are afraid of hurting him. Most men, however, prefer a firm strong grip on the penis, and fairly vigorous strokes. He may have particular preferences on how he likes the pace of masturbation to progress; whether he likes to start off slowly and then speed up, or enjoys to tease himself towards an orgasm by taking the heat off just before the ejaculatory process begins and then resume his strokes. He can also show you exactly where the most erogenously sensitive parts of his penis are and which areas respond most to your touch. By clasping your hand over his while he masturbates, you can learn exactly what brings him the most pleasure.*

Sharing Sexual Fantasies

Sexual fantasies are common to many people and provide a rich resource of aphrodisiac material which contributes towards their heightened sexual arousal, either during masturbation or intercourse. These fantasies can be extremely diverse, even bizarre by real-life standards, but very erotically imaginative. Whether the content of someone's sexual fantasy is lurid or mild, it is deeply personal to that individual's sexual psyche and private world of erotic imagery.

Some people have a consistent theme to their fantasies, other people change the material, adding new detail, new scenarios and different characters to their fertile sexual imagery. Studies show, however, that there are certain common patterns of imagination prevalent in people's fantasies, such as themes of domination, submission, being forced into sex against their will, making love to a stranger, an ex-lover or a favourite film star, or being watched while having intercourse.

Sex researchers believe that for many people fantasies are formed in substance from their earliest associations with sexual feelings, while others are constantly updating their erotic imagery to reflect the changing circumstances of their lives. Fantasies based on primal experiences can explain why, for some people, themes such as spanking, or other punishment from an authority figure can feature so strongly.

In another circumstance, a fantasy involving forced sexual compliance, such as a rape scene, may be just a creative way of permitting intense feelings of sexual arousal without having the burden of guilt. In the imagination, that person has no control over what is happening and therefore carries no responsibility for the ensuing erotic feelings.

It is important to realize, however, that fantasies involving forced sex, however descriptive on an imaginative level, will bear little relation to an individual's real-life behaviour or desires, and so do not necessarily indicate that a person has masochistic tendencies. The fantasizer is always in control of events within the fantasy, because he or she is the creator of those images and can carefully manipulate them to bring about the desired result: that of increased sexual response and orgasm. This scenario is totally different from a real-life event, during which a person would have absolutely no control over an incident involving aggressive behaviour resulting in forced sex, and from which they would derive no sexual pleasure at all.

Many people love their sexual fantasy world, using these mental images to enhance and enrich their sex lives and sexual responses. Their fantasies seem to have a life of their own, emerging and existing within a vivid arena of sexual imagination. Some people, however, may feel guilt and anxiety associated with them, fearing that the erotic and extraordinary content of their mentally created eroticism reflects a deep inner psychological disturbance. This anxiety may be compounded when the fantasies contain material which is strongly in contrast to their normal moral values and sexual behaviour.

Members of both sexes may have sexual fantasies, although some

A View to a Thrill
▼ *Making love in the doggie position in front of a mirror can give you both a good view of your sexual activity, including the excitement of watching your expressions while becoming aroused, and being able to witness your movements. As the man, you are also able to see your partner's breasts in the mirror as you fondle them from this rear position.*

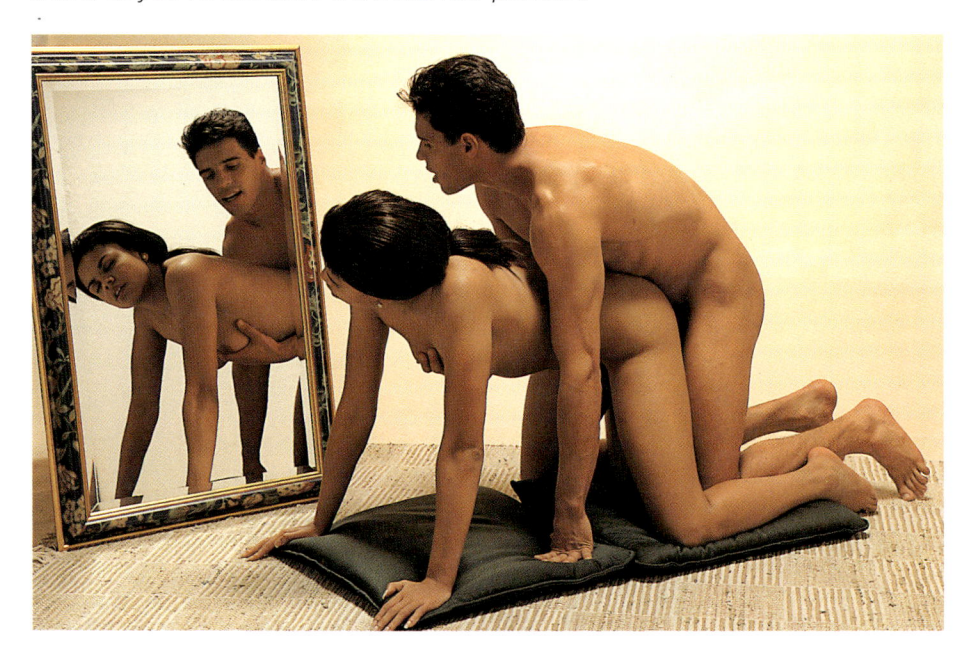

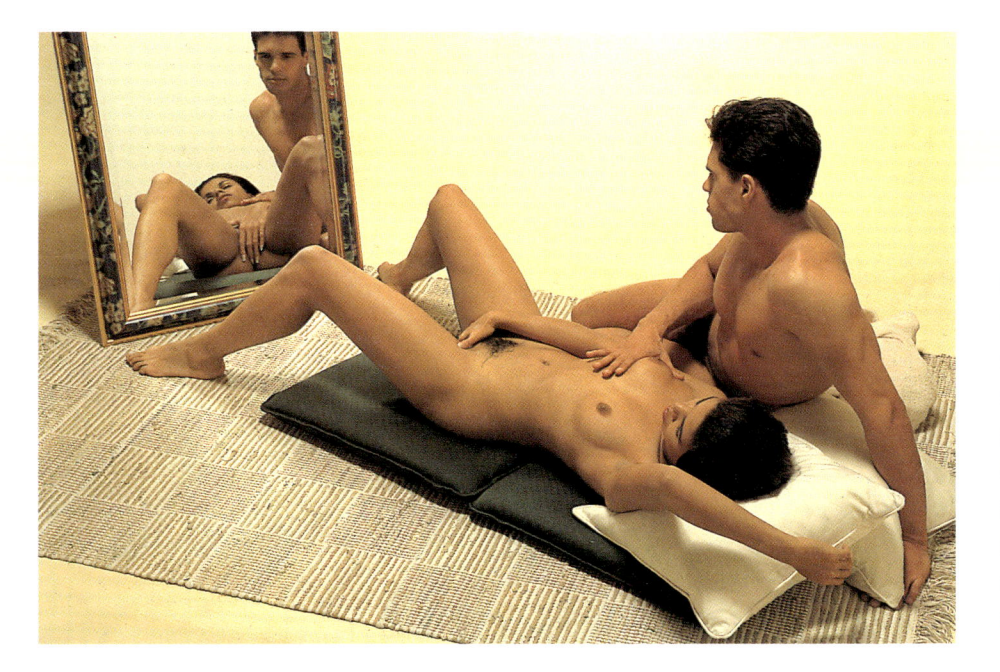

Sharing Sexual Fantasies

Images of Passion
◀ *Watching each other masturbate is another highly erotic way to use the mirror. You can sit beside your partner, stroking her and touching her body and breasts, while being able to see exactly how she likes to arouse herself. The mirror will provide a very clear view of her vulva and the way she stimulates her clitoris.*

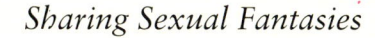

people do not have them at all, and cannot see any value in this mental erotic resource. Such couples may regard fantasy as a mental distraction which will prevent a truly spontaneous interaction between the lovers – a flight into cerebral sex rather than an ecstatic surrender to the physical sensations of the body.

Most sex experts agree that sexual fantasizing is normal behaviour, and can be an important and useful way for people to explore their capacity for sexual arousal and response, either during masturbation or lovemaking. Sex therapy can help, however, if sexual fantasizing has become disturbing to an individual, or is having a serious adverse effect on a sexual relationship.

A sex counsellor or therapist will talk over the issues with the person concerned, helping the client to change the undesirable and habitual patterning of his or her erotic thoughts, or enabling them to accept and integrate it into the context of a loving and fulfilling sexual relationship.

Sharing Sexual Fantasies

Many people who enjoy using sexual fantasy to induce sexual arousal or orgasm would never consider revealing the content of these mental images to anyone else, not even a partner. For them, the fantasies must and do stay within the realm of privacy. They may feel that once a fantasy has been verbalized or shared it loses much of its power and impact.

Other couples discuss their fantasies with each other, and even describe them openly during lovemaking to increase mutual sexual excitement. Some people even feel safe enough within their relationship to act out their fantasies with each other.

Not every person is able to understand or tolerate the erotic imagery that may be part of a partner's sexual consciousness. You need to know and trust your partner's ability to handle this information before revealing your fantasies, or discretion may be a wiser course of action. Your partner may be less than thrilled to know that during lovemaking you have been fantasizing about having sex with your favourite film star or a stranger.

If fantasy is not part of your partner's sexual agenda, then he or she may have no comprehension of your need for it and may even regard it as a personal rejection. In that case, it may be better just to enjoy your fantasies as your own private creation.

This section explores some of the sexual fantasies which can be shared and played out between couples. Some of them are mild and teasing and generally involve a playful content which would probably be viewed as unthreatening and fun by both partners. Other fantasy games, such as domination and bondage, or even cross-dressing, would need to be revealed or acted on only when a relationship is strong enough to withstand their impact.

No one should ever try to impose a private sexual fantasy on another person, or coerce them into acting it out against their will. However, as a loving couple, if you can enjoy sharing each other's fantasy world in a context of trust and mutual exploration, then your erotic imagination can add a new and exciting dimension to your love-life.

Mirror Fantasies

Some people like to use mirrors when they make love because the thrill of watching themselves in different sexual positions increases the excitement of intercourse. It adds a voyeuristic element to their lovemaking because they can actually see themselves making love, as well as watching their partner's body from a different vantage point.

When a mirror is strategically placed, the couple can see the more erotic and intimate parts of the body in action, such as the vulva, the scrotum, and particularly the buttocks and anus, and they can even witness the

83

Adventurous Sex Techniques

process of penetration and thrusting. It can seem as if you are watching yourself and your lover acting the part in a blue-movie, which is an added turn-on to those couples who enjoy watching pornographic films together.

Another fantasy that can arise through the use of a mirror is a sense that other people are copulating alongside you while you are making love. This can provide a safer and less emotionally damaging way of acting out a group orgy sexual fantasy rather than actually doing it for real.

Some couples are fairly blatant about their mirror fantasies, and have one permanently fixed to the bedroom ceiling to provide them with a bird's eye view of their love-making activities. You may not want to go as far as this, and perhaps the use of a mirror during sex is just an occasional fantasy. In that case, a transportable mirror which is easily moved to any part of your bedroom or home to provide a good reflecting angle is the answer.

Strip-Tease Fantasy

It has been said, in a tongue-in-cheek way of course, that inside every woman there is a stripper trying to get out. Not all women are going to agree with that, but it is true that, even among the most reserved, the idea of doing a strip-tease can hold a certain allure. It may even provide material for a sexual fantasy.

There can be something very exciting about the idea of performing an exotic strip-tease dance. If you are confident and extrovert enough, you could have a lot of fun displaying your body to the man you love in such a bold and tantalizing way – and it can be very rewarding to have him adore your every revealing move.

If you do a strip-tease then you must be the one who is in charge of your sexual exhibitionism, and during it your partner is in your control and at your command. He can watch and relish the sight of you, but he must not touch you unless you so desire. The tease is the main point of the exercise so you are allowed to arouse and play with him, showing yourself off little by little, promising hints of your naked body, but you alone must decide when and how to take off your clothes, and how much he can touch you.

Perform your exotic dance for your own pleasure as well as his. You are celebrating your own eroticism,

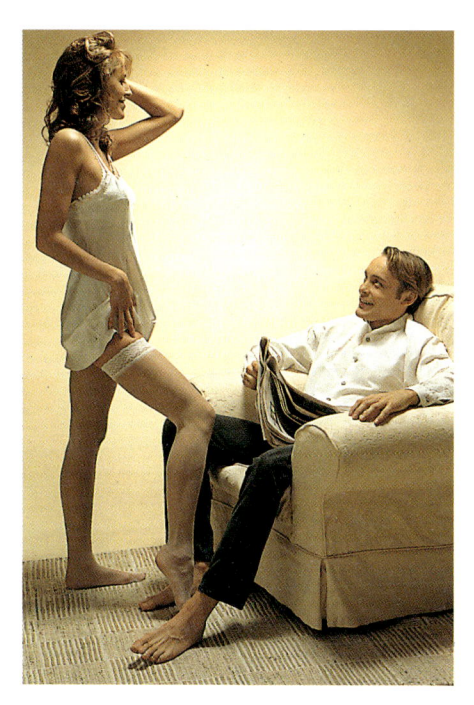

Build the Suspense
▲ One of the more fun ways of acting out your strip-tease is to perform for your partner when he is least suspecting it. Or you can set a date for it to build up his eager anticipation. Put on some of your prettiest lingerie, but make sure you have a few layers on top so you can take your time peeling them off, so keeping him in suspense. White underwear is a particularly good choice – the combination of snow-white innocence and your sexy routine will add extra appeal and excitement. Also, wear pretty stockings which you can roll sexily down your legs, or you can add a suspender belt to the strip-tease kit.

Shimmy and Shake
▼ Once you have got his interest, begin your strip routine. To the sound of raunchy music, start to move and sway in front of him. Motion is important in strip-tease, because the sight of your swaying body will be arousing and it should be executed as a dance and a performance. Tease your petticoat straps on and off of your shoulders. Roll down one strap to allow the petticoat to slip slightly off one side of your body. Then haughtily replace it, while you let the other strap fall teasingly off your other shoulder. Keep moving to show him the back and front of your body, and toss your hair with each seductive turn. Then shimmy the petticoat straps down your arms to expose your bra and cleavage.

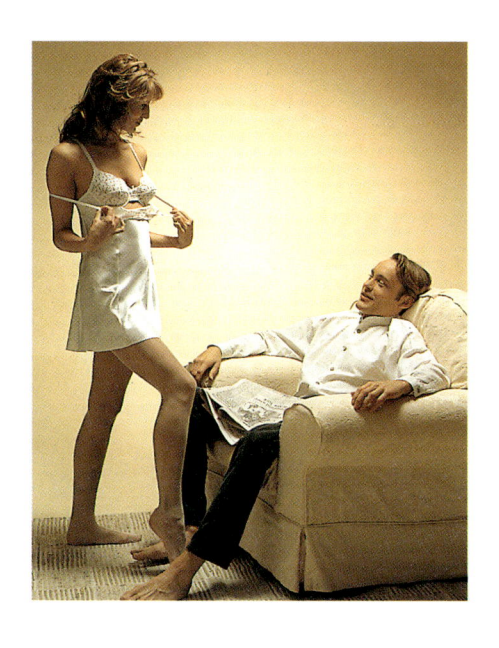

Sharing Sexual Fantasies

and what is more, you are enjoying showing it off.

One of the more fascinating aspects of performing strip-tease is that it allows you to counteract an aspect of your gender conditioning. While women are often portrayed as objects of desire, society also expects them to behave in a demure and chaste manner. Stripping for your lover helps you to challenge that restraint, and you can flaunt your body in such as way that you are making a statement about your own sexuality.

If it is your fantasy to do a strip-tease, then pluck up the courage to do it for your lover. It could be one of his fantasies too, but he may have been too shy to ask you to do it. Visual arousal is an important part of male sexuality, and he is sure to enjoy the invitation to become your captive audience. Devise your own dance routine, and if you need to build up some confidence, practise your steps in front of a mirror when you are alone. The illustrations and further suggestions shown here should provide you with some inspiring ideas on how to turn your strip-tease into an art.

The Art of Strip-Tease

Good strip-tease should be an art, a dance and a performance, so it is worth preparing properly to do it. If you have practised a few routines on your own, you should, by now, have built up your confidence. The two most important props for your show are the right music and sexy underwear. You might like to use additional accoutrements like a feather boa or silk scarves which you can stroke and trail all over your skin, and which you can use to reveal a glimpse of your body.

Seductive Sex Kitten

▼ *Allow the silky petticoat to slide slowly down your body so that you begin to reveal more and more naked skin. Gradually expose your chest and belly but for now do not let the petticoat fall any lower than your hips. The main idea is to keep him in suspense. Pose and move in such a way that you accentuate your curves. In a playful game like this, you can adopt the classic "sex-kitten" postures of movie starlets in the 1950s. Flexing your knee to balance one leg on the ball of your foot will define its shapely contours, and tilt your pelvis back seductively. In strip-tease, you are totally in control of the situation, as you send out inviting come-hither looks. At this stage, though, the man should look but not touch. The whole purpose is to tease him.*

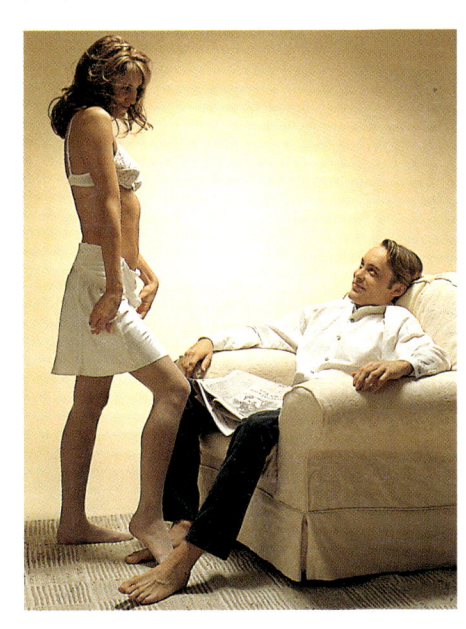

The music you choose should be sexy, or slow and sensual, depending on your dance routine. Or select songs which hold romantic memories for you and your partner. Whatever music you pick, it should have just the right rhythm to put you into an arousing and playful mood.

Concealing and Revealing

▼ *Very slowly let your petticoat slide over your hips and down your legs to reveal your buttocks. You can tantalize him further by letting it slip a little and then re-adjusting it several times before you are ready for full exposure. Sway your hips seductively from side to side, and then rotate to the beat of the music so that the whole of your pelvis is in constant motion. Then turn a little to the side, so that he can see the profile of your body, and enjoy its undulating contours. Panties that are saucy and skimpy will show your buttocks off to their best advantage. For most men, the sight of a woman's bottom is very visually stimulating. When you are ready, turn your back to him so he can enjoy seeing it in full-view, then bend over to allow him a closer look.*

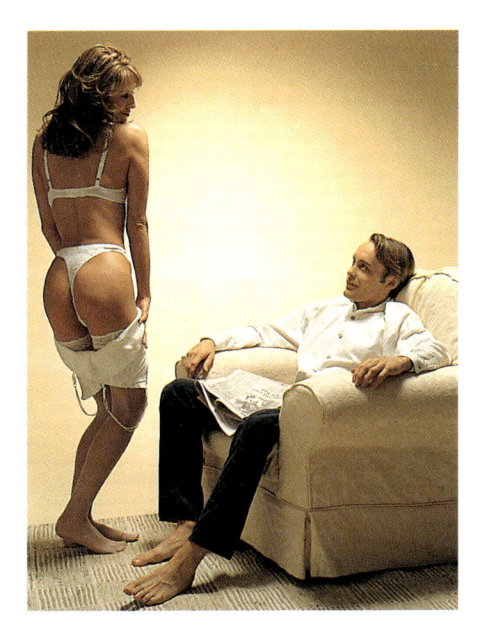

If you want to make strip-tease a regular part of your fantasy play to enjoy with your lover, it is worth investing in several sets of lingerie. Select different colours and styles, and save them for these occasions as well as for your most romantic nights. You need a bra and panties of

Adventurous Sex Techniques

matching colours and soft fabrics. Silk and lace items always look wonderful. You might like to wear a suspender belt, or choose stockings which cling to your legs. You then need a sexy petticoat, or a slinky dress, so that you are fully covered when you first appear. The fun of strip-tease comes from peeling off the layers piece by piece. You can go for the vamp look, dressed all in black, and even wear high-heeled shoes. Red is exotic and brazen, while white is pure and innocent.

The correct actions during the strip-tease are very important if you are to create the right alluring effect. They should be slow and sexy but slightly exaggerated. Your aim is to pose and move your body as erotically as possible. Lots of pelvic gyrations will excite him and you.

However, you should let your dance be an expression of your own inner sexuality. Do what feels good to you and what turns you on. Find that sex queen part in yourself and act it out to the full.

While you tease your partner and peel away your clothes, stroke and caress your own body as if you are making love to yourself. You can run your hands sensuously over your breasts, along your inner thighs, and in between your legs.

Although the aim of the strip-tease is to excite and tantalize your partner, it should be done for your pleasure too. Love your body and have fun showing it off, and let your liberated eroticism turn you on too. Enjoy the thrill of your sexual power.

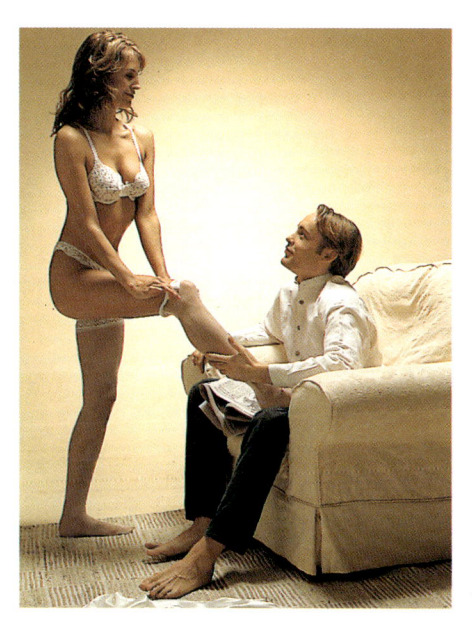

Involve Your Partner
▲ Now let your petticoat slip to the floor, and begin to remove your stockings. Like everything else in strip-tease this should be done slowly with a constant "Will I? Won't I?" tease. You can roll your stockings down your legs – one at a time – either by yourself, or involve your partner in the action. Before, he had simply been a spectator, but now he gets a chance to touch. However, you must stay in control, and allow him to touch you only to help you undress – part of the fun of strip-tease is that he knows you have the upper hand.

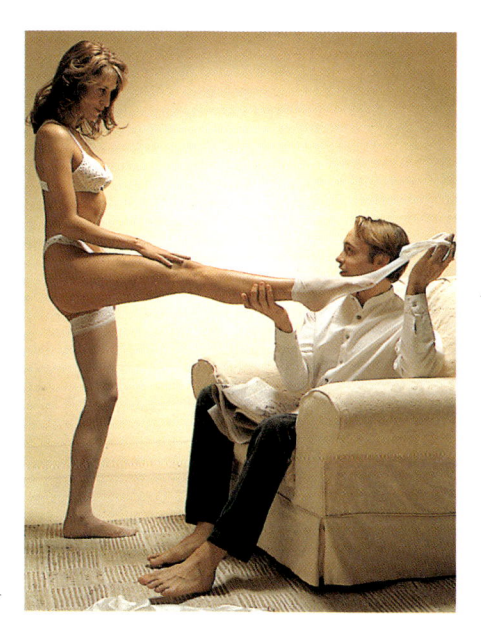

Peel to Appeal
▲ Everything about your movements should be seductive, sensual and erotic, but it needs to be graceful too. So when it comes to taking your stockings off completely, you should enlist your partner's help. Otherwise, you may be struggling in this position, unless you put one foot on the chair or sit on the floor. One way is to give him your leg to hold and have him peel the stocking right off your foot. At the same time, you can sexily stroke over your own leg, thigh and buttocks. Self-caressing is an alluring aspect of strip-tease.

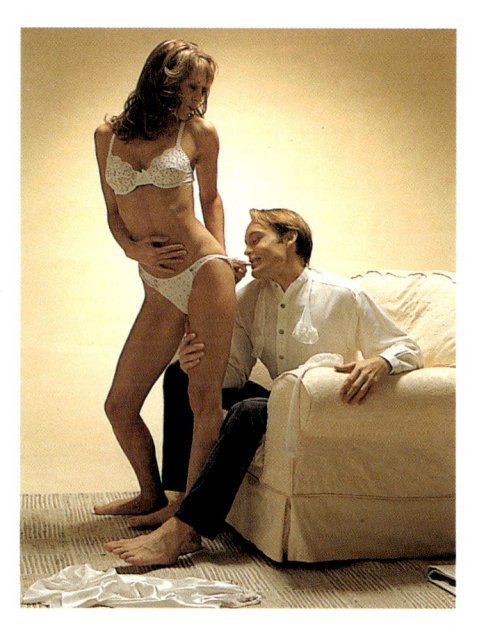

Teasing Touches
▲ The show goes on – and you can now get down to the nitty-gritty of your strip-tease. When you are just wearing your panties and bra, take lots of time to remove them. Move and dance around his chair, coming in close enough so he can give you a fleeting touch, and then moving slightly out of his reach. Start to turn up the heat in your act, by rolling your panties down just enough to give him a little peek. Stand close enough that he can begin to touch and caress you, and even let him tug at your panties with his teeth.

Sharing Sexual Fantasies

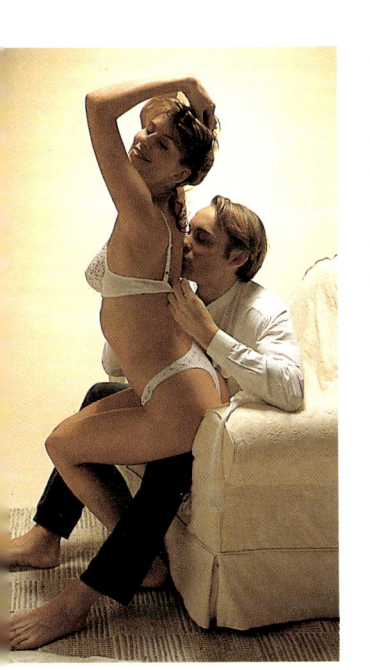

Unsnap the Strap
◀ You can enlist his help to undo your bra fastener, especially if undoing it yourself would prove too awkward. Perch saucily on his lap with your back to him and stay in your performance mode, gyrating your pelvis subtly on his knee. If you have long hair, sweep it sexily away from your shoulders and back to expose more bare flesh to him, and if he wants to, let him plant little kisses on your skin. It is too soon to let the bra slip off, so once he has undone it, cup it to your breasts with your hands. The point of the exercise is to keep him wanting more.

Caress Your Breasts
▶ Let the rounded swell of your breasts begin to show, but don't expose your nipples yet. Turn to face your partner, and incline towards him so your breasts come close to his body. Gently palpate your breasts with your hands as if caressing them, and let the bra material stroke across their skin. Don't let your partner touch your breasts yet – at this point you are using visual stimulation to arouse him – but you can move your leg closer to him so he can stroke your thighs. Gradually let your bra slide down from your breasts, to expose the edge of your nipples.

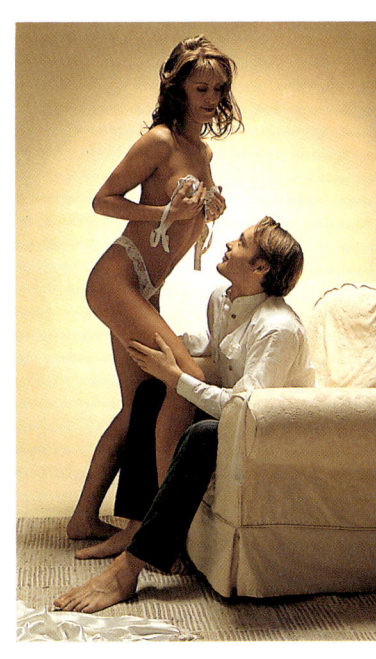

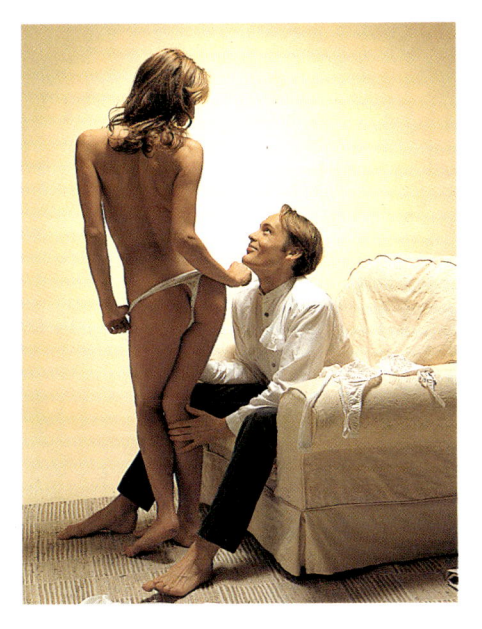

Panty Time
▲ Now comes the really sexy part, as you start to peel off your panties. Keep the movement going in your body as you turn from side to side and back and forth, sometimes leaning your hips or buttocks within reach of his touch. Begin to edge your panties very slowly downwards. Turn around sometimes to give him a little glimpse of your pubic hair, but change angles constantly so he gets an all-round view of this very erotic part of your body.

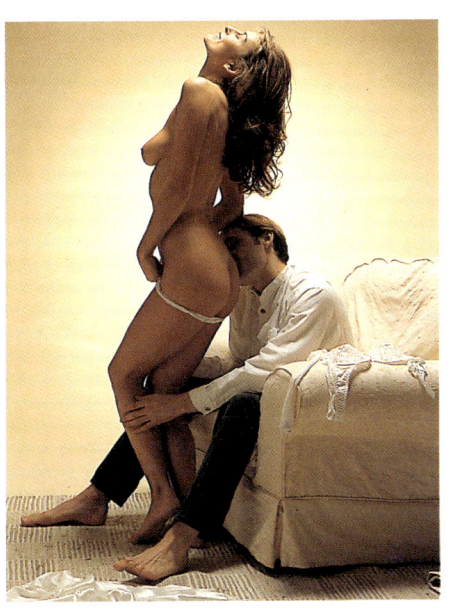

Move in Close
▲ Still holding on to your panties, languidly roll them over the curve of your buttocks so they rest on the top of your thighs. At this point, your whole body is almost entirely naked. Make the most of these last tantalizing moments of your strip-tease, but moving very close to your partner and dancing erotically in front of him. Let different parts of your body brush and rub against him, and then allow him to reach out and caress you a little more.

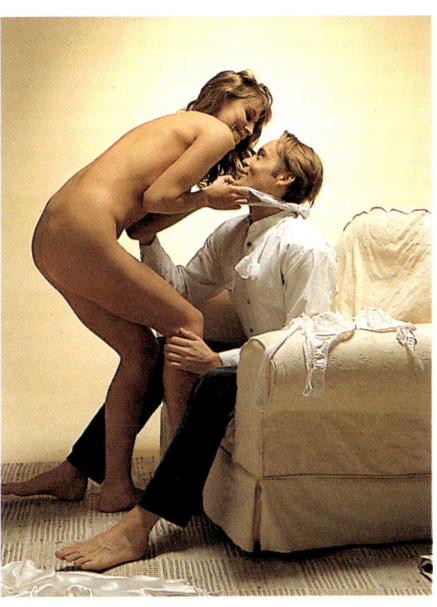

Fun Finale
▲ Find an easy way to roll your panties down your legs so you remove them completely from your body. If necessary, you can rest one foot on the chair for easy manoeuvring. Then use your panties as part of your dance. Stroke them softly over your skin, between your legs, against your partner's face, and hook them around his neck to pull him playfully towards you. The strip-tease is over, what you do next with all that smouldering sexual excitement is up to you.

Adventurous Sex Techniques

Feeding Frenzy

A fun fantasy to share with your partner is to prepare a sumptuous banquet of delicious desserts, only instead of laying the food on a table, you spread it on each other's bodies – and then have a wonderful time nibbling and licking it off. You can gather around you all kinds of delicious ripe fruits – tropical mangoes are an exotic choice. Or you may

Cream Stream

▼ When she is lying down, pour the cream or sauces, or rub the juicy fruits on her body. If you are pouring a liquid cream, let it trickle out slowly so she feels its cool sensations running down over her skin.
(If you are worried about making a mess, cover your mattress with a washable sheet.)

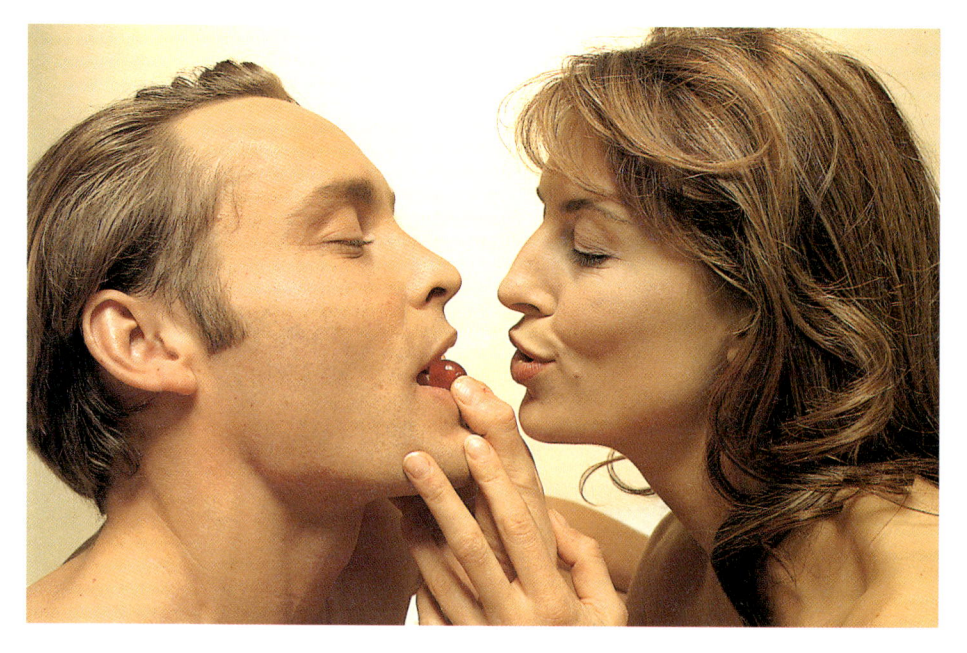

Fruity Fiesta

▲ Start off your bacchanalian feast with a fruit cocktail for the hors d'oeuvres. Feed each other juicy pieces of exotic fruits to excite your taste buds and make your mouths water. Be sure, though, to spice up your snack with plenty of kisses and cuddles.

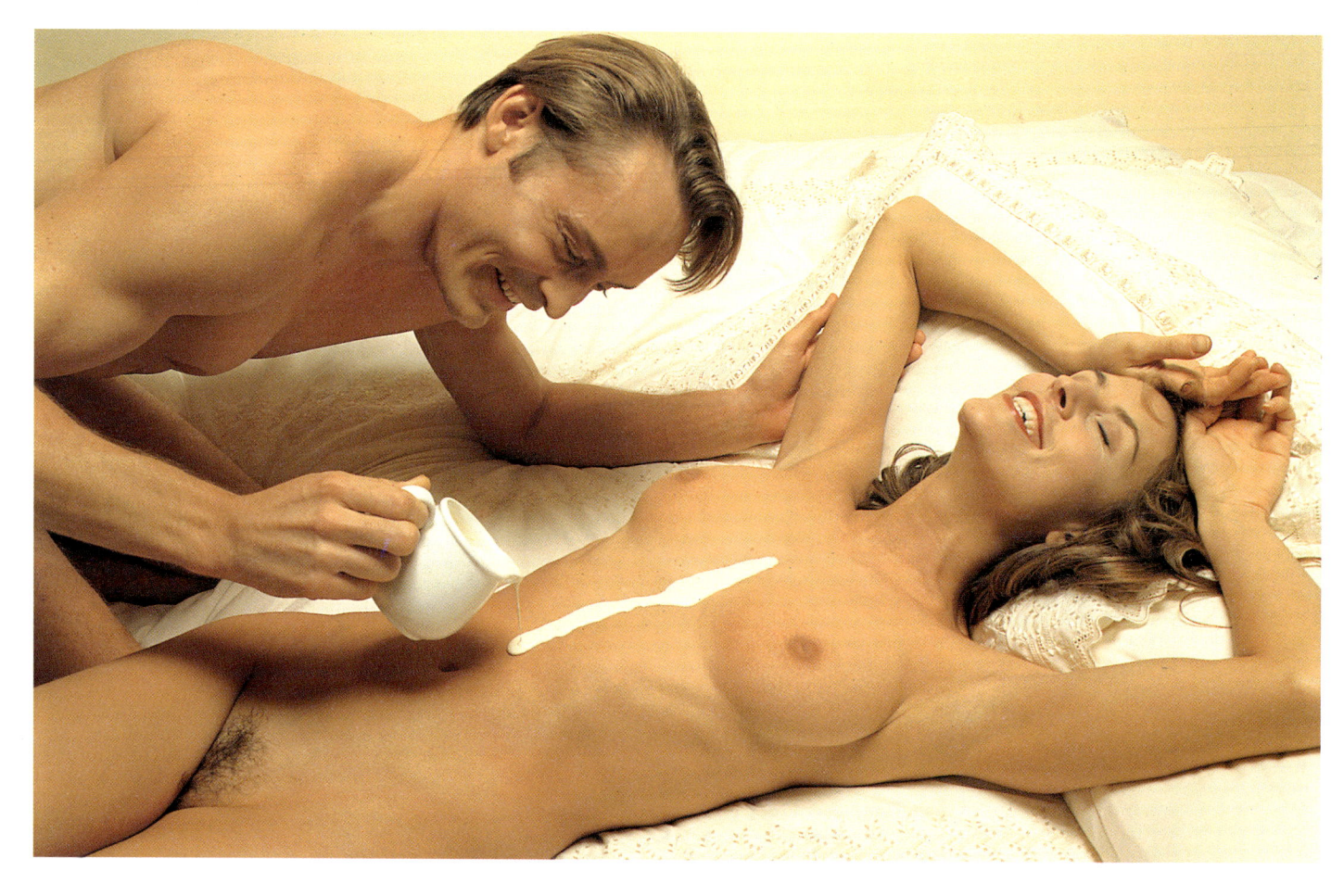

Sharing Sexual Fantasies

Taste Sensations

▶ Begin to lick the cream from her body. Slow, languid licks of your tongue, and then some darting motions, will thrill her skin and delight her. Spend extra time on the most sensitive areas, such as her belly. Run your warm tongue around and around her navel and tell her that she tastes delicious.

want to go for the smoother tastes of icecream, honey, chocolate sauce, cream, and yogurt.

This is a sensual and hedonistic feast in every way, so make sure you pick the most mouth-watering foods you can find. If you want to make the event simpler, go for one type, such as cream, which has a soft consistency and can be easily poured over the skin.

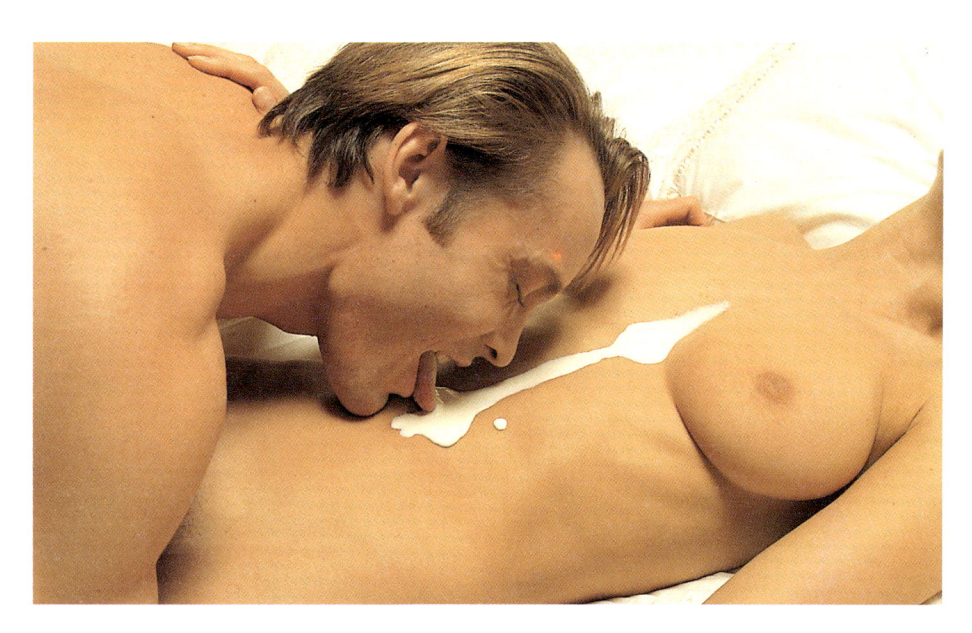

The idea is to let your tongue travel slowly around your partner's body so that you lick off the food in such a slow, sensual and titillating way that you drive your partner into a frenzy of arousal. Linger awhile over the more erogenous zones of her body, teasingly nibble around the breasts and nipples, or seductively run the tip of your tongue over her belly, or along the inside of her thighs. Sup on the succulent juices and creams, telling your partner that she is "good enough to eat" whenever you reach certain pleasure spots on her body. Let yourselves luxuriate in an epicurean orgy of sensual taste and skin pleasure. No need to hurry over this feast and, at this banquet, seconds and dessert are definitely in order!

Feast on Her Breasts

▼ Pour drops of the cream onto her breasts and take as long as you like to savour its taste. Work your tongue slowly around the circumference of her breast, before adding a little more cream to her nipple. Suck and lick her nipple teasingly, relishing in the erotic feast.

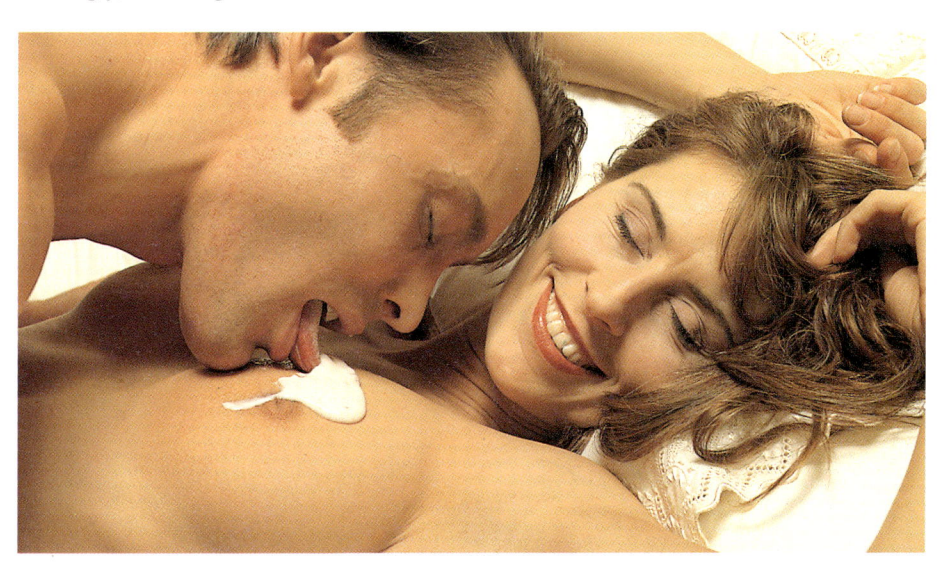

Just Desserts

Gerry, 32 years, a masseur and keep-fit trainer: "My girlfriend, Nicole, and I made love one time covered from head to foot with fruit pulp and cream. It was a totally spontaneous event, though we were at home and just in our underwear at the time. It started out as a joke, her flicking a bit of the food at me, and then me retaliating. One thing led to another and we ended up smearing our dessert all over each other's bodies and then licking it off each other. The whole thing just got more sensual and erotic by the moment. We were slithering all over each other in the end. I can definitely recommend it. It was yummy!"

Adventurous Sex Techniques

Dressing-Up Fantasies

While most of us present a particular personality to the outside world, with which we predominantly identify ourselves, within us all there are many other character traits which weave together to create the rich tapestry of our human psyches. At best, the varying shades of our personalities can mingle with each other and become integrated, each part having an opportunity to express itself at an appropriate time.

Occasionally, though, certain aspects of our internal world become suppressed or denied, perhaps because of moral conditioning, fear of judgement from others, or through self-censure. Sometimes it is just a lack of opportunity that forces us to resign some of our more colourful internal personality traits to the back shelf. This is particularly true in regard to our sexual consciousness, and one of the reasons that fantasy can often be so helpful is that it enables us to access those more obscure parts of ourselves.

In a close and loving relationship, where two people trust each other and are willing to share each other's fantasies without condemnation, there is a tremendous opportunity to play-act roles which allow them to express and have fun with some of their sexual identities. One way to do this is by dressing up, thereby allowing your hidden sexual fantasies to emerge in full regalia.

You can even dress up to be theatrical, turning your bedroom into a fantasy land where you act out heroes and heroines from the movies, the stage, literature – or even those from your imagination. You can turn yourselves into Heathcliff and Cathy, or Romeo and Juliet for the night. Or perhaps one or the other of you has a favourite film star – so why not be Humphrey Bogart, or Marilyn Monroe, or whoever else you admire, and play-act the part for the night for your favourite audience? Or, if you trust each other, dress up to manifest your sexual secrets and fantasies. Raid your wardrobe, or scour the sales for items of clothing which will help you to fulfil your complete sexual personality.

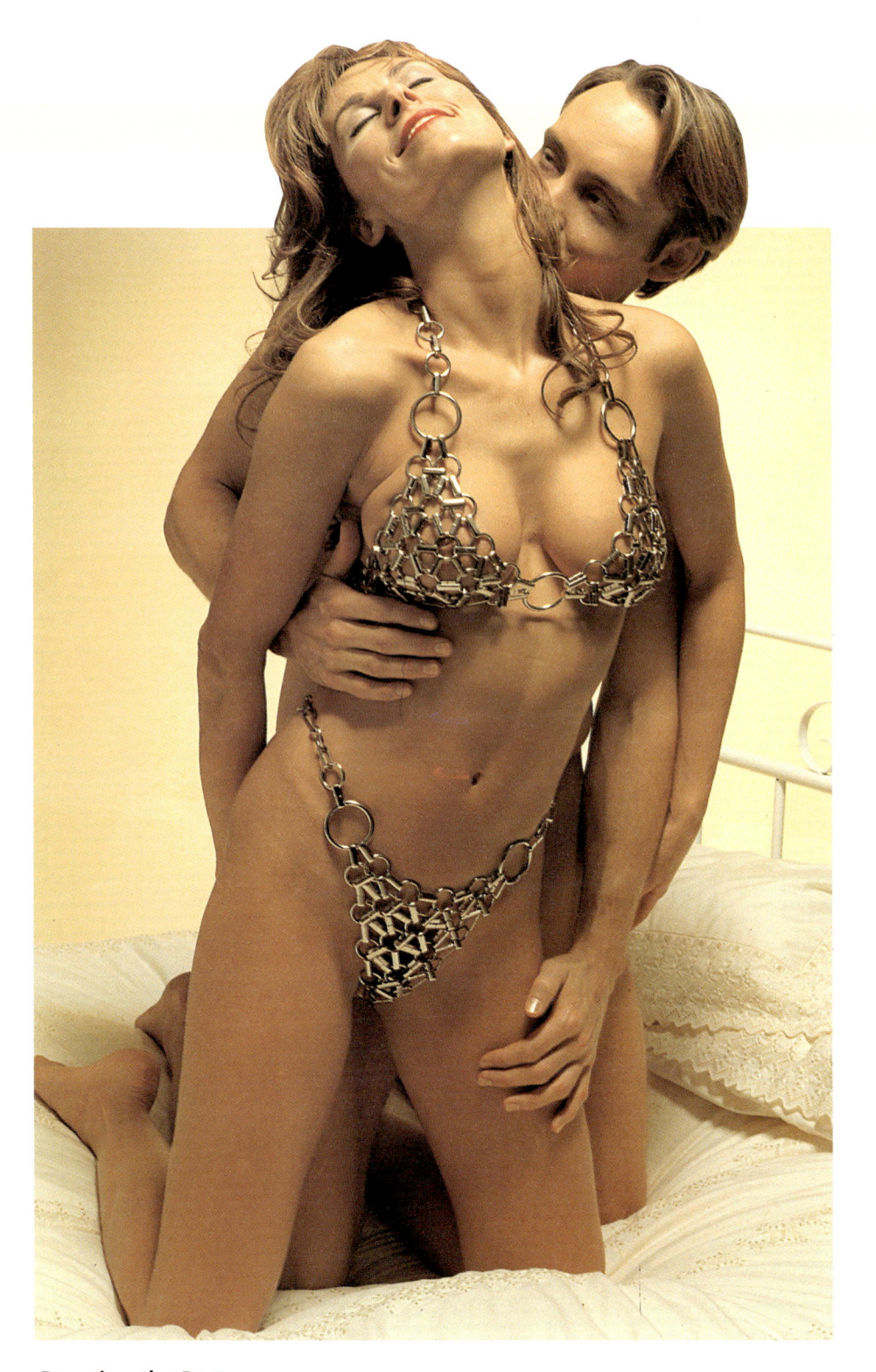

Dressing the Part

▲ *Look for the kind of outrageous outfit or underwear you would never normally wear. It should be pure show biz or downright sexy. If you want to be a James Bond girl or an Amazon Queen, leather, latex, rubber or chain mail will give you the tough, sexually assertive look to help you play out your fantasy role.*

Sharing Sexual Fantasies

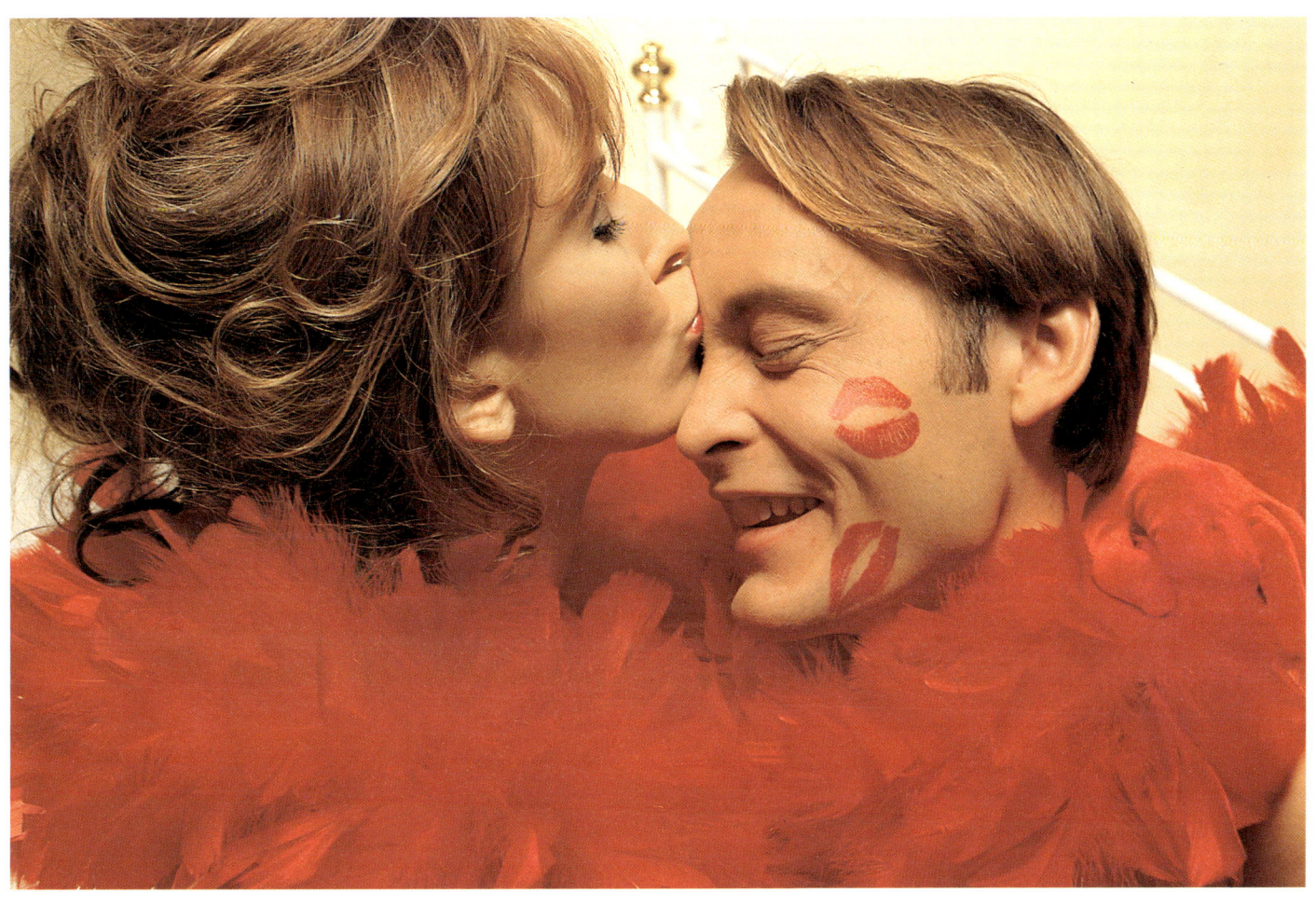

The Temptress

So you have a respectable job, your life is well-organized, you may be a mother and have a secure long-term relationship. Or you have strong feelings about sexual equality, support the feminist movement, and hate to see women portrayed as sexual objects. There is, however, a part of you (it may be a very small part!) that has an on-going fantasy about being a scarlet woman, a femme-fatale, a bordello queen, or a temptress.

If you give yourself permission to allow that side of your nature to come out once in a while, it does not mean to say that your whole value system and way of life is about to change. Dressing up and play-acting your sex queen or brazen woman fantasy in the safety of your bedroom

Lavish Your Attention
▲ *You have succeeded in winning over the man and now he is putty in your hands. Wrap him up in your feather boa and pull him close to the warmth of your skin and into the soft curves of your body. Now that you have him in your arms, you are going to lavish attention on him. How about planting kisses from those full red lips of yours all over his face.*

An Offer He Can't Refuse
▶ *Pose yourself to look alluring, and make the most of your feminine curves. For extra effect, drape your feather boa around your body. Learn to pant seductively. Let everything you do signal a hint of promise and pleasure. Then pat the bed beside you expectantly and invite him to join you.*
How can he refuse?

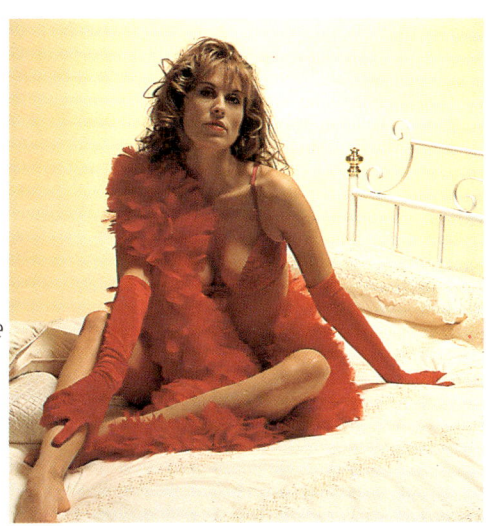

Adventurous Sex Techniques

and together with your partner will just be an exciting and fun way to express a certain side of yourself. You may feel enriched by it too, because an important aspect of who you are can claim its place in your life.

Cross-Dressing

Nobody knows for sure how many men enjoy cross-dressing or even fantasize about it. The subject is still taboo in our society, although transvestite issues are now being discussed more openly. However, research shows that a considerable number of men do cross-dress and become sexually aroused by wearing, or thinking about wearing, women's clothes, and especially women's underwear.

The reason why this is one of the most secret fantasies of all is that many men, who clearly identify themselves as heterosexuals and who only want to make love to female partners, are afraid of the ridicule and condemnation that cross-dressing invariably causes. Studies conducted on men who cross-dress, show that over 75 per cent of them are married and have children. Their sexual orientation is towards the opposite sex, and they clearly identify their gender as male.

There are various reasons why a man may fantasize about cross-dressing. It may be due to curiosity and the desire to discover how it feels to "be like a woman"; soft, feminine or exotic underwear may appeal to him, or he may even need to wear female underwear or other clothing to become sexually aroused. In the latter case, this can be termed as a transvestite fetish, as the man is reliant on these objects to become sexually fulfilled.

Having fantasies, or wearing female clothing, is not a problem in itself, unless the man feels confused or unhappy about his sexual identity, is plagued with guilt about it, or his female partner feels distressed, offended and threatened by his transvestite tendencies. (Some sex counsellors specialize in cross-dressing, transvestite, or transsexual issues and are able to help the individuals concerned to talk through any problems that may result.)

Many wives and girlfriends, who discover their partners are cross-dressers, find it almost impossible to accept or understand their behaviour.

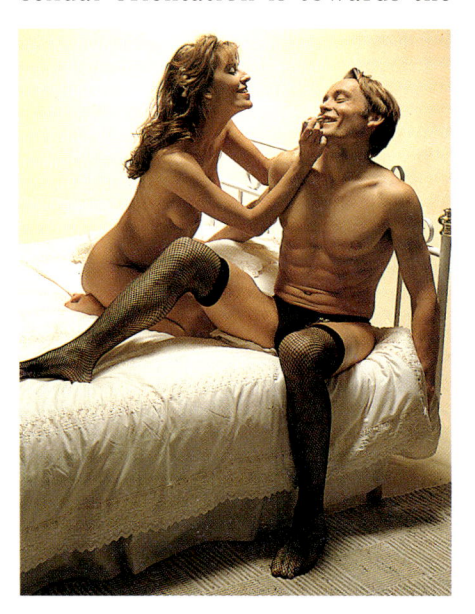

Fantasy Femme Fatale

▼ *Is there a temptress or a femme fatale inside you waiting to express herself? Do you have a fantasy about being a Mata Hari, a high-class courtesan, or an expensive mistress? Enjoy playing your role. Go for the glamour look, and keep it totally feminine. Choose passionate red, lace, and feathers, and lots of make-up. Go all out to seduce your man.*

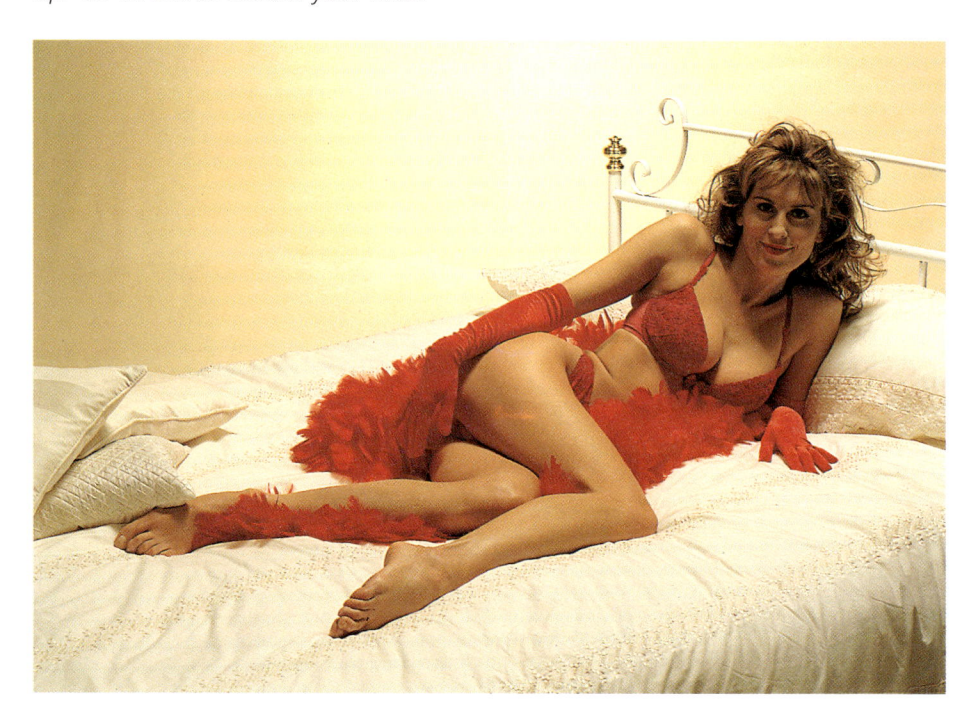

Enjoying His Fantasy

◄ *Not all women are disturbed by a man's cross-dressing fantasy. She can be happy to join in, selecting items of her clothing for him to wear, or taking him out on a shopping trip to choose his female underwear. In fact, her role of dressing him up may be an acted-out fantasy for her too.*

Sharing Sexual Fantasies

> ### Coming to Terms With Cross-Dressing
>
> *Melanie*, 42 years, has been married to Tom, also 42, for 14 years:
>
> "We had been married for about nine years before I discovered that Tom liked to wear women's underwear. I found out because I walked into the bedroom one afternoon and found him wearing a pair of my best knickers – a black, silky pair that I kept for special occasions. I don't know who looked more shocked – Tom, for being found out, or me.
>
> "We had a terrible scene about it, during which he confessed that he often fantasized about wearing women's clothing, and that he did sometimes dress up as a woman, whenever he was alone in the house. I went a bit hysterical, and I said some awful things to him, accusing him of all kinds of perverted behaviour. He said he had always felt guilty about this trait, and he was obviously very distressed about me knowing about it.
>
> "On my side, I felt he had turned into a stranger in a second, that he was no longer the man I knew, and I even wondered if he was actually a real man at all. Our relationship went through a very rocky patch, but somehow we managed to keep talking it through because the bottom line was that we really loved each other, and we had a good relationship. We were lucky because we met some people who knew a great deal more about cross-dressing than us and we were able to get advice from them.
>
> "Slowly, Tom felt less guilty, and I came to accept this side of his sexuality. I became less suspicious and judgmental about the whole thing. In the end we even started to use his cross-dressing as an occasional 'extra' in our sexual relationship. When he feels the need, and I am ready for it, I dress and make him up. We don't discuss this with our friends, but it has become our special secret and we even make it fun."
>
> *Tom*'s response:
>
> "All I want to add to what Melanie has said is that none of this ever had anything to do with how I felt about her because I have always really loved her. At the end of the day, it was a relief that she knew. I am very lucky to have someone like Melanie who could eventually accept and understand this part of me."

They may fear that their partners have homosexual tendencies, are effeminate, or they may regard the behaviour as a perversion. Some female partners, though, are happy to comply with this aspect of the man's personality, and even enjoy dressing him up, putting make-up on him, or choosing his specialized items of clothing. It is their secret, and it becomes part of their sexual agenda – an important feature of their relationship, even if it is something that is hidden from others.

Perhaps your dressing-up fantasies might include cross-dressing. This could be a response to the man's real desire to sometimes wear women's clothing, or it might just be a one-off game to act out the opposite-sex gender role. If this is acceptable to both people involved, and you feel your relationship is strong enough to withstand the implications, cross-dressing can become a shared fantasy game involving you both.

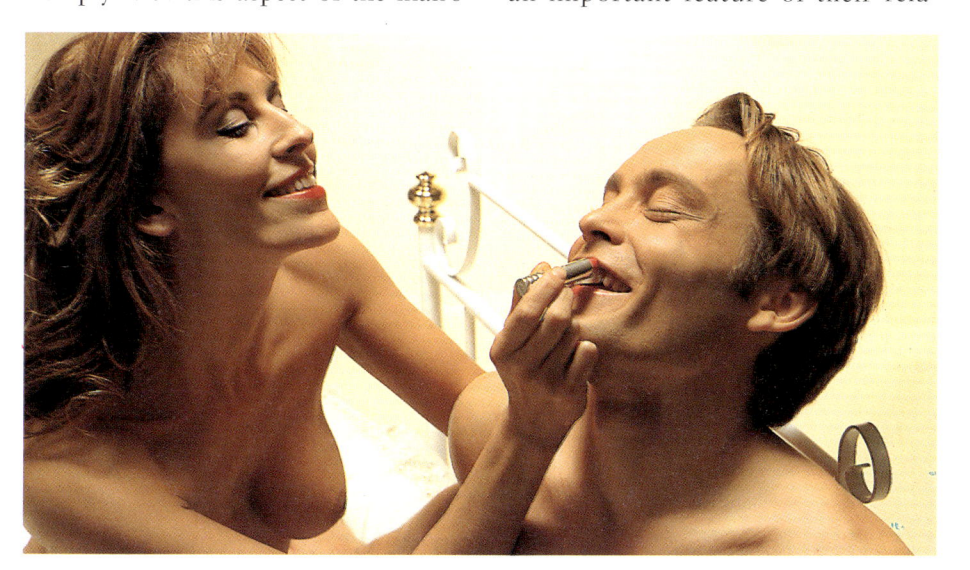

Feminine Role-Play

◀ *He may just want to wear women's panties or stockings, but he might also want to dress up completely as a female and play-act the role of a woman for a while.*

Getting Turned On

Some people are very turned on by the idea of skin teasing, where they are stroked all over the body with the lightest of touches and using all kinds of textures which can result in an almost unbearable intensity. At the other extreme, so long as both partners are willing, lovers can find it stimulating to act out fantasies that involve bondage and domination.

Skin Teasing

It is not a fantasy for the ticklish, but if the idea of a session of skin excitation appeals to either of you, then gather around you all kinds of sensual materials so that you can enjoy a variety of tactile sensations. Find out from each other if either of you has a particular tactile fetish – perhaps you love the feeling of feathers, or of soft, luxurious silk on your skin, or even the firmer texture of leather or rubber being stroked against the surface of your body.

Even more exciting is to use different materials and different touches, perhaps even blowing or licking the body all over, or trailing your fingers very lightly over the most sensitive parts of the skin. Erotic touches on

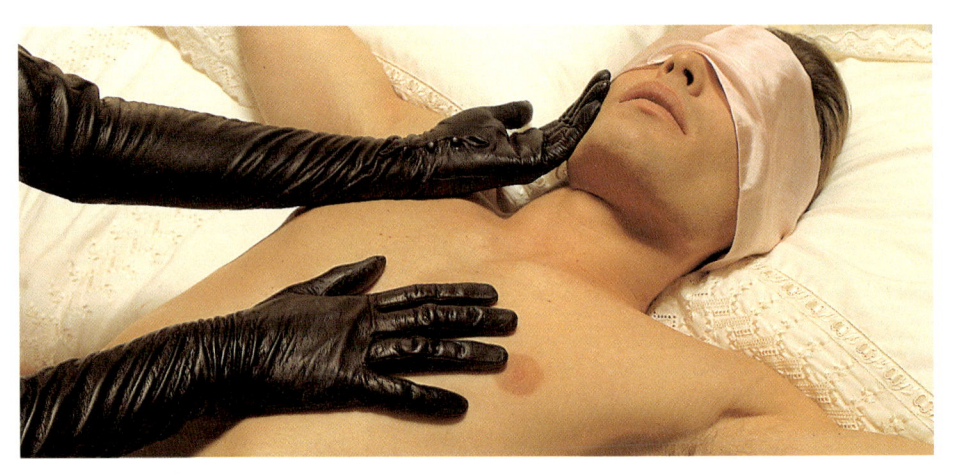

Feel of Leather

▲ *If your partner is turned on by the idea of black leather, find a pair of erotic-looking soft leather gloves to wear and begin to stroke very lightly but slowly over his whole body. Blindfold him loosely with a silk scarf so he doesn't know where your touches will go, or exactly what you are planning to do, and this will add to his excitement. Stroke all over his face so he can take in the smell of the leather, and then draw one hand after the other lightly on the surface of his skin down over his body to the tips of his toes.*

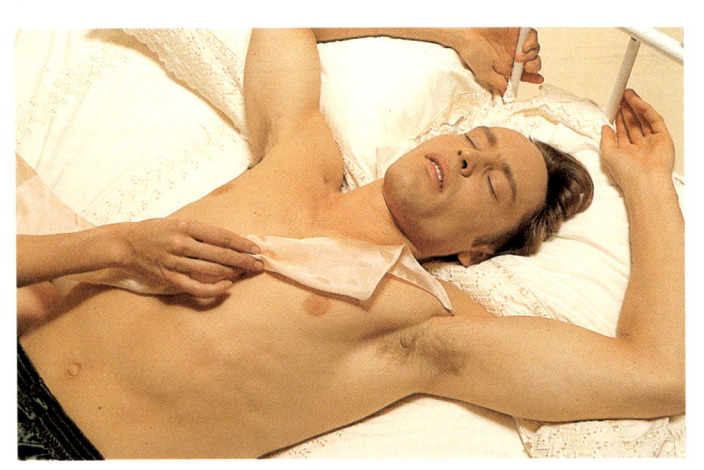

Caress of Silk

▲ *The soft caress of a silky scarf will create a contrasting skin sensation compared to the feel of leather. Its light sensual texture will barely put any pressure on the skin at all. This will heighten the nerve sensation, drawing your partner's feeling senses out to the very surface of his body. Silk can produce a wonderful sense of luxurious caress, particularly when trailed over areas of highly sensitive skin. Velvet or chiffon are also texturally sensual materials.*

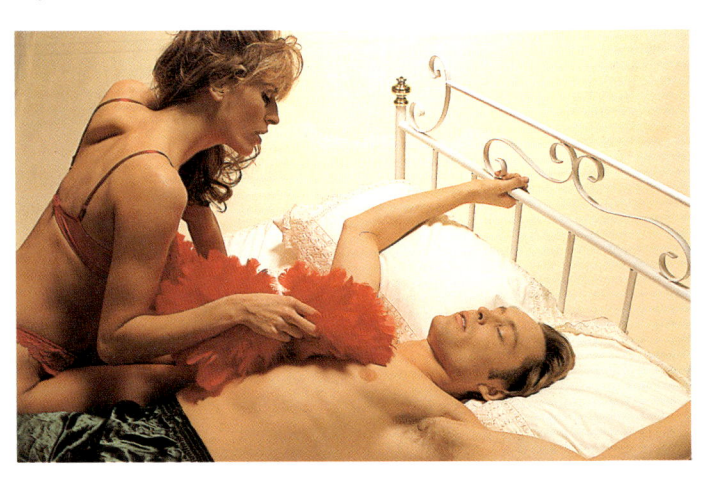

Featherlight Touches

▲ *The ruffling of downy feathers against the skin will tickle and tease it pleasantly. Feathers are even softer than silk, so light they can fly away. For the tantalizing effect of many feathers stroking the skin, loosely bunch up an ostrich feathered boa, and rub it back and forth gently across his chest. Then you can loosen it and trail its length all over his body, asking your partner to turn over at some point, so it can caress the back of his body.*

Getting Turned On

Plumes of Pleasure

▼ *Lots of people fantasize about having their skin teased lovingly by peacock feathers. The rich colours and beautiful designs in the peacock's plumage give them a very exotic appearance. Then the fan-shaped top of the feather and its delicate quill make it a perfect tool for exciting the skin if it is stroked very lightly all over the body. Give your partner a feathery thrill, running the peacock feather over the surface of her skin with almost imperceptible pressure. It will make her whole body tingle and shiver with pleasure.*

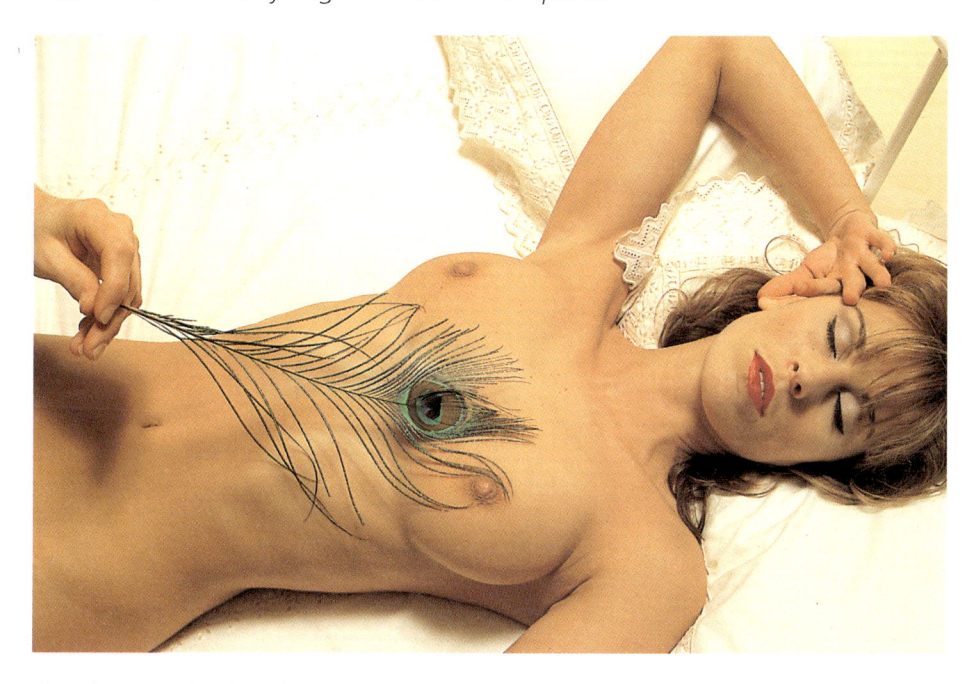

the skin involve brushing its surface, with almost no pressure, so they enliven the skin's most peripheral sensory nerves. All the hair follicles that cover the skin are packed with nerve endings that are stimulated by these erotic caresses. Sometimes your whole body is left tingling and quivering to the point that you are tempted to beg your partner to stop. Yet the pleasure is in being taken right to the height of skin sensation.

There are several ways to enjoy this fantasy game. You might want to try all the different kinds of skin stimulation in one session, so that you experience a whole variety of touches and textures. You can enjoy the caress of any material including leather, silk, satin, chiffon and feathers. Or you might make it a totally feathery event, tantalizing the skin with delicate caresses from a whole variety of exotic plumes. Perhaps you prefer to be excited by the warmth of your partner's touch. Your skin can be stroked all over with the light brush of fingertips, the sensual moistness of the tongue, or the caressing breeze of the breath.

If you are being skin teased, try to relax as much as you can into the intensity of your skin responses. While the touch is exquisitely light, your sensory nerves will be in a state of high excitation. If you tense up it will become too ticklish, but if you surrender to the tantalizing touches, it can become an extremely pleasurable sensation.

Ticklish Delight

▼ *Barely any weight at all, a single boa feather feels like a breeze whispering over the skin – watch the goose bumps come and go! Sweep this lovely, delicate feather over all her erogenous pleasure zones. Run it around her nipples, under her arms, along the side of her neck, and over her belly, groin and thighs. When she turns over, skim the feather over the soles of her feet and on the very sensitive spot at the back of the knees, and then circulate it over her buttocks. See how she squirms with this ticklish delight.*

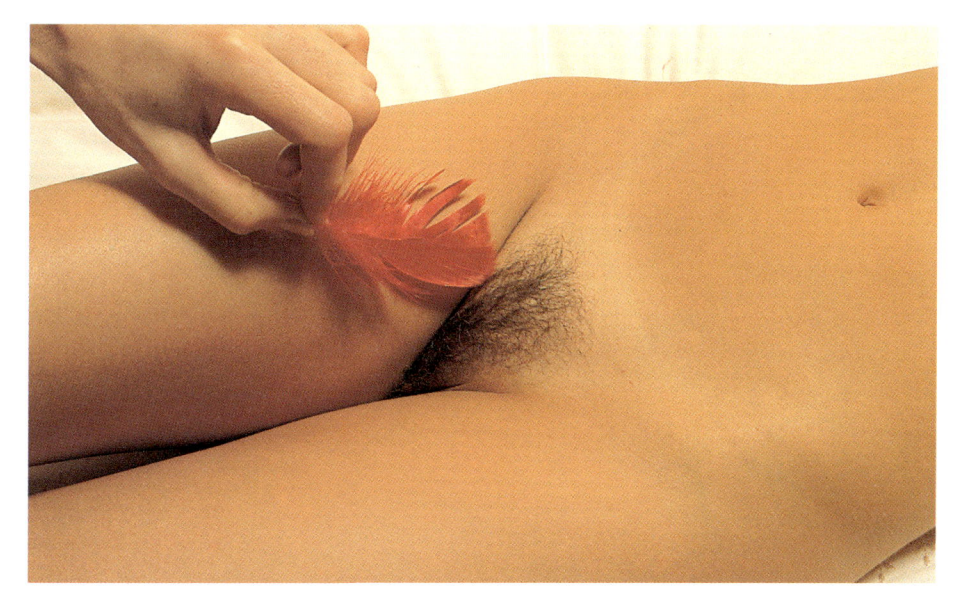

Adventurous Sex Techniques

Tongue Teasing
▼ Bathe the whole body with the warm, moist sensations of your tongue, flicking it and licking lightly over the surface of the skin. This is a very erotic form of skin teasing, inciting his sensual and sexual feelings to fever pitch. Languidly roll your tongue around and around the surface of his lips and the rims of his ears. Then dart it back and forth over his nipples and further down, circle it around his navel. Let your tongue travel down lightly over his genitals, but try not to over-excite him here. Continue running your tongue over the whole of his body, to keep him on the sensory edge.

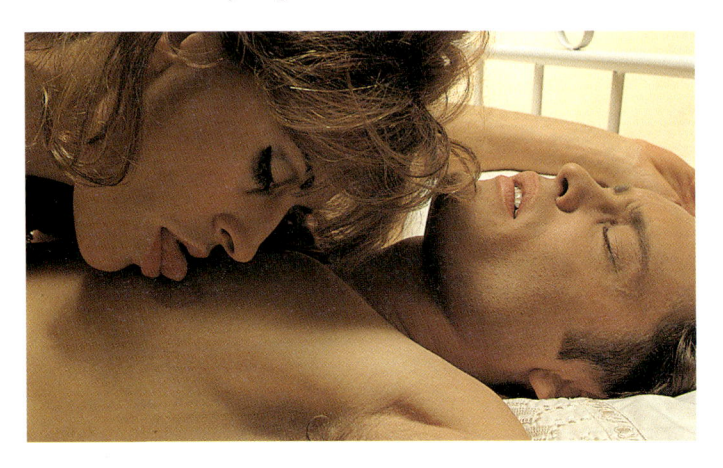

Sensual Breath
▼ When the skin has been moistened by the tongue, blow gently over the wet areas. The warmth of your breath against the damp of the skin is particularly sensual. Brush his whole body with sweeps of your breath, sometimes caressing his skin like a gentle breeze, and sometimes blowing a little stronger in circular motions so it seems as if you are creating a mini-whirlwind on the surface of his body. Breathe on his nipples for a special effect.

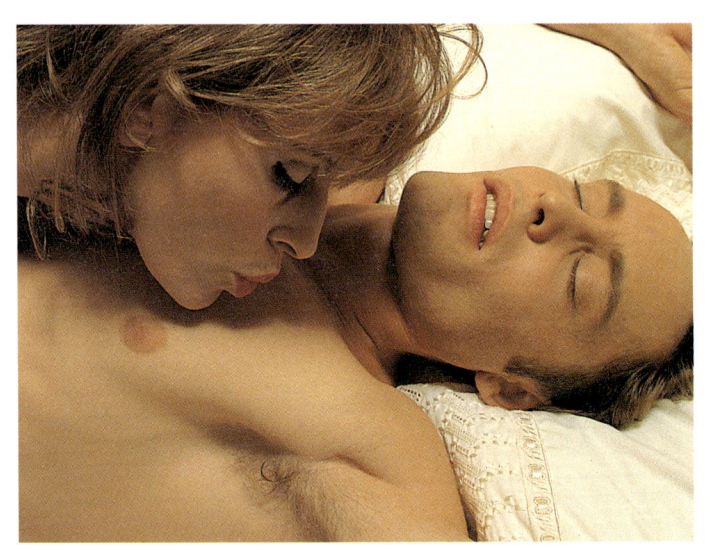

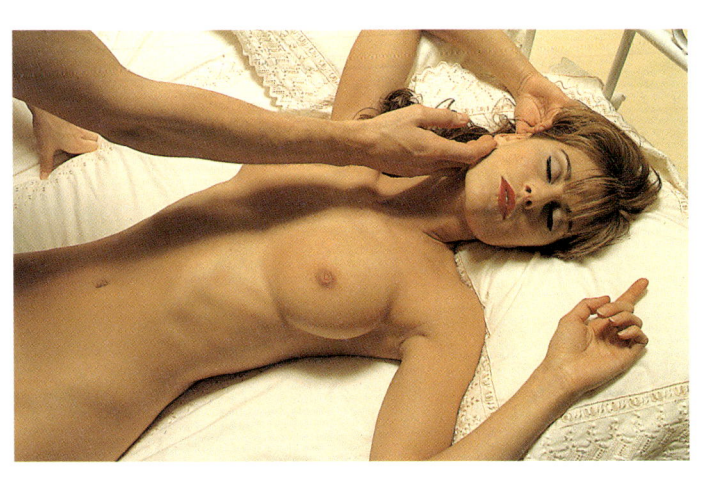

Stroke Play

Patsy, aged 33: "When we were little, my sister and I used to spend hours tickling each other and I loved that very light touch on my skin. I had special places where it felt particularly pleasurable, like my back, my underarms, and most especially my feet.

"In all of my relationships since becoming an adult, I have always wanted a boyfriend to touch and tease me in that way. I just want to lie there, and be lightly stroked all over – the more subtle it is, the more exciting I find it. It is not always sexual, but it is immensely physically pleasurable.

"Now, finally, I have a boyfriend who loves it too, so we spend quite a bit of our physical time just teasing, tickling and stroking each other's skin with all kinds of things. We always take it in turns, so one of us can just give in to enjoying the pleasure of all those lovely skin sensations. To me it feels like luxury and my dream come true. Sometimes I enjoy it as much as making love."

Tracing Her Contours
▲ She can lie back and surrender to the gentle touch of your fingers running softly over her face. There should be no pressure at all in your hands, just a feathery motion that will awaken the most peripheral of her skin's sensory nerves. Let the feeling in your fingers be tender and loving, and move them flowing down over her face, tracing the contours of her features. Run your fingertips delicately over the edge of her eyelashes and over her lips. Try to see how light you can make the touch.

Linger Lovingly
▶ Use the back of your fingers, your fingertips, and even the edge of your nails to heighten her skin senses. Linger sensually over the most sensitive places where the skin is particularly soft and defenceless to tease and excite it. Stroke over her belly and along the sides of her ribcage and then slide your fingers along the inside of her thighs with these teasing and pleasing touches which bring the warmth of your skin to the surface of her body.

Dominance and Bondage

Domination and bondage are common themes in sexual fantasies. Images of being tied up, spanked, or even "forced" (albeit erotically) into having sex are typical fantasies which can run through some people's minds while having intercourse. More often than not, these day-dreams remain in the mind as a private fantasy and are never actually acted out in reality.

A lot of people would never even discuss these fantasies with their partners, either because they feel too shy, or just because they want to keep them in their own private world. However, for many, the fantasy of being the dominant or submissive partner in a sexual scenario, or being restrained while being slowly teased into an orgasm, is an imaginative way to become erotically aroused.

Some couples even like to play out their sexual fantasies together in the bedroom, switching between the dominant and submissive roles from time to time, or settling into a particular routine depending on which excites them most. Bondage, discipline, or dressing up in leather and other fetishist gear may be a big turn-on for some people but abhorrent to others. The major rule of these sex games is that both partners are happy and willing to give them a go. No one should ever pressure his or her partner into this kind of fantasy sex play, nor should anyone submit to it just to please a demanding partner. However, if you both enjoy a little rough play in your sex life, and the idea of taking your eroticism right to the edge excites you, then there is no reason at all why you should not add these saucy alternatives to your sexual repertoire.

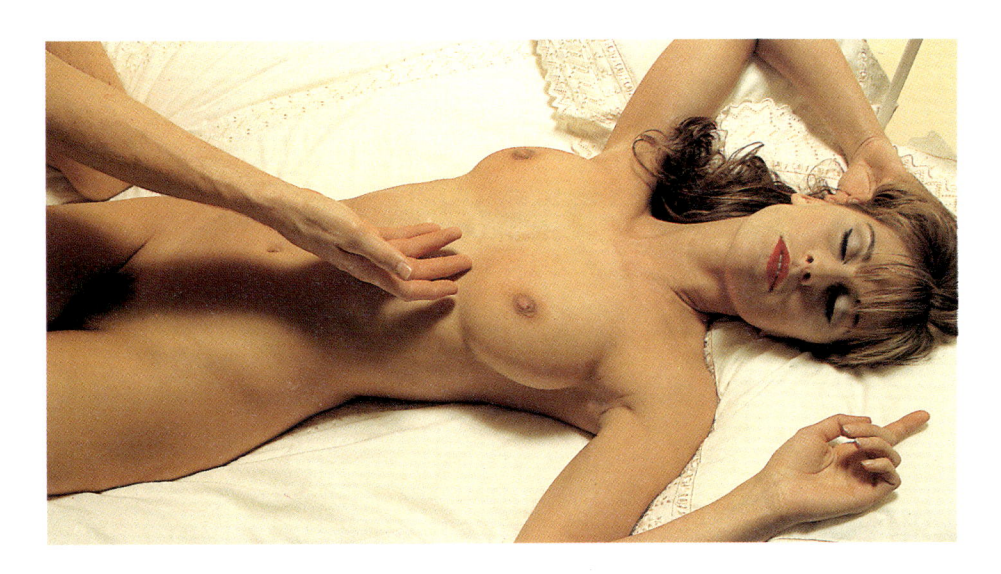

Rules of the Game

Some people fear that their tough love sex play could mean that they are bordering on sado-masochism. There is no need to worry unless you are actually hurting your partner or you feel you are receiving real pain and abuse. What we are discussing here is pretending to use domination and force and playing with these concepts because you find them sexually arousing and enriching to your sex life. So where do you draw the line?

First of all, these fantasy games must always be by mutual consent. Then make some rules and stick by them. Only act out domination and submission games when you are in a relationship you trust, and you know your partner well enough to be sure he or she would never hurt you, or ever force you into something you do not want to do. If spanking the buttocks is part of your play, then only take it so far as you find it fun and exciting.

Don't cause real pain, cause bruises or break the skin. You can pretend you are humiliating your partner, but you should know the boundaries between play and offence. Don't say things you may regret later or which will emotionally scar your partner. Talk over exactly what kind of fantasy behaviour turns you on, what your limits are, and what you do and do not want to happen, and then stick within these guidelines.

Make sure you have a signal or code word which you both recognize as the sign to stop the game immediately. The moment one or the other of you says this word or gives the sign, you must stop!

If being tied to the bed post while your partner makes slow, tantalizing love to you, or gives you orgasmic

Adventurous Sex Techniques

oral sex (research shows that restraint is probably the most popular fantasy) interests you and you plan to act it out, then make sure he or she does not tie the knots too tight, and that they can be undone immediately if you request it, or whenever necessary.

You can restrain the wrists and ankles, but you must never tie anything around the neck, and covering the mouth can also be dangerous. If your partner is restrained, do not leave him or her alone – even for a short time. You need to be conscious and present during the whole time your partner is tied up.

Some people may fantasize about restraint, and even desire to act it out, but are simply too afraid to be tied up. Respect that anxiety and just pretend he or she is tied up. One way is for that person to grip the headboard so the arms are spread-eagled, and the legs are splayed out wide in the posture of restraint.

Master and Slave

▼ *Some men can be very aroused by playing a submissive role in a sex game, especially as a release of tension if they otherwise hold powerful positions. Some couples enjoy a "master and slave" game, where the woman plays a dominating role and disciplines her partner. If you are acting this out as the dominator, dress up to look sexy but stern and severe. Thigh-length black leather boots will put you in the mood for the part. Assert your dominance over your partner, threatening to discipline him if he does not follow your every wish and whim.*

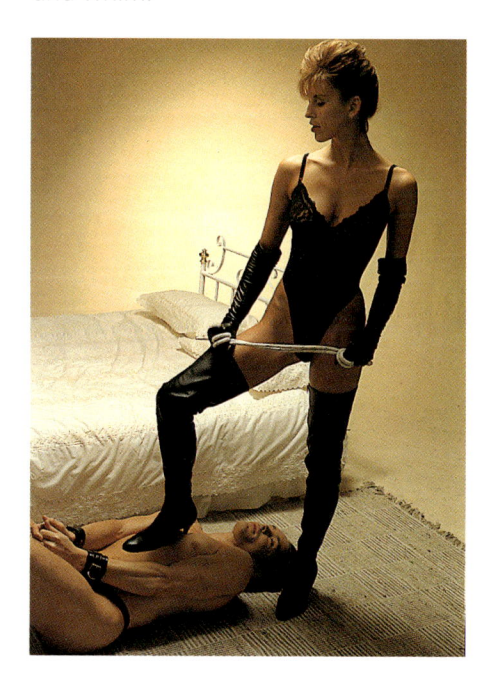

Getting the Gear

Fetishist tools may be in order for these games, and you can get these from a good sex shop. Black outfits

---

Playing Power Games

Jonathan, aged 33, a salesman has lived with his girlfriend, Anja, for five years. "It was Anja who first suggested that we should introduce some domination and submission games into our sex life. She said that in her last relationship, her boyfriend would sometimes tie her arms and legs to the bed posts, and then make love to her, and that she found it to be incredibly sexually arousing. I was more than happy to give it a go because I had always wanted to do something like this myself, but my last girlfriend would have never agreed to it. Now, once in a while, we take it in turns to be tied up. Sometimes I do it to her, and she just goes wild, especially if I am giving her oral sex. She says that this kind of sex game gives her the most intense orgasms. It's the same for me, because there is something incredibly erotic about having to absolutely surrender and be helpless while she is making love to me. She does everything very slowly, and takes me almost to the point of an orgasm, then cools it down, and then starts again. In the end, I feel like I am going to explode – and I usually do."

Clara, aged 27, a landscape designer, has shared a home with her fiancé for two years. "Jack and I enjoy all kinds of sex games, and we are pretty hot on the ones with domination themes. He is the dominator, and I get turned on by the submissive role. We do all kinds of things, and I am sure people who know us would be quite shocked about what we get up to on some weekends because we look so normal. I trust him completely because I know he loves me and he would never do anything that would actually hurt me. I have my code word, and if I say it, he always stops. We also make love in all the more normal ways too because we don't want this to be our only sexual theme. The interesting thing is that it is only in our sexual relationship that Jack's domination fantasy comes out. In every other aspect of our relationship, we are absolutely on equal terms."

Kirsty, aged 26, a teacher, has been married for two years. "This kind of sex play is definitely not for me. I don't even have fantasies about it, though I know that some of my girlfriends do. I can't relate to it at all. For me, making love is all about just that – it's a way of expressing all our loving and tender feelings for each other. I just want to be me in bed and there's no room for fantasy. I think it would make us feel as if we were having sex with a stranger."

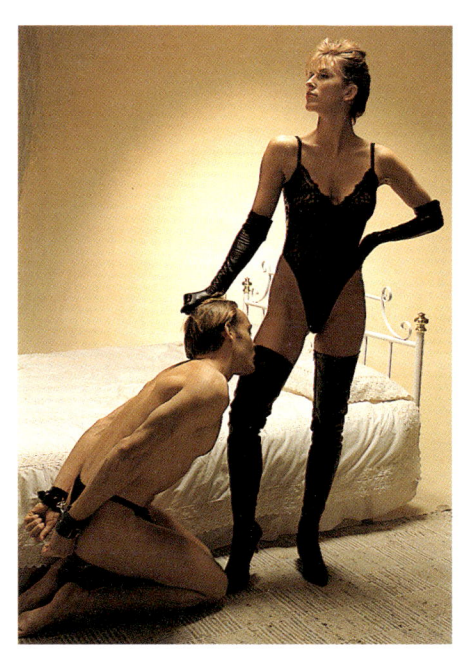

Demand His Obedience
◀ Stay haughty and proud as he grovels at your feet. Let him adore you from his lowly position. He must touch, kiss or caress you in any way you command, but you must appear to be above feeling excited by his attentions. Complain and make him do more. The fun is in acting as if you have total control and can demand complete obedience from him.

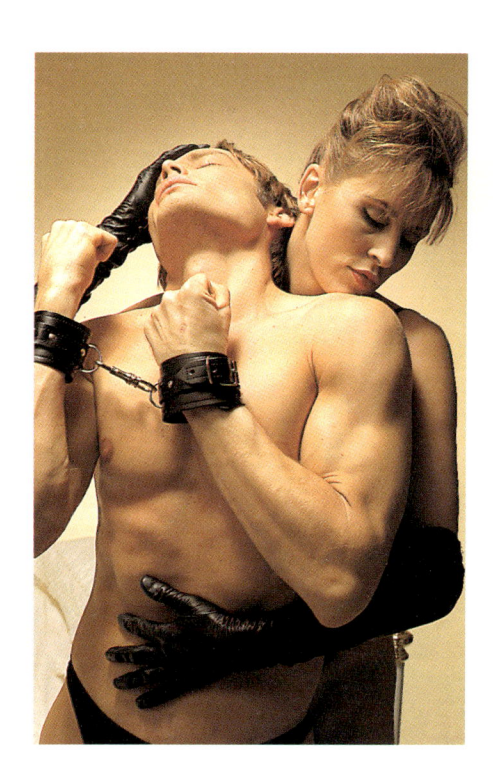

Assert Your Sexuality
▶ If you think he has been "bad" or is showing too much will of his own, you can rough him around a little. Or you can display your assertive sexuality, pulling him to your body and holding his body tight to yours. You can even make love to him, but you must stay in charge.

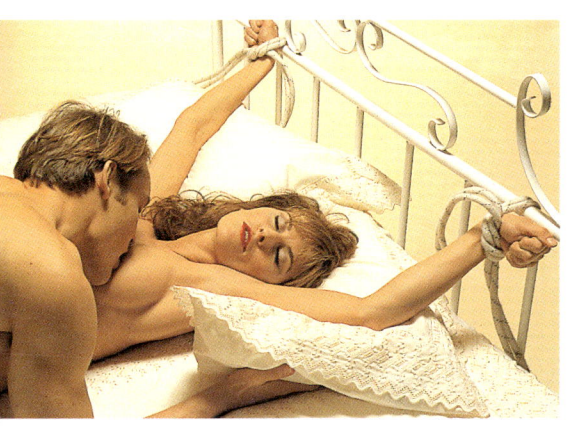

are a popular choice for bondage and domination games. Boots, corsets, armbands, and elbow-length gloves in leather, latex or rubber are the normal gear that turn people on. Men are more visually stimulated than their partners by these outfits, but women can enjoy dressing up to arouse their men. (Some women might find the whole idea chauvinistic and absurd!)

Soft ropes, silk scarves or strips of cotton material can all be used for restraint, but make sure that nothing you use will burn or chafe the skin. If you want to use more serious-looking equipment, there are sexy handcuffs available which both of you can undo, if necessary. Don't use real handcuffs which are too threatening and may be difficult to release.

Helpless to Resist
▲ Restraint, or being softly tied to the bed post, and having your lover slowly, tantalizingly and deliberately turn you on while you pretend to be helpless can be extremely arousing. The added thrill is the restriction on movement which can take your excitement right to its peak. He should pay attention to every part of your body. If he licks and kisses your breasts and nipples while you are tied like this, you may feel as if you are going to explode with erotic sensation. He should deliberately do everything slowly, taking his time to keep you dangling at this almost excruciating pitch of excitement.

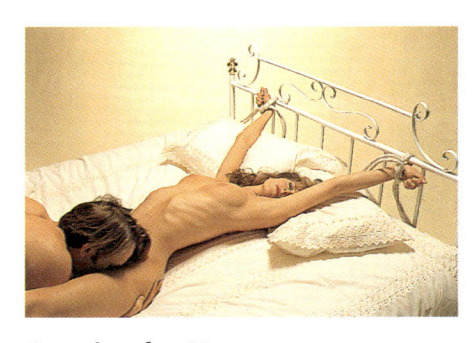

Begging for More
▲ Slow, erotic oral sex while being restrained can be an amazing sexual experience. Again, he should take his time, doing everything in a teasing and super-sensual way. If he is sensitive to your responses, he will know just when to slow down to delay your moment of orgasm, so that you beg him to go ahead.

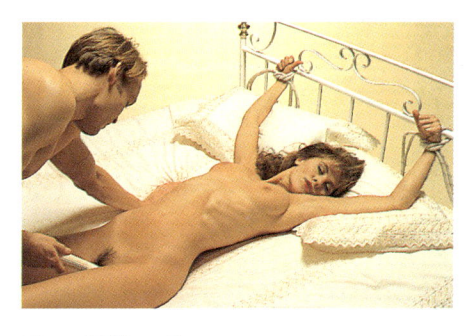

Good Vibrations
▲ Another variation to add to your fantasy play, is for him to use a vibrator to bring you to orgasm. After kissing and stroking every part of your body, and waiting till you have reached a peak of arousal, he can use a sex toy and vibrate it against your vulva. At the same time, you can let the fantasies in your mind run riot.

Spontaneous Sex

Spontaneous sex refers to the proverbial "quickie". It is the stuff of best-selling airport novels, full of erotic heaving, panting and writhing bodies, bodice-ripping sex scenes and exotic or, at least, unusual locations. It is not slow and sensual, or particularly intimate, but it is hot and passionate and deliciously primitive. When spontaneous sex happens it is the meeting of the "wild" man and the "wild" woman – there are no formalities to play out and clothes are cast aside along with inhibitions.

Does spontaneous sex have any place in a loving and intimate sexual relationship? Yes, it certainly does, if the two people concerned are equally eager for the action. It is sexual appetite at its most voracious, a hunger immediately satisfied by two consenting partners.

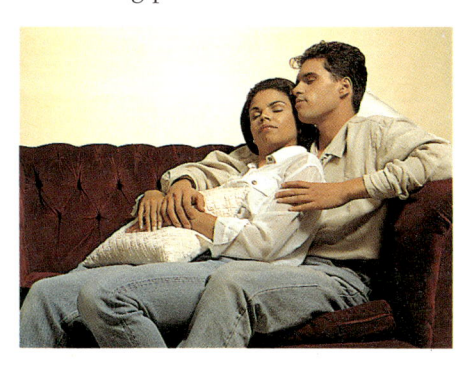

Spontaneous sex can be extremely exciting and exhilarating, affirming a mutual physical attraction and enlivening any sexual relationship with its raw and untamed content. It can happen anywhere, and when least expected, because by its nature it does not run to a schedule.

The one thing you must guarantee, though, is complete privacy, with absolutely no one else in sight, because neither the law, nor your family, nor your neighbours will applaud you if you are caught in the act.

Spontaneous sex rarely happens in the bedroom, it is much more likely to occur in the kitchen, the living room, the bathroom, or on the stairs. It may be even more licentious – forbidden moments in the office basement, on a bed of

Change of Mood
▲ *Sexual arousal can happen when you least expect it. You may be planning simply to relax with your partner after a tiring day at work and watch a little television before going to bed to sleep. The two of you snuggle up for a cosy but quiet evening, then suddenly the mood changes, and your bodies become electrified just from their closeness to each other.*

Desire Takes Over
▶ *A sense of urgency rises. You don't even feel you have time to go to the bedroom. Most of your clothes are hastily removed, either by yourself or your partner. Now you can make better use of that comfortable old settee. As the woman, you can climb astride your partner's lap and mount him immediately.*

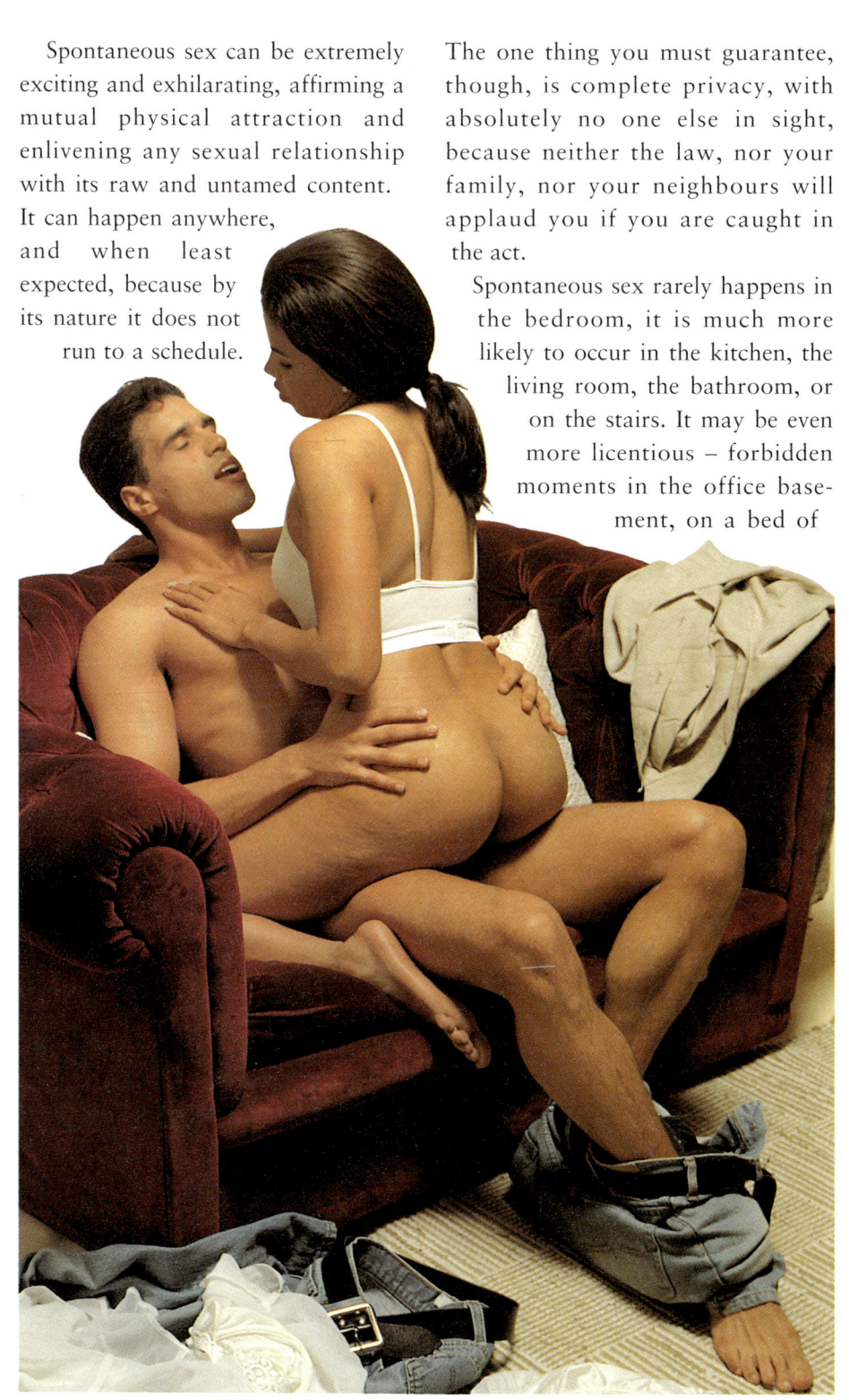

Spontaneous Sex

Sexual Heat is On
◀ Both of you can let go into a passionate session of lovemaking, using the settee to its best advantage. The back of the chair is a good place to sit if your partner wants to perform cunnilingus on you. The heat of the moment will increase the arousal and excitement for both of you and you can let go into waves of pleasure.

Primal Passion
▼ Making love in the doggie position, with the male partner entering the vagina from behind, will add to the primal intensity of your spontaneous sexual happening. You can lean your weight onto the back of the settee, and while he is thrusting, he can also stimulate your clitoris with his fingers.

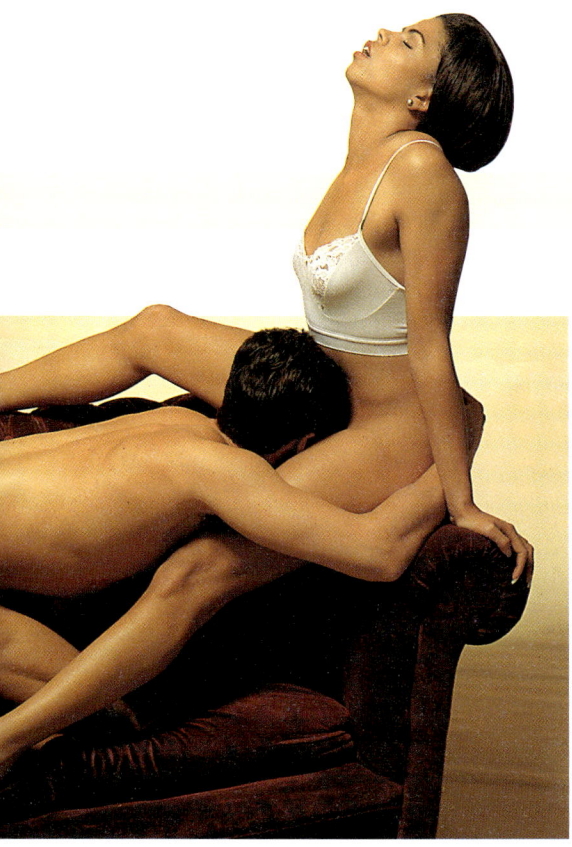

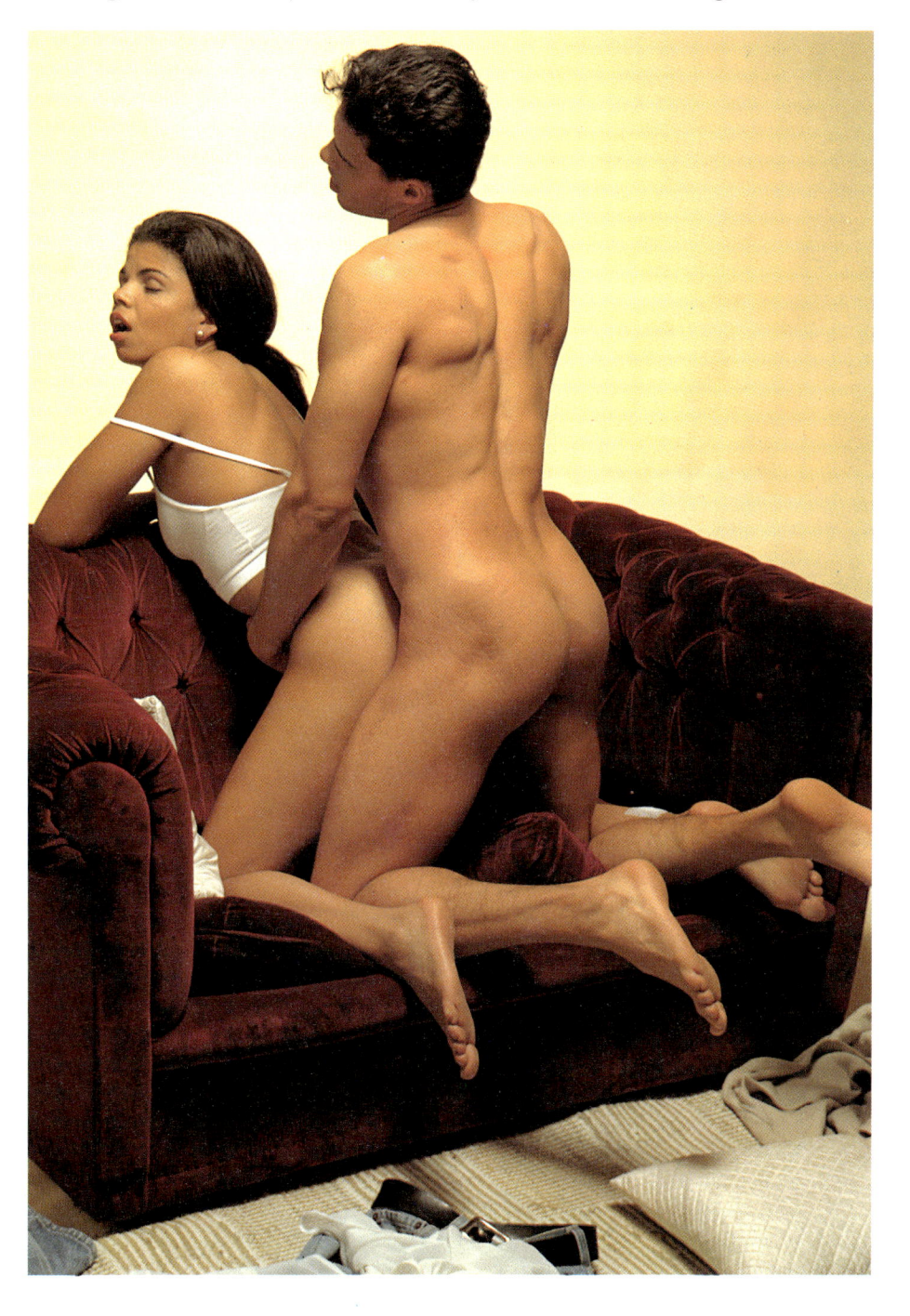

soft grass, against an inviting tree, or on a windswept beach at night.

The wonderful thing about this kind of sex is that it can recapture the excitement and spontaneity of your early days of romance, when your sex hormones were rampant and the two of you could hardly wait a second longer to make love. A "quickie" is the pep pill which can put the zest back into your sexual relationship.

Standing Up
Standing up is a classic but awkward position for the "quickie" way of having intercourse. It usually implies fast and furious sex, with no preliminaries, but it is hot and impetuous and therefore probably very exciting. If you do it standing up, it is best to have something to lean on, such as a wall or a tree, and it definitely works better if the partners are a similar height and weight. The main problem is that the penis can easily slip out of the vagina, and the vertical position makes it difficult for deep thrusting. However, the impulsiveness of the situation usually indicates that the man is so aroused he is likely to ejaculate very quickly.

Adventurous Sex Techniques

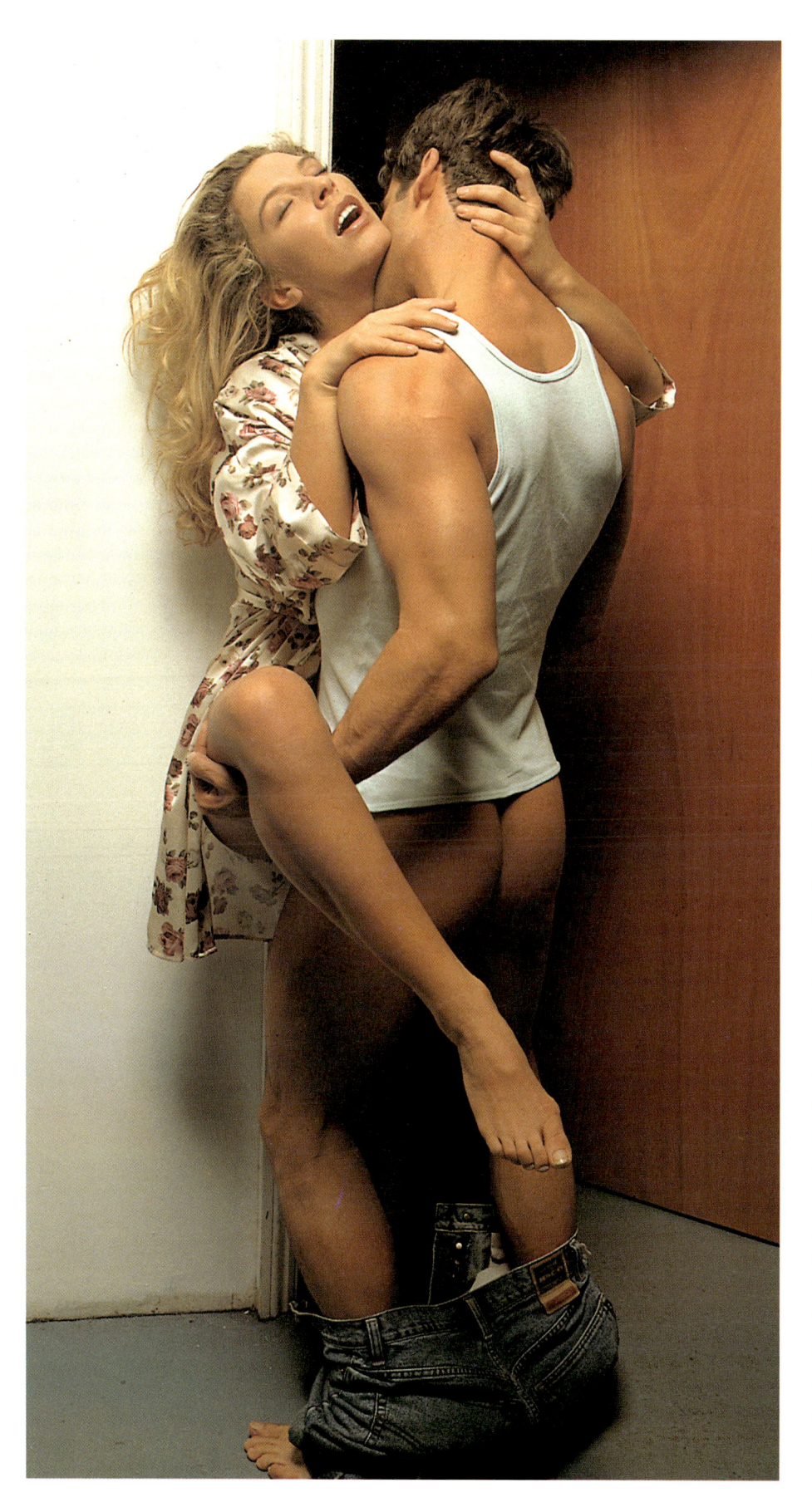

Standing Sex
◀ You can't wait to make it to the bedroom so, pressed against the wall, you make love to each other in the standing position. Your partner will be able to penetrate you deeper if he elevates you slightly, and you curl one leg around him. He must take care not to push you too hard against the wall while he is thrusting.

This is not an uncommon position for young lovers to take when first exploring their sexuality, perhaps because they cannot take their partner home and so have to resort to more furtive methods of sexual contact. It may also be a natural follow-on from a heavy-petting session. However, in these situations, penetration does not necessarily take place, but the female may close her thighs around the penis, allowing it to rub against her genitals. In this way, both people can gain a quick release from their sexual excitement and tension.

Passion and Lust
Passion is the spice of life – it's sexuality in Technicolor. It fascinates and frightens us a bit, because under its spell we temporarily lose our minds, while our emotions and bodies take over. Lust is a sign of a healthy libido racing along in top gear, and life would be pretty boring if we never encountered it at all.

The main thing about sexual passion is the intensity and the speed with which it can come and go. While in the throes of a passionate love affair, all other areas of life pale by comparison. What else would drive politicians, amongst others, to risk their careers, marriages and reputations which they have spent years meticulously building up?

Spontaneous Sex

Passion is the source of inspiration for a thousand songs and poems – the story line for most of the successful movies. It seems as if we need to have passion in our lives, even if we are not the ones actually experiencing it.

Passion and lust inevitably burn themselves out, but in a stable relationship they can leave in their place the warm glow of intimacy and companionship. Sexual love can grow instead, and a physical relationship can become more harmonious and compatible, integrating itself within the context of everything else that is meaningful in life.

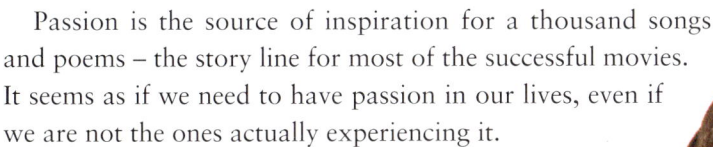

Yet even within the most contented relationships there is often a secret yearning for the flame of passion to be lit again. We miss the excitement, and the thrill of the unpredictable and uncontrollable experience

Business Suitors
▶ *Full spontaneous sex may be out of the question, especially if you are in a business situation, but if you and your partner meet up somewhere at work, you may not be able to resist a surreptitious petting session behind closed doors. There is something especially exciting about this kind of erotic encounter because it will be in strict contrast to your professional persona.*

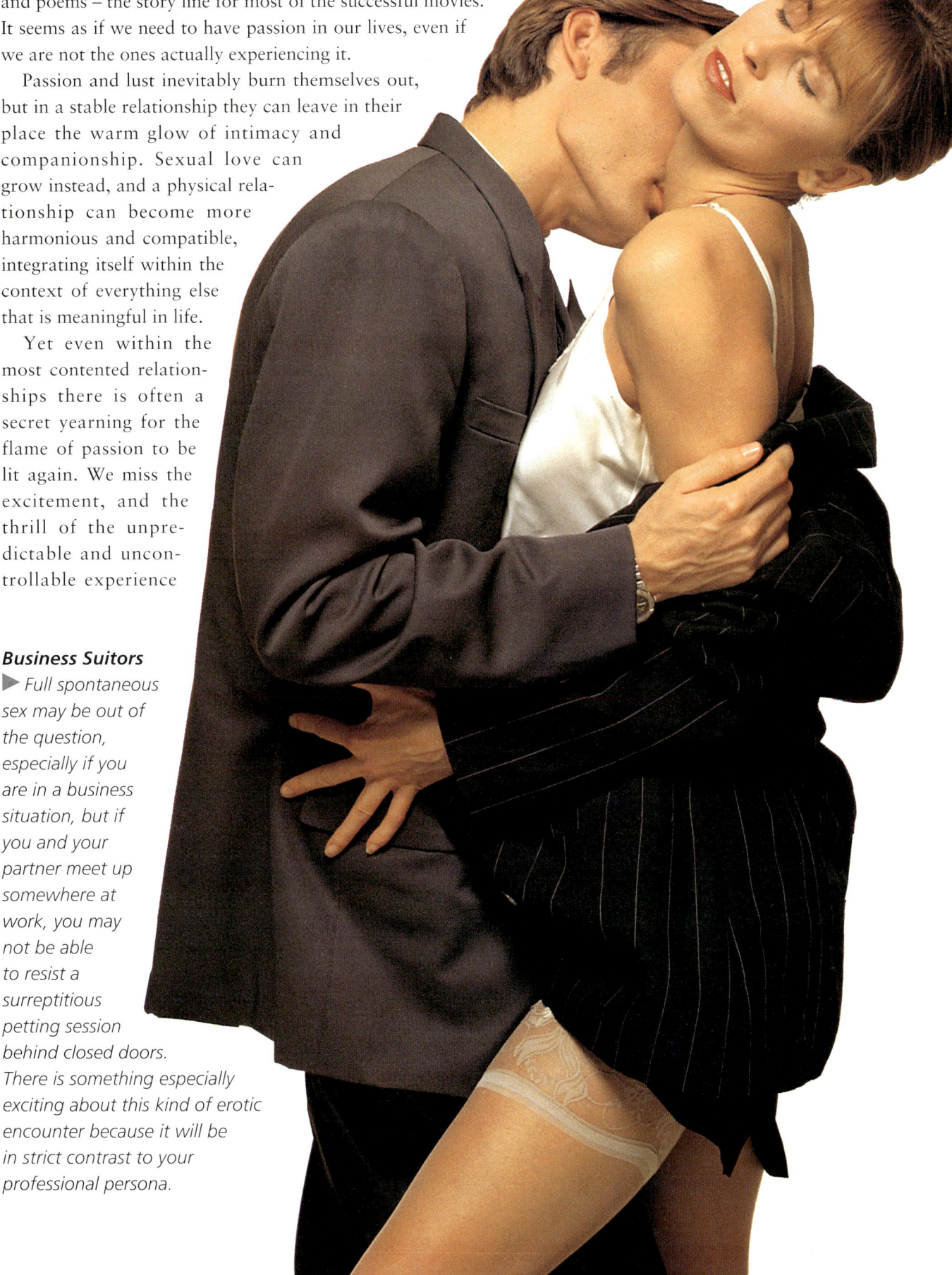

Adventurous Sex Techniques

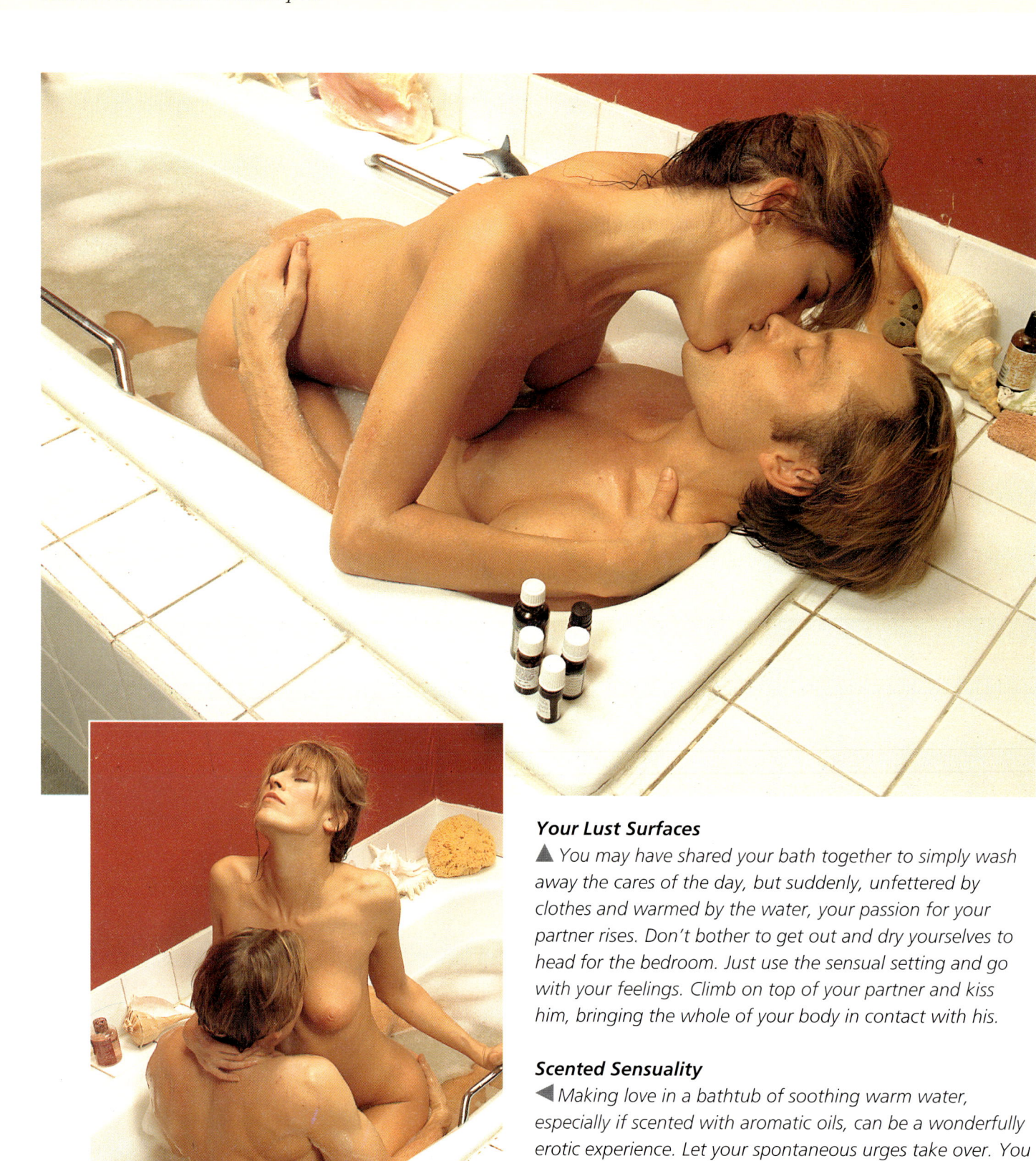

Your Lust Surfaces
▲ You may have shared your bath together to simply wash away the cares of the day, but suddenly, unfettered by clothes and warmed by the water, your passion for your partner rises. Don't bother to get out and dry yourselves to head for the bedroom. Just use the sensual setting and go with your feelings. Climb on top of your partner and kiss him, bringing the whole of your body in contact with his.

Scented Sensuality
◀ Making love in a bathtub of soothing warm water, especially if scented with aromatic oils, can be a wonderfully erotic experience. Let your spontaneous urges take over. You will need to straddle across his lap, but you can use the bath rail for levering your body up and down while he kisses and caresses you all over.

Spontaneous Sex

of overwhelming physical and emotional sensation. Most of us would become exhausted if we lived in a state of passion all the time. However, it is a lucky relationship which can retain its elements, for if a couple can relive those moments of passion and lust and magical chemistry which drew them together in the first place, the mantle of complacency and boredom which can descend on any relationship would have difficulty taking hold.

So spontaneous, wild and lustful sex has a therapeutic place within a relationship. When the mood takes you, you can be creative with it. Let go into it, and allow your erotic fantasies to come true immediately. Don't worry about the time of the day, or what part of the house you are in – let your mutual passion surface unbridled, and use whatever props you have around you, such as the chairs, stairs or bathtub to their best advantage.

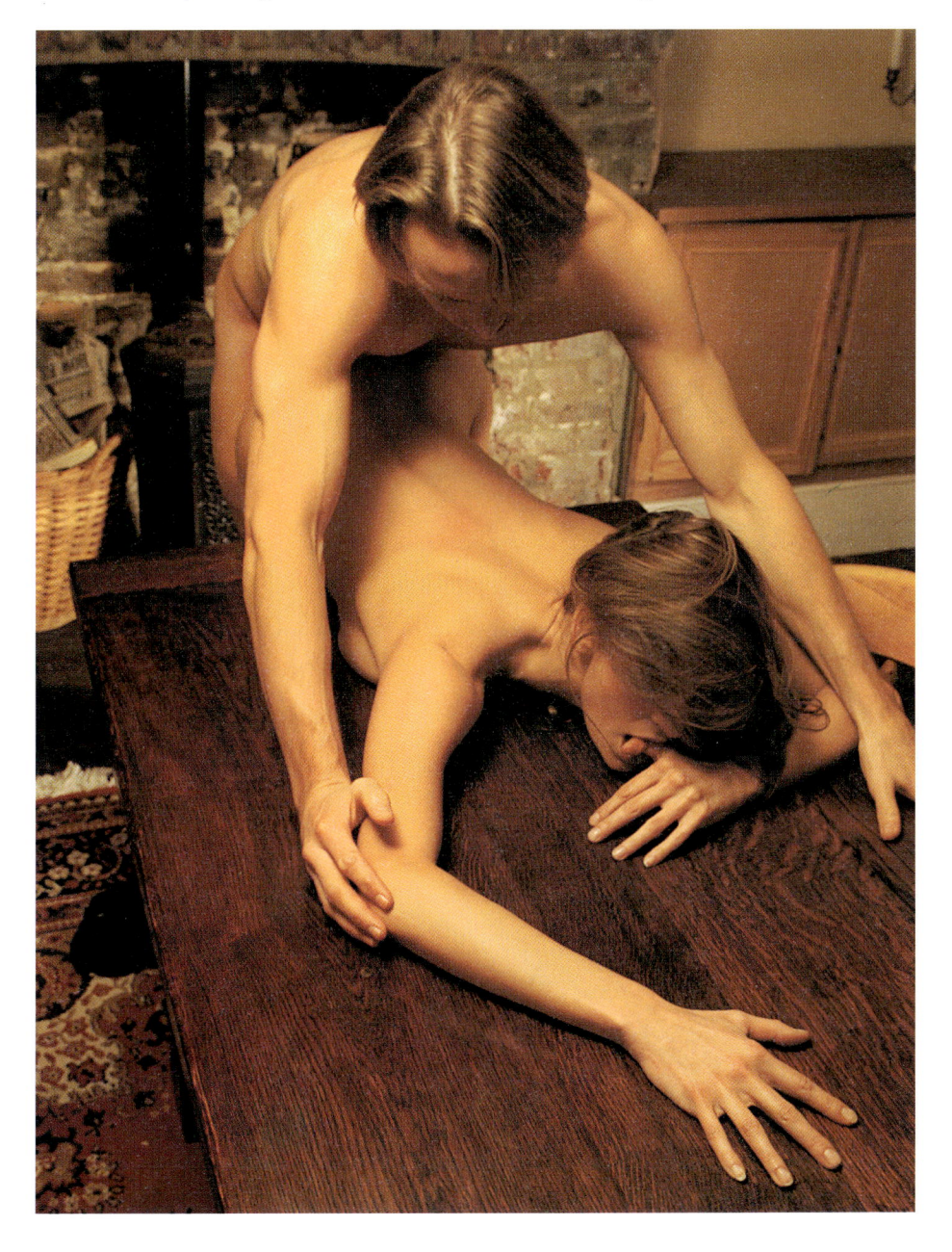

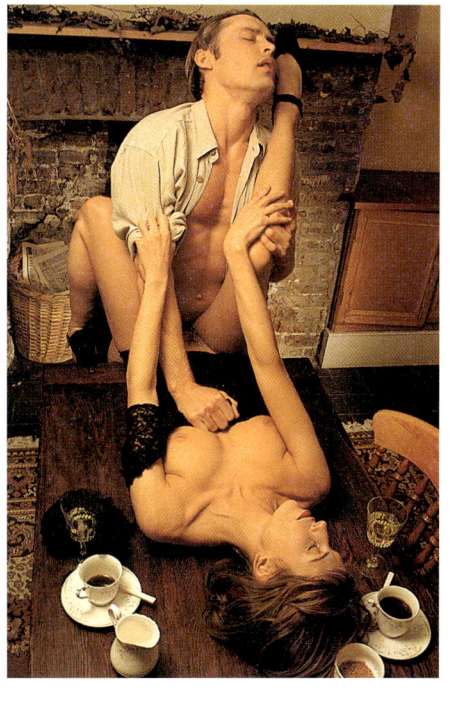

Arousal on the Boil
▲ You can even go for the bodice-ripping "take me-I'm yours" scenario if the urge takes over. Neither of you should hold back; let lust command you. The kitchen table will do, even if you don't have time to clear it. Don't even wait to take your clothes off. You might not be able to wear that dress again, but you can hang it in the wardrobe as a glorious memento!

Torrid Table-top Sex
◀ This could be an extremely lustful episode of spontaneous lovemaking. You have torn off each other's clothes and she is laying face down across the table. You can enter her from the rear position, and make love to her passionately, but take care not to press her too hard against the surface of the table.

Overcoming Difficulties

Lack of sexual interest shown by one or both partners is the most common form of sexual problem occurring within a relationship. There may be a number of factors that block the sexual response. Sometimes stress at work or in the home can cause fatigue or anxiety and consequently a diminished libido. If there is anger or other negative feelings between the partners, and a lack of clear communication skills, then the sexual relationship is ultimately bound to suffer.

Sadly, in many relationships, once the first flush of passion and excitement has subsided, lovemaking can become perfunctory, focused mainly on penetration and thrusting, and regarded more as a relief from sexual tension than a sensual, nurturing and fulfilling encounter. In these circumstances, either partner may withdraw from the sexual arena, and this can lead to a buildup of frustration within the relationship.

Sensate focus exercises are the backbone of psychosexual therapy, enabling couples to overcome their sexual difficulties and regain, or even discover, a more sensual and intimate side of their physical relationship. They work by helping the couple to change their focus away from penetrative sex, performance and sexual obligation. While a couple are working through these exercises, they make a commitment to ban all intercourse until the very last stage.

The point of sensate focus is to help people break old habits and patterns of sexual behaviour which have proved unsatisfying. The pressure is taken away from the need to initiate or respond to sexual overtures, giving the couple an opportunity to relax with each other's bodies and to recreate their sexual relationship in an entirely new way.

Sensate focus exercises, originally devised by sex researchers, William Masters and Virginia Johnson, are based on encouraging couples to discover the joy and pleasure of sensual touching for its own sake, and not for an end result. This is a very important factor which may be missing from a sexual partnership. Sex is often directed towards penetration and thrusting and can become a way of using another person's body for self-gratification.

In their haste to reach a climax, many individuals may not actually experience their own sensual pleasure and may completely miss their partner's sensual responses. If the sexual relationship falls into this mode over a long period of time, it is hardly surprising if one or other partner becomes disillusioned or resentful and eventually withdraws from physical contact.

The human body has an enormous capacity for sensual joy and pleasure, especially that experienced through the medium of touch, but this fundamental sense is often suppressed within us from an early stage of life. Young children are frequently told "not to touch" either their own bodies or the objects around them, thus inhibiting the development of their sensory perceptions. Touch, in western cultures, is generally associated with sexuality once we have reached adolescence. We forget how to communicate and feel through touch, how to enjoy its nurturing qualities and, by doing so, cut ourselves off from a vast dimension of tactile sensory awareness.

If you and your partner are experiencing serious or long-term problems within your relationship, or your communication has begun to break down so that conflict ensues whenever sexual or emotional issues are discussed, you would probably benefit from seeking professional help from a qualified psychosexual therapist. The therapist will be trained to deal with a whole range of sexual disorders or dysfunctions, including premature ejaculation, loss of desire, erectile dysfunction, inability to achieve orgasm, fear of penetration, or intercourse avoidance.

He or she will also help you to improve your communication skills,

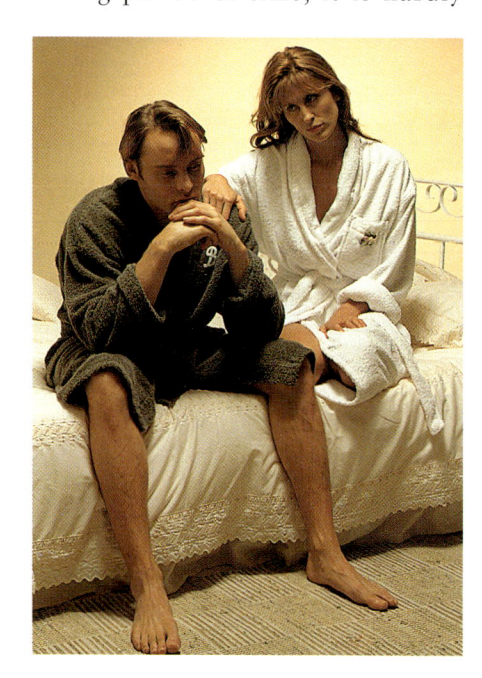

The Effect of Stress
▲ *Sometimes a man can go through a temporary period of impotence due to factors such as stress or anxiety, but with the understanding and loving support of his partner, he should eventually recover his enthusiasm and ability to achieve an erection.*

Overcoming Difficulties

so that you are able to relate to each other and negotiate solutions on difficult issues. It is very difficult for any couple who are experiencing relationship or sexual difficulties, to gain a clear perspective of the situation for themselves, simply because they are too emotionally involved in the issues. A psychotherapist or sex counsellor will act as a mediator, providing practical advice, and helping you reach your own understanding of the problems.

When a couple work through the sensate focus exercises with a therapist, the professional will be able to help them resolve physical and emotional conflicts which may arise between them at any stage of the process. What follows here is a programme of sensate focus exercises, adapted from the therapeutic model, but designed for couples to work with by themselves. They are based on Masters and Johnson's sensate focus self-help programme. You can use them to enhance your relationship, especially if you feel you are able to work on your sexual problems with your partner without professional intervention.

The success of these exercises depends upon a genuine commitment that you and your partner will make to follow the rules of each stage of the process, and your mutual dedication in setting aside a regular time to carry them out.

Choose a specific time during the week when you can both give your full attention to the exercises and decide which partner should initiate the session. Try to choose a time when you both feel generally relaxed and agreeable towards each other. Allocate 40 to 60 minutes per session, and ensure that you have complete privacy, picking a time when there will be no interruptions from the children, or visitors, and remembering to take the phone off the hook.

You need a warm room as you will both be naked, and a comfortable mattress or base to lie on. If possible, choose a room in the house other than a bedroom – somewhere where you are not reminded of the charged issues of your sexual relationship. You are trying to create something new between you, moving away from past patterns, expectations and memories.

Stage One: Non-Sexual Touch

During the first weeks of your sensate focus exercises, you must refrain from sexual intercourse. This is the period when you will, instead, explore your sensual receptivity to one another's bodies, and develop your tactile communication. You will take turns to touch each other, as if you are discovering and exploring the human body for the first time. The person who is touching must remember that he or she is not aiming to arouse the partner, but is simply dedicated to developing his or her own sensory awareness.

You can touch anywhere on your partner's body except the genitals or other erogenous areas, such as the woman's breasts. You should allow yourself to feel through your hands and fingers all the different sensations of touch, texture and temperature of the skin. Vary how you apply your tactile contact, using your palms, fingertips, or even the backs of your hands.

You should experiment using one hand at a time, or stroking with both hands, and keep taking note of the

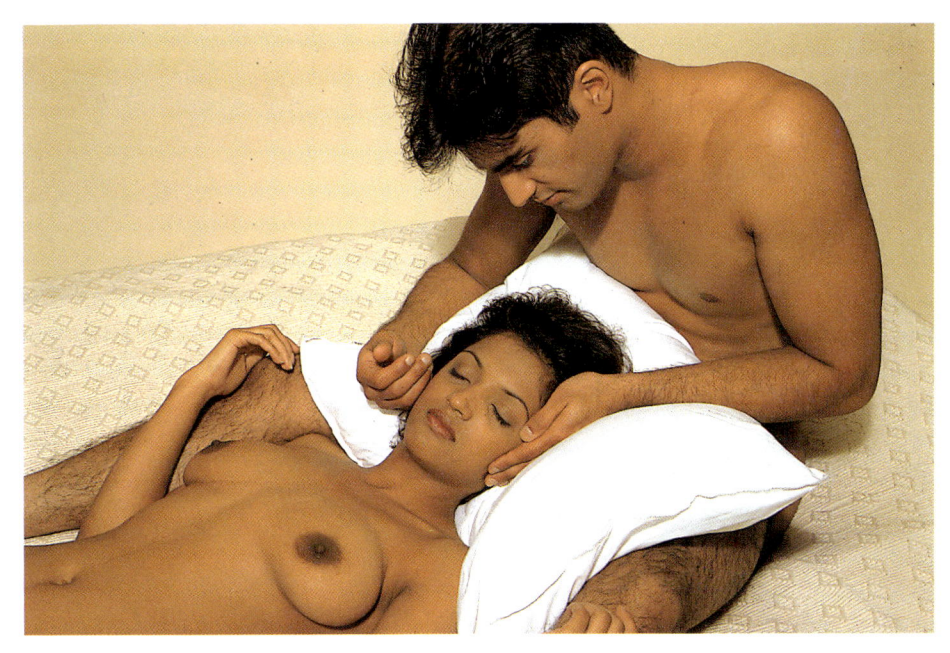

Explore Her Face

▲ *Carefully, you should explore the angles and contours of her face, feeling the difference between the firmness of the bones and the softness of the skin and muscles. The whole point of this touching experiment is for you to increase your sensory awareness and your sensitivity of touch.*

Overcoming Difficulties

different sensations as they occur. The passive partner has only to lie there and focus on the sensation of being touched.

Do not try to reciprocate touch, or go into any sexual fantasy. Both of you should try to avoid analysing the situation or making judgements, such as "this feels good" or "am I doing it right". All you have to do is focus your whole attention on the physical sensations you are experiencing, whether it is through touching or being touched.

Agree beforehand that if the passive partner is uncomfortable about the type of touch he or she is receiving, they can say so and the session can stop, to be resumed at another time. Each partner should spend up to 15 or 20 minutes giving and receiving touch before swapping roles. Do not go on for so long that you become bored or tired. When the exercise is over, you can share with each other what each of you has experienced.

Stage Two: Adding Lotion

You can continue to touch in the same way as before, but now, if you want, you can add oil or lotion. This is still a touching exercise, not a massage. The aim is to experience

Vary the Contact
▶ Take it in turns to become the first active partner in each session. Touch and explore every nuance of his body as before, only this time use a lotion or other lubricant for a different quality of contact. Let your hands touch his skin with varying degrees of pressure, and mould over the rounded curves of the body, such as the buttocks, hips and waist.

Experiment with Touch
▼ Take the time to touch and feel your partner's body in a way you have never done before. You are not trying to please him or turn him on; this experiment is purely for your own sensation. Run your fingers around his nipple, and along the soft skin at the side of the ribcage, feeling the difference between bone and skin. Explore his body with your touch, feeling each and every part, except for the genital area. Move his joints, wiggling his fingers and toes. Notice the skin's temperature changes and its rougher and smoother parts.

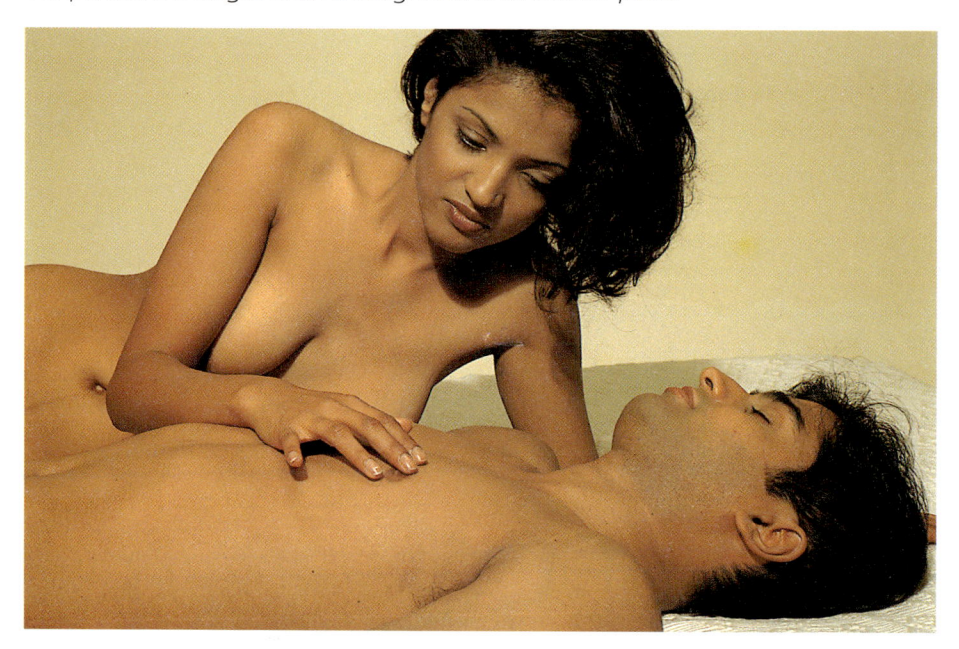

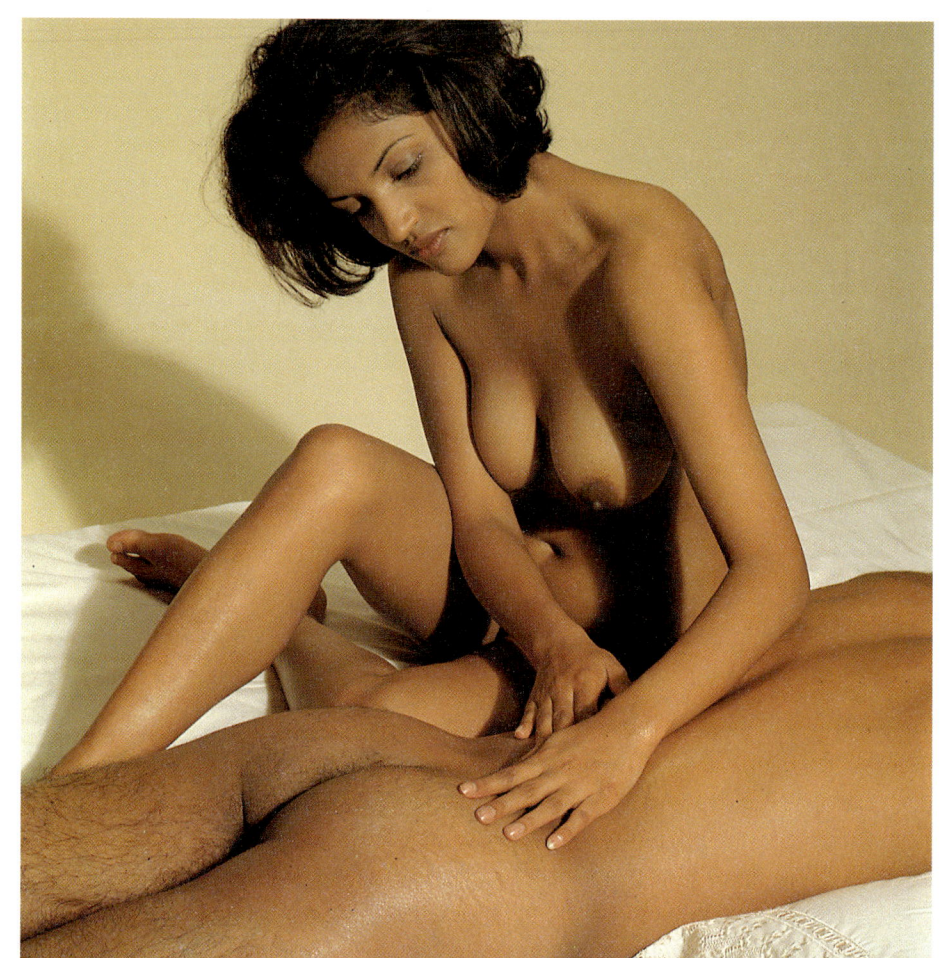

Overcoming Difficulties

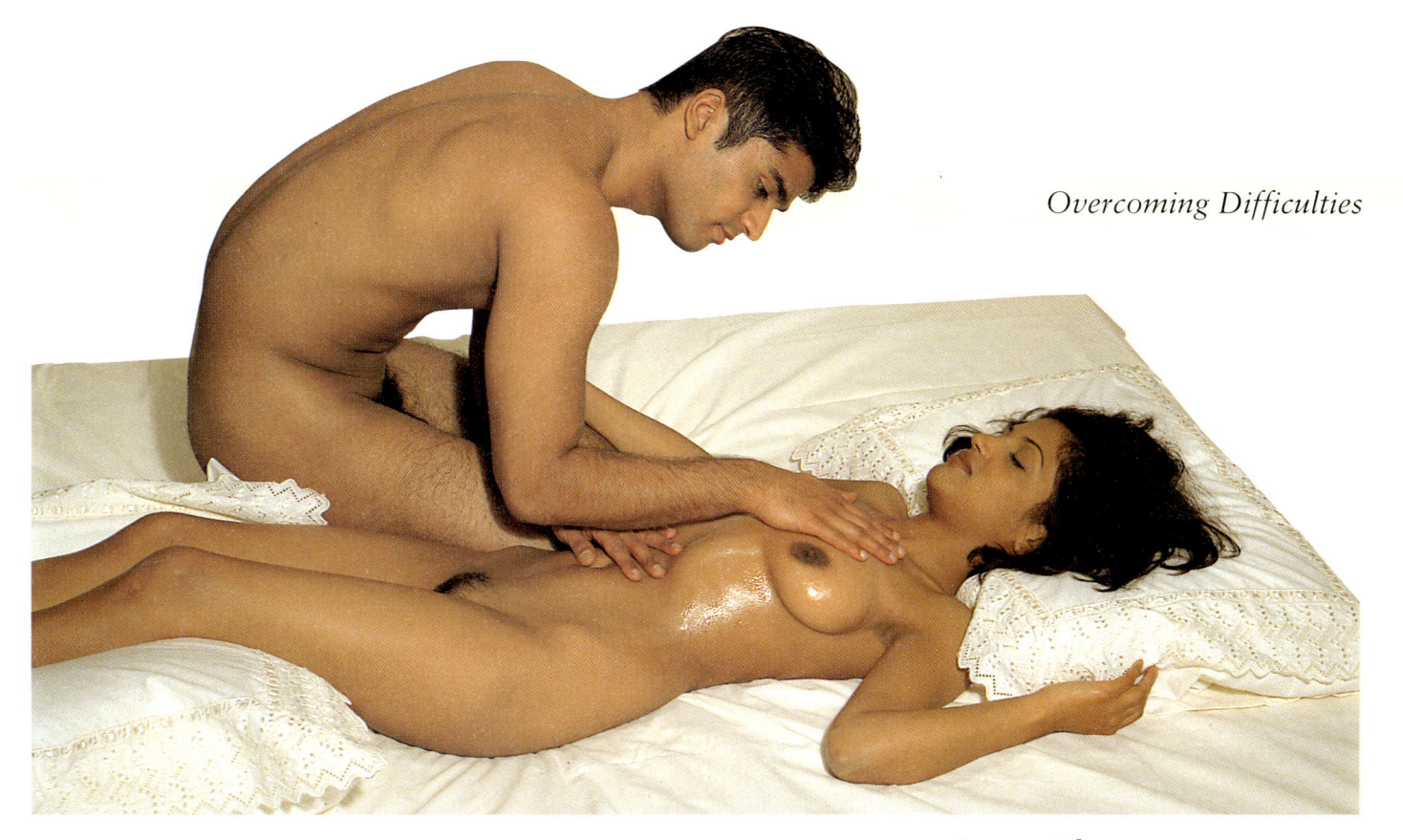

Let Your Hands Flow
▲ *Try to continue to touch in a sensual but non-sexual way when it is your turn to spread lotion over your partner. Feel the fluid quality of your hands as they slide over her skin and around the curves of her body. Use your fingers, thumbs, and the heels of your hands to make varying levels of pressure in your strokes. Stop moving occasionally, letting one hand rest on the heart and the other over the belly. See if you can feel her heartbeat under your hands, and sense the movement of breath in her body.*

yet another dimension and aspect of touch, which may become more smooth and sensual, more flowing and soft with the addition of lubricant. Remember, the purpose of these exercises, at this juncture, is not about pleasing the other person but about discovering new tactile responses for yourself. Stroke, knead and press the flesh, each time becoming aware of the different sensations of movement and touch, especially now that you have added the oil or body lotion.

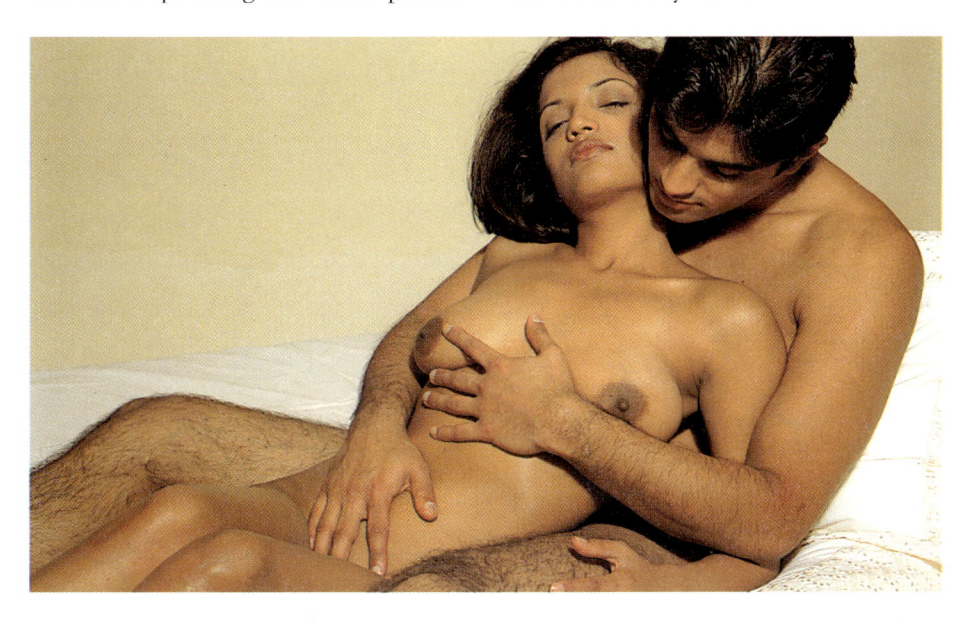

Stage Three: Touching the Genitals

Once you both feel ready, you can progress to the stage of these exercises where you are allowed to include the genitals and breasts into your programme of exploratory touch. However, your tactile contact should not be intended to create sexual arousal, although this may happen inadvertently. Do not zone onto the erogenous areas immediately but start with all-over-body touch as before, with or without lotion.

There is still no goal in mind except to experience fully the present moment of tactile awareness. If you find yourself becoming too excited, then move on to another area of the body, as you

Keep Touches Innocent
◀ *Even though you can now make tactile contact with her more sexual areas, such as her genitals and breasts, you should be stroking and caressing her erogenous zones in the same manner as you have been touching the other parts of her body – with a sense of wonder and innocence. This sitting position can be adopted during this stage when the man is the active partner.*

109

Overcoming Difficulties

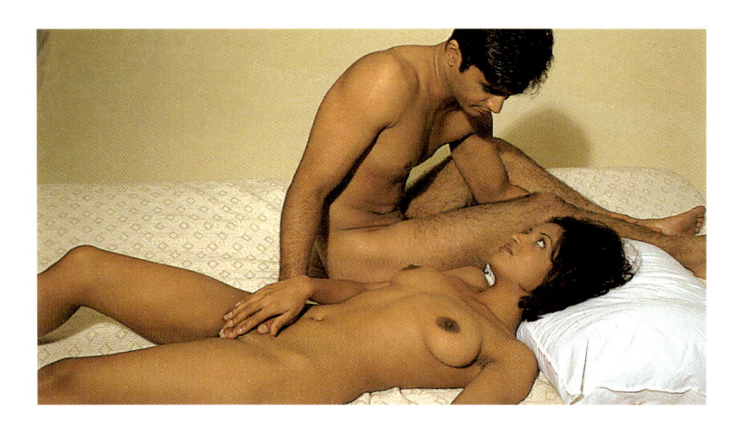

Let Yourself be Guided
▲ She can lay her hand over yours and, through her touch, give you a gentle direction of where to go, how firm or soft your pressure should be, when to move your hand to another place and when to return. See if you can pick up her signals through the receptivity of your skin. In this way, you are becoming more deeply attuned to her physical messages. You can also reverse the position of your hands, so that your hand lies on top of hers.

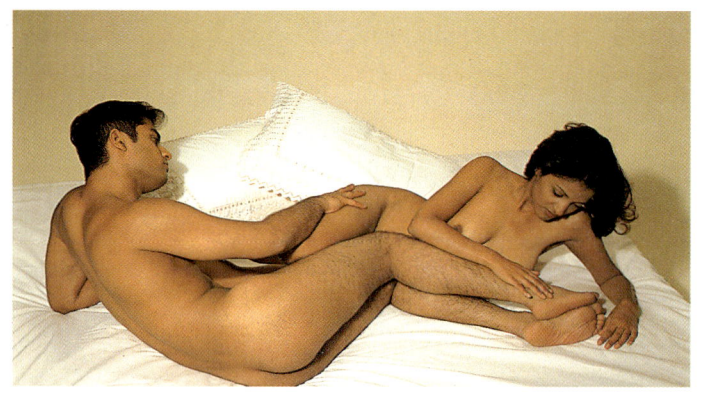

Simultaneous Sensations
▲ Once you begin the mutual touching exercise, you must be very careful not to turn the episode into a session of foreplay or full lovemaking. Lie comfortably close to each other so that you can simultaneously touch and explore each other's bodies with the sensual awareness that you have steadily been developing through this programme. Focus all your attention on the sensations that you are experiencing of touching each other and of being touched.

did in the first stage of this exercise. If you are the male active partner, you can use a sitting position during this phase, so your partner's back is leaning against you. Prop yourself against some pillows and reach comfortably around to touch the front of her body. Also, become aware of the feel of her back as it nestles against your skin. As the woman during the active phase, you can kneel between your partner's legs to gain easier access to his genital area.

Once you are touching the genitals, the passive partner can also guide you by laying his or her hand over yours, and giving you silent cues as to how he or she likes to be touched there. Move your hands with synchronicity, and try to remain receptive to the passive partner's subtle directions. You can even swap the position of your hands, so that at some point, your hand overlays the hand of the receptive partner. Follow their movements, gauging how your partner likes to stroke himself or herself and what variations of pressure he or she may like to apply.

Your intention is not to arouse each other to orgasm, as your focus is still on gaining a greater sense of tactile awareness. Do not concentrate only on the genitals, but continue to touch other parts of the body as before. You should not kiss at this stage, or pursue any activity which may lead to intercourse. If, however, either partner does become orgasmic while being genitally stroked, you can continue your manual touching, with just your own hands, or your combined hands, to allow orgasm to happen.

Stage Four: Touching Each Other

Mutual touching is now the new phase in your sensate focus programme. Here you begin again with your sensory awareness exercises, but this time you are touching each other simultaneously. There is still a ban on kissing and sexual intercourse, but you can now use your tongue to explore one another's bodies, although not with the purpose of arousal. Now you must simultaneously focus your attention on touch and on the sensation of being touched. Explore each other's bodies with different types of strokes, using fingertips or palms, just as you have done in the previous exercises.

Stage Five: Making Love

Begin this stage of the programme with your whole-body touch, including sensual touching of the genital regions. However, during this phase, you can now move onto the first steps of resuming sexual intercourse. The man should lie on his back and, as the woman, you should climb on top of him so that you are kneeling across his hips.

Carry your sensual awareness with you, and begin by just letting your genitals make contact. Absorb these

Overcoming Difficulties

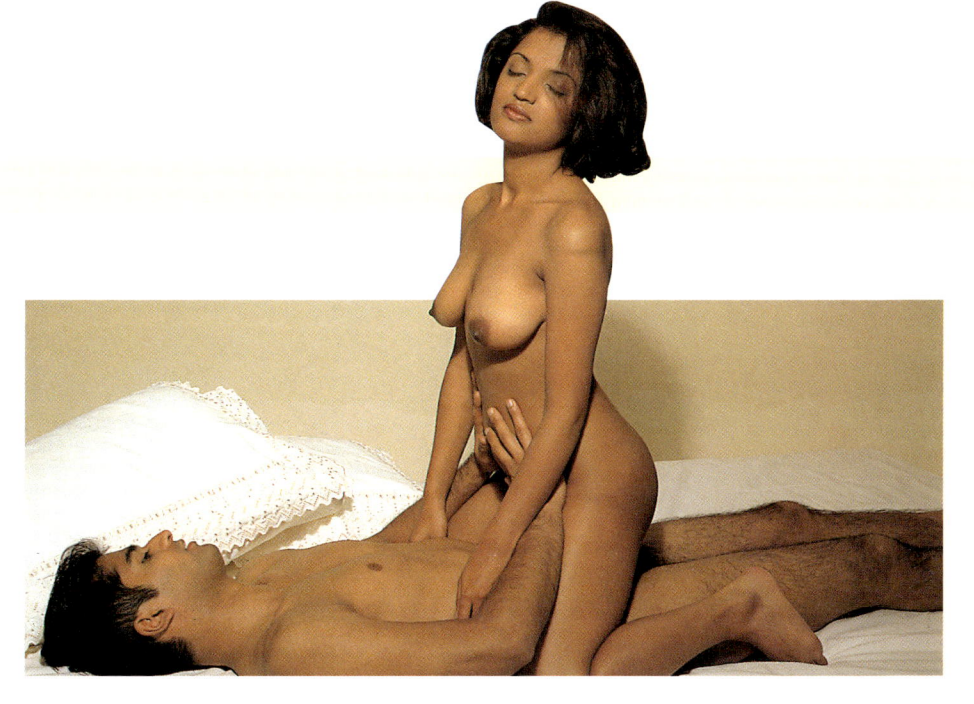

Gentle Penetration
▲ When you are ready, take your partner's penis and very carefully slide it just inside your vagina so that only its head nestles within you. Both of you should now fully experience this sensation and refrain from thrusting movements or deeper penetration. Try also to feel what your partner is experiencing. When you are ready, you can allow the penis to penetrate a little further into your vagina and then, once again, stop and concentrate on how this feels.

sensations into yourself. Then, as the woman, take your partner's penis and gently guide its head into your vagina. Avoid any thrusting or deep penetration. Explore the different feelings which arise with each motion that you make. Gradually, you can deepen the depth of penetration and begin to move very slowly and gently, continuously focusing on your immediate physical experience, while having a greater awareness than ever before of the sensations your partner is experiencing.

You are now ready to resume your full sexual relationship, but with a completely heightened sensual awareness. This does not mean you cannot have passionate and wild sex again, but every once in a while, go back to the exercises to enrich your intrinsic feeling senses.

Overcoming Erection Failure

A failure to get an erection or to maintain one during sexual activity happens to most men at some time in their lives. This may be the result of stress and tiredness, sexual boredom, lack of attraction to a partner, or ill health. This is usually temporary, and the man's arousal response will improve by itself, or when circumstances and events change for the better.

Erection failure, which is also called impotence, can have psychological or physiological causes – or a combination of the two. Erection failure often has an organic basis, so if the condition is a persistent problem it should be investigated by the man's doctor, or a medical expert who specializes in sexual dysfunction. Possible physiological causes include diabetes, neurological and vascular disorders, a side-effect of certain medications, abnormal hormone levels, or alcohol- and other drug-related problems.

For many men, though, it is the fear of impotence and anxiety over performance that most often lead to consistent erection failure. A man may be putting himself under a lot of pressure to achieve super-stud status every time he makes love. Sometimes, a bad sexual experience, perhaps compounded by the unsympathetic comments of a sexual partner, has increased his anxiety about how well he is going to perform. This worry may then become a self-fulfilling prophecy in all future sexual relationships. If the man does not have a secure relationship, and so is constantly involved in new sexual situations, his fears about his performance in bed may become so extreme that the tension makes it virtually impossible to get an erection, or to keep one once he has started penetrative sex.

Alternatively, if a man has been orientated solely towards thrusting, penetrative sexual intercourse, driven along by high levels of excitement, and his relationship then becomes more companionable, he may be unable to achieve or sustain arousal in this new climate of intimacy.

When a man is struggling with the emotional and physical factors of erection failure, for whatever reasons, the best thing he can do is to take the pressure off the situation. Temporary abstinence from sex will give him the time he needs to unlink the connection between anxiety and performance. If he has a sympathetic partner, who is willing to assist him at this time, they can benefit from the sensate focus exercises described previously.

They should work through the programme step by step, not reaching the last stage until the man has been able to relax totally into sensual touching and receiving touch for its own sake, rather than to achieve a climax. Once the woman has started to touch his genitals, she should avoid focusing on them too closely. If an erection occurs it should not

Overcoming Difficulties

become central to the sensory experience of whole-body touching.

When the man begins to relax into his whole-body sensuality, the woman can stimulate him to an erection, either manually or orally, but should then allow the erection to subside while she concentrates on other areas of his body. When his penis has become softer, she can again stimulate him to an erection. At this stage, she should not try to bring him to an orgasm.

In this way, the man begins to realize that he can have an erection, lose it, and then regain it at a later time. The couple should practise this phase of the exercises for about three weeks, or for however long it takes for the man to accept the fluctuations of his erections without anxiety.

As the couple progress through the mutual touching and genital-to-genital contact stages of the sensate focus exercises, the man should continue to involve himself totally with touching and caressing the woman's body, and avoid focusing on whether or not he has an erection. The woman can help by continuing to touch and stroke his body and genitals without expecting something to happen. When the couple are able to reach the sensual lovemaking stage, the woman should begin by taking her partner's penis slowly into her vagina as described. If the penis becomes soft at any stage, both partners should simply continue with their sensual touching, allowing the erection to return later, or not as the case may be.

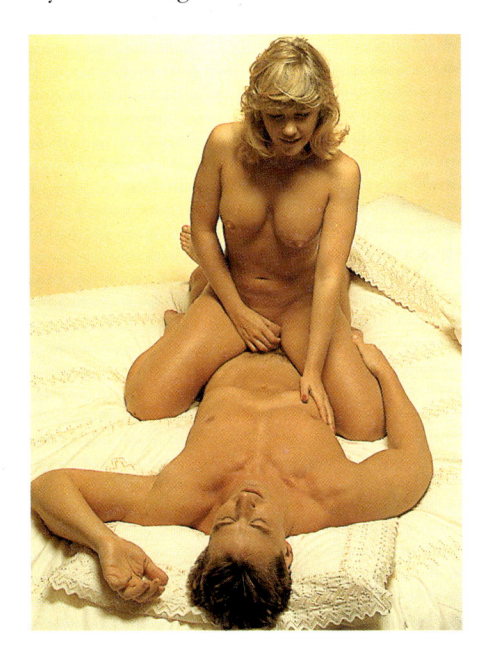

Gradually, with patience and loving support, the man may be able to break the cycle of anxiety which has inhibited his responses. By becoming less focused on his penis, and more involved in the pleasures of sensual contact with his partner, he will be able to relax and gain a new confidence in his sensuality and sexuality.

A single man who has anxieties about his performance should try to avoid casual sexual encounters which may confirm his insecurity. It is better to develop a secure and loving partnership where the sexual relationship has time to build slowly and where his sexual confidence is not immediately challenged.

Overcoming Premature Ejaculation

Premature ejaculation is fairly common in younger men who have not yet learned to control and extend the plateau phase of their sexual response, which occurs just before orgasm. In all men, there is a point when ejaculation is inevitable. However, some men ejaculate almost immediately upon genital-to-genital stimulation, or even during the initial stages of physical contact. This is disappointing for both partners, but is particularly frustrating for the woman if she has no time to achieve orgasm herself.

A consistent pattern of premature ejaculation will cause anxiety because the man feels unable to control his bodily responses, and fears disappointing his partner. Such anxiety can lead to erection failure, or sex avoidance, especially if he is regularly criticized for "poor performance" in bed.

Fortunately, premature ejaculation can be successfully treated by sex therapy. Ideally this should involve both partners. If the couple have a good basis of communication, and are mutually willing to explore new sensual techniques to help change the man's habitual patterns of sexual response, they can benefit from the following self-help exercises using the "squeeze technique" (see opposite).

However, if there are other fundamental problems within the relationship, the couple are better advised to seek professional help to improve their communication, and resolve the emotional or sexual problems involved. In the self-help method, the couple must agree to abstain from intercourse during the period of time they are following the exercises until a certain stage of progress has been reached. However, the man can help his partner climax through oral or manual stimulation whenever she wants him to.

Having committed themselves to this programme, which should be practised at least three times a week, the couple begin with manual stimulation. The woman masturbates the man, applying the "squeeze" to the

Applying the Squeeze
◀ *Whenever you feel your partner is close to ejaculating, you can apply the squeeze technique so that his erection subsides slightly. Then you can begin to stimulate him again.*

top of the penis whenever he begins to approach his orgasm threshold. Once the erection has subsided slightly, she stimulates him again by hand, repeating this procedure up to three times. He is then allowed to ejaculate. After several sessions, which ought to be no more than two days apart, the man should begin to feel more confident in his ability to delay ejaculation.

At this point the couple can progress to genital-to-genital contact. The woman sits astride her partner and uses her hand to move his penis around her vaginal lips and clitoris, while applying the squeeze technique as necessary. Once both partners feel confident that the man has achieved some control over his ejaculatory process in this more intimate situation, they can apply the squeeze technique to the first stages of intercourse. The woman should position herself astride her partner and then guide his penis into her vagina. They should both then remain still.

If the woman senses her partner is close to ejaculating, she must lift herself off of his penis and apply the squeeze technique. The couple can then repeat this procedure at least three times before allowing ejaculation to occur. If the man ejaculates prematurely, despite their efforts to delay it, neither partner should regard this as a disaster. Anxiety, expectation or criticism all work against the possibility of overcoming premature ejaculation. By patiently persevering with the exercises, and with the loving support of his partner, the man gradually builds up his confidence and ability to delay ejaculation.

If good progress is made after three or more sessions in the penetration phase described above, the woman can begin to move very gently while his penis is inside her. Again, as she becomes aware that her partner is reaching the point of no return, she should stop moving, lift up from his penis and apply the squeeze technique before resuming penetration and gentle movement.

The Squeeze Technique

The basic squeeze technique is useful in helping a couple tackle the problem of premature ejaculation. The squeeze is applied by the woman who simultaneously presses her thumb pad against the frenulum, just below the head of the penis, and the pad of her first finger just above the coronal ridge on the top of the glans, while her second finger rests parallel to the first on the shaft of the penis. Pressure must come directly from the pads of the fingers and thumb (avoid a grasping squeeze) and needs to be maintained firmly for at least four seconds. It should not be applied to the sides of the penis. The man can indicate how much pressure feels comfortable if his partner is unsure. This pressure should cause the erection to subside slightly and delay the ejaculation. The procedure is carried out at least three times in one session, always just prior to the ejaculation phase. The woman should learn to recognize the signals that indicate when her partner is close to this level of arousal, or he can let her know himself.

The couple should continue with these exercises until the man is able to sustain his erection for up to 15 minutes inside his partner before ejaculating. The more the couple engage in this phase of the exercise, the more likely it is that the old patterns of sexual response will dissolve. They should not worry if the man occasionally ejaculates too soon, but should persevere with continued good humour and optimism.

Once the partners are able to sustain a longer period of intercourse, and feel confident enough to increase thrusting and movement, they can start to apply a different form of squeeze which does not necessitate the woman dismounting from the penis. The pressure is now applied, by either the man or the woman, to the base of the penis, with the thumb pad pressing on the area just above the scrotum, and the first two fingers parallel, applying pressure on the opposite side of the penis. Again, the penis should not be squeezed at the sides.

Eventually, the couple can experiment with other lovemaking positions, using the squeeze technique when necessary, especially if the man resumes the on-top position, which is more likely to lead to premature ejaculation. The squeeze technique can also be incorporated into the sensate focus exercises and applied throughout each stage whenever necessary.

Many men may wish to prolong lovemaking without ejaculating before either they or their partners are ready. The sensate focus exercises will help them to relax more into sensual touching and leisurely intercourse and are bound to enrich their sexual relationship.

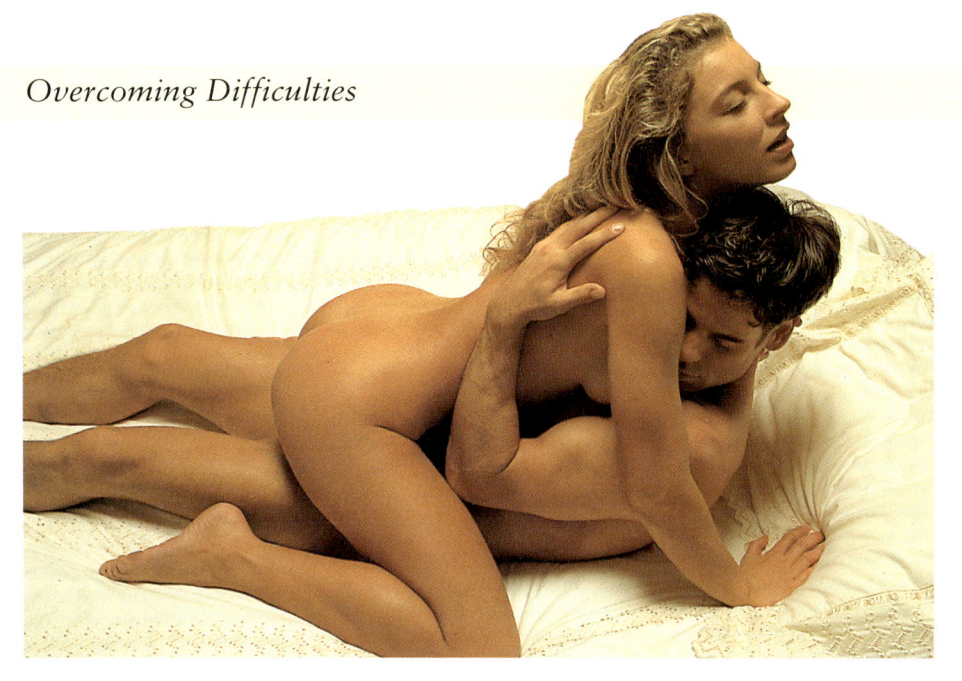

Overcoming Difficulties

Learn to Relax
◀ *Once you are able to fully relax into your own body and sensual and erotic feelings of pleasure in touching and lovemaking, without worrying about performance or results, you may find that your orgasmic capacity increases.*

Overcoming Orgasmic Difficulties

There are many reasons why a woman may have difficulty in reaching an orgasm, but most of these can be overcome by creating a new and more sensual attitude towards her body, and by the willingness of her and her partner to explore more mutually satisfying forms of lovemaking.

For a woman who has difficulty in achieving an orgasm, or who has lost this capacity altogether, the following self-help suggestions may enable her to attain sexual fulfilment.

She should learn to enjoy self-pleasuring, not only through masturbation, but also by becoming more sensually aware of her whole body. Self-massage, stroking and caressing herself, applying aromatic moisturizing creams to her skin, and learning to love her own body, will help to boost her body image and self-esteem. If she is shy, or has negative feelings about her genitals, exploring herself, using a mirror and her fingers, will help her to accept these most intimate parts.

Once she has established a better body image, she will benefit from self-masturbation, allowing herself to stroke, caress and rub her vaginal lips and clitoral area to find out which pressures and motions that are most arousing. The more sensual she makes this experience, the more enhanced her responses are likely to be. She should dedicate time to regular self-pleasuring, letting her strokes involve her whole body, including her face, neck, breasts, belly, thighs, buttocks, mons and vulva.

To put herself in the right mood, she can bathe in an aromatic bath beforehand so that she feels totally relaxed both mentally and physically, and then moisturize her skin with lotion to leave it soft and glowing. She can then retire to a warm and private setting, perhaps lit by candles and with relaxing or sexy music playing in the background.

The woman can begin to let go into erotic fantasy, conjuring up whatever sexual pictures help to arouse her. Some women find it difficult to allow sexual fantasy, either because of guilt feelings, or because they do not have an adequate source of erotic mental images. Women who feel guilty about having erotic fantasies should read Nancy Friday's book *My Secret Garden*. Here, the author's careful research reveals the rich diversity of women's fantasies, some funny, some bizarre, some lurid, but all giving testimony to the fertile, erotic female mind. The woman can also use a vibrator to explore her sexual responses.

Sometimes, a woman may block her orgasmic reactions because she is reluctant to really let go, fearful of losing control over her body. Enacting out an orgasmic response to the full, breathing deeply, writhing on the bed, sighing and crying out will give her more confidence to abandon herself freely when she is orgasmic with a lover.

Self-stimulation techniques allow the woman to become familiar with her own unique sexual responses, so she can regard herself as orgasmic in her own right, rather than as a result of what someone else does to her. She can then use this greater understanding of her own physical and mental erotic responses in a sexual relationship.

When a woman is experiencing orgasmic dysfunction within her sexual relationship, both she and her partner will benefit from the sensate focus exercises. They can learn or rediscover how to touch each other's bodies in a sensual rather than immediately sexual way. They can also benefit from the non-demanding genital contact exercises, during which the woman shows her partner how she prefers to masturbate herself.

Leisurely foreplay, including kissing, caressing, manual clitoral stimulation and oral-genital contact, all enjoyed for the sheer sake of pleasure, rather than focused purely towards orgasm, will help the woman to feel cherished and become more fully aroused before penetration occurs.

The woman should not feel she has to have an orgasm to soothe her partner's sexual ego, or to prove herself to be sexually responsive. This demand can create a mental and physical tension which is likely to block her natural responses.

It is also important for the couple to resolve their relationship conflicts before making love, because hidden resentments, and other negative feelings may also affect the woman's ability to relax sexually. Choosing the right time to make love, when neither partner is tired or under stress, or when they are unlikely to be interrupted by their children, will enhance the sexual responses of both of them.

A woman who is unable to come to an orgasm by any means of stimulation – a condition known as anorgasmia – will benefit from the guidance of a qualified sex therapist if she wishes to become orgasmic.

Treating Vaginismus

For some women, penetrative sex can be an uncomfortable, or even painful experience. In rare cases, intercourse may be impossible because of involuntary contractions of the muscles surrounding the vagina – a condition known as vaginismus. Many sufferers may otherwise have completely normal sexual responses, and may easily attain orgasm through non-penetrative sex such as masturbation or oral-genital contact.

Vaginismus occurs most commonly in young women. However, a woman may suffer this disorder throughout her sexual life, and it can cause great distress to both her and her partner who may, in every other respect, enjoy a close relationship. The problem can be so serious that the woman is unable to insert a tampon, a pessary, or even her own finger into her vagina, and a pelvic examination is an impossibility without sedation.

If the woman has never been able to experience vaginal penetration, the condition is known as primary vaginismus. If she has had penetrative sex in the past, but has consequently developed these distressing symptoms, the condition is called secondary vaginismus.

Vaginismus can result from a number of complex causes. If it is primary, the problem may stem from early childhood or adolescent conditioning, possibly due to parental or religious influences, which have created negative feelings about sexuality in general, or her genitals in particular.

Other causes include trauma due to rape or childhood sexual abuse, a painful and insensitive gynaecological examination in adolescence, or an exaggerated fear of becoming pregnant or of contracting a sexually transmitted disease. Secondary vaginismus may occur as a result of a genital infection, a difficult childbirth, or other pathological causes which previously made intercourse painful and have consequently precipitated the involuntary muscular response. The woman may then become fearful of further pain on penetration.

Whatever the reasons for vaginismus, and sometimes they are complex and indefinable, a woman must first be examined by a sympathetic gynaecologist to discover whether there is an identifiable underlying cause, such as a physical abnormality or infection.

Vaginismus is almost always treatable once the woman, and her partner, if she has one, decide to seek professional advice and receive sex therapy. The complexity of the psychological issues involved in vaginismus, and the need to ascertain whether the condition is a primary or secondary one, makes it advisable that the woman's circumstances are assessed by a psychosexual counsellor. The therapist will then be able to guide the woman and her partner through the treatment strategy that is most appropriate to her.

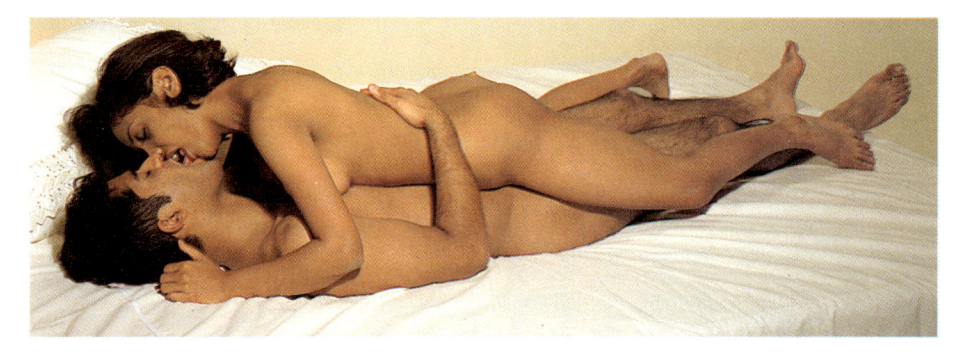

Mutual Understanding
▲ *Through loving care, mutual support, and the changing of existing patterns through simple exercises and techniques, problems such as premature ejaculation and vaginismus can be understood, coped with, and hopefully overcome, especially with the aid of sympathetic counselling.*

Contraception

Contraception is an important consideration for most sexually active people, as a way of avoiding unwanted pregnancy or as an aid to family planning. It is important to keep in mind, however, that no method is 100 per cent reliable, and some forms of contraception do not protect against HIV or other sexually transmitted diseases. Condoms have been shown to be effective against these risks and to play an invaluable role in safer sex, as well as guarding against conception.

There is now a much wider choice of contraceptive methods than ever before, and most are readily available. The various forms are discussed below, and their suitability for you can best be determined by consulting a health practitioner. Changing lifestyles or needs, or relevant health issues, may require that you re-evaluate the type of contraceptive you are currently using. This is easily done in consultation with your doctor or local family planning clinic.

It is important, as a sexually active person, to take a responsible attitude to contraception and to avoid spreading sexually transmitted diseases. Some forms of contraception carry health risks, which you should take into account when choosing the most suitable method for you, bearing in mind factors such as your medical condition, weight, age and lifestyle.

However, it is worth bearing in mind that pregnancy and childbirth also involve slight risks, to say nothing of the distress of an unwanted pregnancy. The various methods now available should make the decision on these matters easier and ensure your choice is best suited to the specific needs of you and your partner.

The failure rates quoted in this section are based on the theoretical number of pregnancies that can be expected within one year among 100 couples having regular sex and using the particular form of contraception mentioned. The risk of failure is obviously increased if a contraceptive method is used incorrectly.

HORMONAL METHODS

Oral Contraceptive Pill

The oral contraceptive pill has been used by millions of women since its introduction in the early 1960s. There are currently over 60 million women world-wide using this method. If used correctly, the pill is a highly reliable form of contraception – up to 99 per cent effective. The advantage of the pill is that couples do not have to think about contraception (so long as it is taken on the days and at the times specified) and so it does not interfere with their spontaneity.

The pill works by suppressing normal control of a woman's sex hormone system, thereby artificially regulating her menstrual cycle. Most forms of the pill contain a combination of progestogen and synthetic oestrogen, which mimic the female hormones progesterone and oestrogen. The effect is to prevent ovulation, make the cervical mucus impenetrable to sperm, and alter the lining of the uterus so that a fertilized egg cannot implant in it.

The combined pill is taken on 21 days out of 28 – with seven pill-free days. It is available in three forms: monophasic, biphasic and triphasic. Monophasic pills release constant doses of hormones. Biphasic and triphasic pills release staged doses – in two phases and three phases respectively – to mimic the normal pattern of female hormone production more closely.

The combined pill may be less effective if it is taken more than 12 hours late, or if there is any vomiting or diarrhoea. Other medications, such as antibiotics, sedatives and some painkillers, may also alter the efficacy of the combined pill. In any of these cases, an additional form of contraception should be used until the end of the cycle.

Studies have linked the combined pill with an increased risk of cardiovascular disease, and liver and cervical cancer, but it seems to offer protection against ovarian cancer, cancer of the endometrium (the lining of the uterus), ovarian cysts, non-cancerous breast tumours, fibroids, and ectopic pregnancy. Medical opinion is divided on the link between hormonal pills and breast cancer.

All women who use hormonal contraceptive methods should have regular breast examinations, cervical smears, and six-monthly check-ups of blood pressure and weight.

The combined pill does have some serious side-effects such as increased risk of blood clots in the arteries and veins. This risk is much greater in women over the age of 35, smokers, and those who are very overweight. It is not usually prescribed for women in these high-risk categories. Some of the other side-effects of the pill reported include breast tenderness, mood swings, weight gain, water retention, and loss of libido. Vaginal infections, such as thrush, are also more common among contraceptive pill users.

Mini-Pill

Another form of hormonal contraception is the progestogen-only pill, or mini-pill, which is taken every day, without a break. It uses only very low doses of progestogen, so it must be taken at the same time each day to prevent fertilization, and never more than three hours late. It has fewer side-effects than the combined pill but there is a higher failure rate (up to four per cent).

Because it does not contain oestrogen, which is the hormone that has been linked to thrombosis, or blood clots forming in the veins and arteries, it may be a better alternative in certain cases. It is associated with a higher risk of breast cancer than the combined pill, particularly among women who have taken the drug for over five years. Some women who use it may have irregular periods, or light spotting between periods.

Implants

Implants are another hormonal method of birth control. Six tiny, flexible capsules are inserted under the skin of the upper arm. This requires minor surgery, which is carried out under a local anaesthetic. Once in place, the capsules release low levels of progestogen directly into the bloodstream. Implants rarely cause discomfort, and they provide contraceptive protection for up to five years. They may cause changes in menstruation, producing either heavier periods or irregular periods, and weight gain. They also require minor surgery to be taken out.

Fertility is restored soon after removal of the implants. As this method does not contain oestrogen, it may be suitable for women who cannot use the combined pill.

Injectable Contraceptives

In this method, an injection of progestogen is given in a muscle during the first five days of menstruation. It provides contraceptive protection for eight to twelve weeks. Though its effectiveness rivals that of the pill, it is mostly prescribed in exceptional circumstances. These include women who have just been immunized against rubella, when pregnancy could result in birth defects in the foetus; women whose partners have recently had a vasectomy, until tests can show there are no longer sperm present; and women who are unable to use other forms of birth control. Once injected the contraceptive action cannot be reversed and there may also be a delay before fertility returns. Menstrual disturbances, weight gain and a delay in fertility are the most common side-effects.

BARRIER METHODS

IUD

The IUD (intra-uterine device, or "coil") is a T-shaped appliance that is inserted through the cervix into the uterus. It is not known exactly how the IUD works. It was previously thought that it prevents a fertilized ovum implanting in the lining of the uterus, but research now suggests its main action is to make conditions in the uterus hostile to sperm.

Many IUDs are made of plastic, or copper wire on a plastic frame. Some have a silver core and there are versions that also release progestogen. IUDs have two nylon threads that hang down into the vagina, enabling the woman to check each month whether the device is still in place. Some forms must be replaced every two to three years, others can be left in the womb for up to five years, and some last over ten years. Regular check-ups will be necessary.

An IUD should only be inserted by a doctor. This is usually done during menstruation because the cervix is slightly dilated at this time, and there is little likelihood that the woman is pregnant. An IUD can, however, be expelled from the uterus soon after insertion or in the first three months. Sometimes, though rarely, the IUD can dislodge and perforate the wall of the uterus. Usually, this is signalled by sharp pains in the lower abdomen and vaginal bleeding. Many users experience heavier, more painful periods, especially in the first few months. It also makes a woman's reproductive system more vulnerable to infections such as PID (pelvic inflammatory disease) which, when untreated, can lead to infertility. It is therefore not advised for younger women, or those who have had no children, or women with a history of sexually transmitted diseases.

The IUD is a very effective form of birth control with a protection rate similar to the combined pill. However, if pregnancy does occur with an IUD in place there is a higher risk of miscarriage, either if it is left in place or at the time of removal. It does not protect against STDs and is better suited to women in monogamous relationships.

Spermicides

Spermicides are available in many different forms, most often as vaginal creams, gels, foams, pessaries and tablets. A contraceptive film is also available, which is packed between squares of silver foil for easy handling. Spermicides are available from the chemist without a prescription and most contain the active ingredient Nonoxynol-9. They usually offer protection for only one episode of intercourse, and must be re-applied before sex is repeated. On their own, they are not highly effective as a contraceptive, with failure rates as high as 25 per cent.

Spermicides are most effective when used in conjunction with another barrier method, such as the condom, diaphragm, cap or sponge (see below). They may cause minor irritations or allergies in either partner. Some spermicides may damage condoms and diaphragms, so only recommended types should be used. Recent tests show that Nonoxynol-9 can kill the HIV virus, the disease responsible for AIDS.

The Diaphragm

The diaphragm is a soft rubber dome, reinforced with a flexible metal spring in the rim, that is placed inside the vagina so that it covers the cervix. It is easily fitted by the user herself, simply by pressing two sides together so it can be inserted. When used consistently with spermicide, placed on the surfaces of the diaphragm before insertion, it can provide a very safe form of birth control – up to 98 per cent effective – and does not interfere with a woman's hormonal balance. However, when used without spermicide, the failure rate can be as high as 15 per cent. The diaphragm must be left in place for at least six hours after sexual intercourse, but no longer than 24 hours. Additional spermicide must be applied before intercourse is repeated.

As the diaphragm is made of a relatively thin form of rubber, it must be checked for signs of deterioration, such as small cuts or tears, before each use. It should also be checked for size every six months as childbirth, miscarriage, or weight gain or loss of more than 3kg/7lb in the user can make it less effective. In such a case a more appropriate size should be fitted. Some women find it difficult to insert, though with practice it usually becomes easier. It can also impair spontaneity for it needs to be inserted before lovemaking. Some women cope with this by inserting it earlier in the evening, but they should keep in mind that spermicide loses a great deal of its potency after three hours and more should be added prior to intercourse.

The diaphragm puts pressure on the bladder and so is not recommended for women who suffer from recurrent cystitis or other urinary infections. A few women are allergic to the rubber of the diaphragm and will not be able to tolerate it. There is a risk of toxic shock syndrome if the diaphragm is worn continuously, especially during a period.

The Cap

The cap functions very much like the diaphragm but is smaller, fitting snugly over the cervix where it is held in place by suction. It has the same success rate as the diaphragm and must be used in conjunction with spermicide to be most effective. It must also be left in place for six hours after sexual intercourse. Additional spermicide should be inserted if sexual intercourse is repeated. Like the diaphragm, its main drawback is that it may detract from spontaneity as it needs to be fitted prior to intercourse.

The Condom

The condom is one of the oldest forms of contraception. Condoms are enjoying renewed popularity for their ability to provide protection against HIV and other sexually transmitted diseases. They are made of fine latex rubber with a teat at the end to collect sperm. To provide maximum protection, the condom should be fitted prior to any genital contact. The condom should be rolled down evenly over the erect penis, taking care to expel all the air from the tip. After ejaculation, the man should withdraw his penis, holding the base of the condom so that no sperm escapes into the vagina.

Only water-based lubricants should be used; oil-based products can cause the rubber to deteriorate. Most condoms contain spermicide and this usually provides sufficient lubrication. Condoms should always be handled with care and checked for signs of damage or ageing. They should not be carried in pockets or wallets where they can get damaged.

Some men complain of a loss of sensation when using condoms, but this is less of a problem nowadays as modern condoms are made of a very thin form of latex. Indeed, any reduced sensitivity may be an advantage for men who suffer premature ejaculation, or who wish to extend lovemaking. Fitting a condom can become part of foreplay so it does not detract from the spontaneity.

Apart from a very small number who are allergic to rubber, there is nothing to prevent most people from using them. Condoms play an invaluable role in safer sex. Their use is particularly recommended with new or casual partners. Used consistently, they are up to 98 per cent effective.

The Female Condom

The female condom, which was developed by a Danish physician in the 1980s, is an innovation in birth control. Like the male condom, it has the added benefit of protecting the user against sexually transmitted diseases, including HIV.

The female condom is a long, loose tube, about 17.5 cm/7in in length, which is closed at one end. It has a smaller fixed ring which is inserted into the vagina and pushed in as far as possible to cover the cervix. A larger ring remains outside and is pushed back against the labia during intercourse. The female condom is pre-lubricated, and made of flexible polyurethane, which is thinner than latex, so there is not so much loss of sensitivity. It is also very loose so it does not have the same constricting feeling as its male counterpart, but is likely to affect sensation nevertheless.

Some women find it rather uncomfortable, but it has the advantage of not requiring the man to withdraw immediately, as is the case with the male condom. Polyurethane is also stronger and more durable than latex, so is less likely to break during intercourse. As it is heavily lubricated, the female condom may be of benefit to women following childbirth or suffering vaginal dryness, around the time of the menopause, for example. Some trials claim a success rate similar to the male condom, though other studies suggest it may be less effective, with failure rates of up to 25 per cent.

The Sponge

The sponge is made of soft polythene foam, impregnated with Nonoxynol-9 spermicide. In order to activate the spermicide, the sponge should be moistened with water before insertion. It is placed as far into the vagina as it will go, and should cover the cervix. It can be inserted any time before sex and must be removed no longer than 30 hours afterwards (but must be left in for at least six hours).

The spermicide component kills sperm for up to 48 hours, regardless of the number of times intercourse takes place. Its major disadvantage is that it has a high failure rate, up to 25 per cent, and should be used with a condom to protect against the risk of pregnancy. A small number of women, between three and five per cent, are allergic to the spermicide.

POST-COITAL CONTRACEPTION

The "Morning-After" Pill

If a woman has had unprotected sexual intercourse, or suspects her method of contraception has failed and is concerned about pregnancy, she can obtain the morning-after pill from her doctor. This emergency contraception is a form of hormonal pill which is taken in double doses – that is, two pills at a time. The first dose is taken within 72 hours of intercourse, and the second dose 12 hours later. Many users experience nausea and breast tenderness.

If vomiting occurs, another dose will be necessary as the pills may not have been absorbed by the body. It does not seem to have any other adverse effects, though it may be unsuitable for women who have been advised not to use other forms of hormonal contraception. Should the morning-after pill fail, it is not yet known what effects there may be on the developing foetus.

Post-Coital IUD

The IUD can also be used as a method of emergency contraception, and has the advantage that it can be used up to five days after unprotected sex, or within five days after the release of an egg. It is not recommended for women who have not had children, or where there is a risk of sexually transmitted disease, for example in cases of rape. As a method of post-coital contraception the IUD is credited with a 100 per cent success rate, to date.

STERILIZATION

Sterilization is a permanent form of birth control, and though it may be reversed, there is no guarantee that fertility will be restored. It is an option that is favoured by people who already have children. It is usually inadvisable in young people, or those who have not had children, for if they have a change of heart later, reversal may not be successful. Counselling is advisable prior to deciding on sterilization.

Vasectomy

A vasectomy is a relatively minor surgical procedure that is usually carried out under local anaesthetic, taking around ten to 15 minutes. It involves cutting and tying back the vasa deferentia, the tubes which carry sperm from the testicles. Most men will need one or two days to recover fully from the operation.

The man's semen may still contain active sperm between six to eight weeks after a vasectomy, so it is important that an alternative means of birth control is used during this time until two separate semen samples have been examined and shown to be free of sperm.

Quick Guide to Contraception

METHOD: **The Combined Pill**
Risks:
- ✗ Side-effects: mood swings, nausea, weight gain, loss of libido, headaches
- ✗ Increased risk of blood clots, especially in the overweight and smokers aged over 35
- ✗ Possible increased risk of cardiovascular disease, and liver, breast and cervical cancer

Benefits:
- ✓ Highly effective as a contraceptive
- ✓ Protection against cancer of the ovaries and endometrium
- ✓ Lighter periods
- ✓ Reduced risk of ovarian cysts

METHOD: **The Mini-Pill**
Risks:
- ✗ Small increased risk of ovarian cysts
- ✗ Less effective than the combined pill
- ✗ Possible increased risk of breast cancer

Benefits:
- ✓ Possible protection against ovarian cancer
- ✓ Side-effects are less severe than the combined pill

METHOD: **Hormonal Implants**
Risks:
- ✗ Complications have been reported in some women during insertion or removal of implants
- ✗ Heavy, irregular or absent periods
- ✗ Weight gain

Benefits:
- ✓ Does not interrupt spontaneity of sexual intercourse
- ✓ Provides effective contraception for up to five years or until removed

METHOD: **Hormonal Injection**
Risks:
- ✗ Heavy, irregular or absent periods
- ✗ Weight gain
- ✗ Delay in return of fertility

Benefits:
- ✓ Reduced risk of ovarian and endometrial cancer
- ✓ Reduced risk of ovarian cysts
- ✓ Does not interrupt spontaneity of sexual intercourse

METHOD: **IUD**
Risks:
- ✗ Increased risk of PID and other pelvic infections
- ✗ Increased risk of ectopic pregnancy
- ✗ Heavier periods in many users

Benefits:
- ✓ Very effective form of birth control
- ✓ Can be removed without delay in return of fertility

METHOD: **Diaphragm/Cap**
Risks:
- ✗ Slight risk of toxic shock syndrome
- ✗ Can interrupt spontaneity of sexual intercourse
- ✗ Not as effective without the use of a spermicide

Benefits:
- ✓ Does not interfere with a woman's hormonal balance
- ✓ Some protection against genital warts
- ✓ Some protection against cervical cancer
- ✓ Some protection against HIV and other sexually transmitted diseases, particularly when used with spermicide

METHOD: **Condom**
Risks:
- ✗ It may break or tear during intercourse
- ✗ Can interrupt spontaneity of sexual intercourse

Benefits:
- ✓ Protects against HIV and other sexually transmitted diseases

METHOD: **The Sponge**
Risks:
- ✗ Relatively high failure rate

Benefits:
- ✓ Once in place it can be left for 24 hours

METHOD: **Vasectomy**
Risks:
- ✗ Psychological regret about loss of fertility
- ✗ Must generally be considered irreversible

Benefits:
- ✓ Freedom from fear of impregnating partner

METHOD: **Female Sterilization**
Risks:
- ✗ Psychological regret about loss of fertility
- ✗ Must generally be considered irreversible
- ✗ Some women experience heavier periods

Benefits:
- ✓ Freedom from fear of pregnancy

METHOD: **Natural Family Planning**
Risks:
- ✗ Without adequate tuition, motivation and commitment, this is an unreliable form of birth control

Benefits:
- ✓ Morally acceptable for couples that don't want to use artificial means of contraception
- ✓ Gives better insight of how a woman's body functions

METHOD: **Coitus Interruptus**
Risks:
- ✗ Too unreliable

On rare occasions, the ends of a vas deferens may rejoin spontaneously, but usually a vasectomy is a highly effective form of birth control. Reversal techniques using microsurgery are becoming increasingly successful, but there is always the risk that anti-sperm antibodies will have been produced that will render the man infertile. Vasectomy should therefore be considered irreversible and only contemplated if the man is sure he has completed his family.

Female Sterilization

Female sterilization is growing in popularity, particularly among those women who have had children. It is a more complicated operation than a vasectomy, and as it is usually carried out under general anaesthetic carries a greater risk. It involves blocking the Fallopian tubes, which carry eggs from the ovaries to the uterus, by cutting, cauterizing or attaching clips to them. This is normally done via a small incision made in the lower abdomen just above the pubic bone.

Sterilization does not usually require an overnight stay in the hospital and its effect is immediate. There may be some pain for a couple of days, while gas pumped into the abdomen during the operation gradually disperses. For many women who have had children, sterilization removes the fear of pregnancy. It is not recommended in younger women or those that have had no children. Some women do experience heavier periods after sterilization. Reversal is a costly and difficult process, and not always effective, though there is a 40 to 80 per cent chance of success. Like male sterilization, it should only be considered if a woman is sure she has completed her family.

NATURAL FAMILY PLANNING (THE RHYTHM METHOD)

Once an egg has been released at ovulation it can only survive for around 24 hours. Sperm have a longer life span, but conditions must be suitable for them. About six days before ovulation, the cervix starts producing a special kind of mucus that provides just the right kind of environment for the sperm. They cannot live long without it, but when it is present they can survive for up to five days, lying in wait ready to fertilize the egg as soon as it is released. Natural family planning is about learning to recognize the changes in a woman's body that indicate her fertile time. Then, unless the couple plan to have a baby, they can abstain from sex during those days or use a barrier method of contraception.

It may be the only option for couples who, for moral or religious reasons, choose not to use artificial means of birth control. It can also be used by women who want to feel they are in tune with their bodies, or who do not find other methods of birth control satisfactory, or who are actively trying to get pregnant.

There are various forms of natural family planning. The most widely practised is the sympto-thermal method, which uses a combination of factors to recognize the fertile stage. These include changes in basal body temperature (her temperature at rest, usually taken soon after waking in the morning), changes in cervical mucus, and changes in the softness, firmness and position of the cervix. Other signs include pain or discomfort in the back, lower abdomen, or breasts. Such changes need to be recorded on a chart, and a woman will usually have to monitor these symptoms and signs over several cycles before she begins to recognize a pattern.

For example, following ovulation a woman's basal body temperature rises by a very small amount and stays at this level until the onset of her next period. This slight change can only be detected by a special fertility thermometer, available from chemists and family planning clinics. Her mucus also alters, from scant, sticky, white or absent, often becoming more profuse, and usually changing to a slippery and stretchy texture that may be clear or slightly cloudy. Some women also experience pain or discomfort at the time of ovulation. Careful monitoring of these various signs should pinpoint the fertile days.

Natural family planning is a complicated procedure that requires motivation, commitment and careful observation of the rules. Women need to learn the correct method from a properly trained natural family planning teacher before they use it as their only form of birth control. When practised conscientiously it has a 97 per cent success rate, which compares with the IUD and hormonal contraception.

COITUS INTERRUPTUS/ WITHDRAWAL

Coitus interruptus, also known as the withdrawal method, is probably the most widely used form of birth control in the world and also the most unreliable. It involves withdrawing the penis from the vagina just prior to ejaculation. As a man's pre-ejaculatory fluid can contain millions of sperm, and accidents are unavoidable, this method has a very high failure rate.

STDs *(Sexually Transmitted Diseases)*

Sexually transmitted diseases (STDs) can have unpleasant and often serious consequences. The world-wide spread of AIDS, a potentially fatal condition arising from a sexually transmitted disease, has highlighted more than ever the need to avoid high-risk sexual practices. If you suspect that you have caught a sexually transmitted disease, it is vital that you seek medical attention at the first opportunity. With all STDs, the infected person should inform all known sexual partners so that they too can be examined and receive the appropriate treatment.

Never ignore the symptoms of a sexually transmitted disease. Most STDs respond well to prompt treatment but delay can allow the disease to spread and risks infertility, crippling side-effects and even death. Medical aid is available from your doctor or, if you prefer, at an STD or GUM (genito-urinary medicine) clinic, where medical staff have specialist knowledge. At such clinics, treatment is confidential and visitors can remain anonymous, if they wish. They will, however, be asked for the names of sexual partners who may be at risk, as the clinic will need to get in touch with them to arrange treatment. They will be contacted in strict confidence. Below, in alphabetical order, are listed the most common sexually transmitted diseases.

Candidiasis (Thrush)

Candidiasis, or thrush, is a common complaint. It is caused by a yeast-like fungus called *Candida albicans* that lives, usually quite harmlessly, in the mouth, intestinal tract and vagina. It is normally kept under control by bacteria that also live in these locations. A warm, moist environment is needed for the fungus to thrive, so the vagina makes an ideal home.

Anything that alters conditions in the vagina can tip the balance in favour of the fungus and enable it to multiply. Tight and confining clothing, illness, or antibiotics, which can destroy the beneficial bacteria, may trigger an outbreak. It is more common in pregnant women, diabetics, and those using hormonal contraceptives. Thrush can also be contracted through sex, and every year thousands of people with the condition visit STD clinics.

Symptoms vary. In women, there may be intense itching of the vulva, with soreness, redness and swelling around the vagina, vulva or anus. They may experience a burning sensation during sex, and when urinating, and some may notice a thick, white, yeast-smelling discharge, which has the consistency of cottage cheese. Not all women show this symptom, however.

In men, a rash may appear on the penis and can occasionally spread to the scrotum. Some may notice a slight burning sensation on the penis during or after sexual intercourse. Thrush can cause considerable discomfort, particularly in those who are prone to recurrences.

The condition is usually treated with antifungal drugs, often as creams or pessaries. The partner should be treated at the same time to prevent re-infection. Other measures may be needed such as wearing loose, natural clothing, and sterilizing underwear and towels. Women who use hormonal contraceptives may be advised to use an alternative form of birth control.

Chancroid

Chancroid is a sexually transmitted disease caused by the bacterium *Haemophilus ducreyi*. It is most often found in tropical countries, mainly through contact with prostitutes, but is becoming more common in the West because of increased international travel. There is an incubation period of up to one week before a painful ulcer forms on the penis or near the entrance to the vagina. There may also be a painful swelling in the groin. If the disease is not treated, abscesses can form in the groin which leave deep scars. Chancroid is usually treated with an antibiotic such as erythromycin.

Chlamydia

Chlamydia trachomatis, a microorganism similar to a bacterium, is the most prevalent STD in the West. It is one of the main causes of a disorder called non-specific urethritis, or NSU (see below) which can lead to infertility. Chlamydia can be transmitted by vaginal, anal, or oral sex, or it can be passed on to a baby during childbirth.

Men may experience a burning sensation when urinating, a whitish discharge from the urethra, and pain and swelling of the testicles, but often there are no symptoms. In women, symptoms are even less common but some may notice pain or a burning sensation when urinating, or a cloudy, white discharge.

If chlamydia remains undetected it can spread through the reproductive tract resulting in a potentially life-threatening condition called pelvic

Sexually Transmitted Diseases

inflammatory disease (PID), itself a major cause of infertility. Chlamydia is treated with antibiotics such as tetracycline and erythromycin. Partners should be treated at the same time, to avoid re-infection.

Genital Herpes

Genital herpes is caused by the *Herpes simplex* virus, which produces painful blisters on or near the genitals. *Herpes simplex* occurs in two main forms. The first, type I, causes cold sores. It is type II that causes genital herpes. The latter form is usually transmitted by sexual contact, including oral sex, and can enter the body through the mucous membranes, or through tiny tears in the skin. It is very infectious and the risk of catching the disease greatly increases if an individual has multiple sexual partners.

There is an incubation period of three to six days, followed by the appearance of a group of small, painful blisters on or near the genitals. These blisters break open and then heal, over a period of 10 to 20 days. The initial attack of genital herpes is usually accompanied by symptoms such as fever, headaches, muscular pain and itching. Further outbreaks will usually cause a recurrence of the blisters.

Once a person has become infected the virus is with them for life, although up to 20 per cent only have one attack. For the rest, the flare-ups usually grow steadily less intense over time. Various factors can cause outbreaks, including stress, anxiety, depression, or illness. Some people are able to anticipate an attack, two or three days beforehand, when they notice symptoms such as tingling, itching, or burning sensations in the genitals. Sexual contact should be avoided during and just before an outbreak, as the condition is highly infectious at this time. There is no cure for genital herpes, but antiviral drugs such as acyclovir can reduce the pain and speed up healing. Genital herpes may play a part in cervical cancer, so infected women should be sure to have annual cervical smear tests.

Genital Warts

Genital warts are caused by the human *papillomavirus*, which is sexually transmitted. The warts are soft and dry, and greyish-pink in colour. Usually painless, they are found on or near the genitals and anus. There is an incubation period of six to eight weeks after exposure. The virus is transmitted by direct contact with the warts, although the virus has also been found in semen. Like genital herpes, genital warts have been linked with cervical cancer, so yearly cervical smears are advisable for affected women.

Genital warts may be destroyed by caustic chemicals, such as podophyllin, or by laser surgery, or liquid nitrogen. As the virus remains in the tissues, however, genital warts tend to recur. Even when warts are not present, affected people should use condoms to avoid transmitting the virus to partners.

Gonorrhoea ("The Clap")

Gonorrhoea is an infection caused by the bacterium *Neisseria gonorrhoea*. It is one of the most common sexually transmitted diseases and is found principally among teenagers and young adults who have several sexual partners. It can be passed on during vaginal, anal, or oral sex, and an infected woman can transmit the disease to her baby during childbirth. Men are more likely than women to show symptoms. They may experience soreness or swelling at the tip of the penis, and a burning sensation when passing urine, often accompanied by a milky discharge from the urethra, two to ten days after infection. The discharge may become thicker, and yellowish in colour, and sometimes contains traces of blood.

Up to 60 per cent of infected women have mild symptoms, or none at all. They may urinate more often, and urination may be painful. There may be a watery, yellow or greenish discharge from the urethra. If the cervix has been infected, there may be vaginal discharge and abnormal menstrual bleeding.

Gonorrhoea is a common cause of infertility and can lead to pelvic inflammatory disease (PID). In a few cases, the infection can spread through the bloodstream, causing conditions as diverse as arthritis, skin rashes, and septicaemia, and even leading to brain damage and death, in severe cases. The disease is easily treated with penicillin antibiotics (or suitable alternatives, for those allergic to such drugs) and, as with all STDs, sexual partners must be contacted so they can receive treatment as well.

Hepatitis

Hepatitis is a serious and potentially fatal disease in which the liver becomes badly inflamed, leading to serious tissue damage. It can be caused by alcohol abuse, drugs, poisons, chemicals, and certain viruses. Of the different forms of viral hepatitis, the two most common are hepatitis A and B. Type A is

Sexually Transmitted Diseases

usually caught from contaminated food or water. Hepatitis B is mainly passed on during sex, or via contaminated needles, particularly among drug users.

It has an incubation period of a few weeks to several months. Sufferers may have a flu-like illness, with nausea and vomiting, followed by jaundice. Some carriers, however, show no symptoms and yet are still be able to infect others. Up to ten per cent of sufferers go on to develop the chronic, or long-term, form of the disease resulting in steadily increasing liver damage.

There is no specific treatment, other than bed rest, a good diet, and anti-inflammatory drugs. However, there is a vaccine against hepatitis B which is recommended for anyone at particular risk, including those with multiple sexual partners (homosexual or heterosexual), intravenous drug users, health care workers, and relatives of carriers.

HIV/AIDS

HIV (human immunodeficiency virus) is a disease that is most often transmitted through unprotected sexual intercourse and by sharing needles and syringes among intravenous drug users. HIV can attack the brain directly, but most often it targets white blood cells called T-4 cells, which are vital to the body's immune system.

Over a period of time, the immune system is so badly impaired that the body becomes vulnerable to a range of opportunistic infections and cancers. This latter, potentially fatal, stage is called AIDS (acquired immune deficiency syndrome). Some of these illnesses, such as Karposi's sarcoma or Pneumocystis carinii, are rare or relatively harmless among non-AIDS sufferers, but life-threatening in those with impaired immune systems.

The rate at which HIV progresses to AIDS is highly variable. Some people develop AIDS within months, while others have milder symptoms for years, a condition known as ARC (AIDS-related complex). They may have periods of good health, interspersed with periods of illness. Some infected people show no symptoms and yet are capable of infecting others. It can take up to ten years or more for the symptoms of full-blown AIDS to develop.

HIV is easily killed outside the body and there is no known risk through ordinary social contact, such as hugging, sharing a meal, or using another person's cups, cutlery, or crockery. The main risk is through the exchange of body fluids. This is why HIV can be passed on through all forms of penetrative sex, especially if there are cuts, tears, or sores in the vagina or anus, or on the penis or cervix.

There is a greater risk if a person has already contracted genital herpes or warts. While HIV is present in all body fluids of an infected person, particularly in semen, vaginal fluids and blood, the risk of transmission in saliva is considered to be minimal. Mothers can transmit HIV to their babies, at birth or through breastfeeding. In the past, HIV has been contracted through contaminated blood and blood products, but this risk is now negligible in the West, with the introduction of screening and heat treatment of donor blood. Health workers can be at risk through accidental injury with a contaminated needle.

Those who suspect they may have HIV, especially people in high-risk categories, can have a blood test to determine whether they have been infected. This test detects whether the body has developed antibodies to try to fight the disease. Those found to have developed antibodies are said to be HIV-positive. A negative result means either that individuals do not have the virus, or that their body has not yet made antibodies, which take two to three months to develop. If you're considering having an HIV test it is vital that you first get specialist counselling to help you understand the implications if the result is positive.

At present there is no vaccine against HIV and no cure for HIV or AIDS, though symptoms and complications can often be treated with antibiotics, anti-cancer drugs and radiotherapy. Anti-viral drugs such as AZT (zidovudine) and acyclovir may reduce the speed at which AIDS develops.

To reduce the risk of HIV infection, individuals should practise safer sex if they are unsure of a partner's sexual history. This means finding safer alternatives to penetrative sex, such as mutual masturbation, or using condoms or other forms of latex barrier. This applies both to casual sex, and sex with long-term partners who might previously have been at risk of acquiring HIV. Intravenous drug users should never share needles and syringes.

NSU

NSU (or non-specific urethritis) is inflammation of the urethra, the tube through which urine passes out of the body, due to causes other than gonorrhoea. It is a fairly common complaint. The main symptom is pain when urinating, which is sometimes, but not always, accompanied by a discharge. There can be over 70 causes of NSU, the most common being chlamydia (see previous page) and trichomonas (see below) infection. It is usually sexually transmitted.

Treatment can be difficult unless the disease responsible is identified. This is usually done by taking samples from the opening of the urethra, or by examining a urine sample (usually taken in the morning when there is the highest buildup of organisms). The choice of medication depends on the underlying cause, although it is most likely to be cured by antibiotics. Partners of those with NSU should also be treated to avoid re-infection.

Pubic Lice ("Crabs")

Pubic lice, *Phthiris pubis*, are a parasitic form of insect. They are more commonly known as crabs because of the crab-like claws by which they attach themselves to hairs. They are most likely to infest the pubic region, but they can be found on all body hairs – even the eyebrows. They do not usually infest the scalp.

Crabs are mainly spread by sexual contact, though they can also be caught from infested bedding or clothing, or from lavatory seats. The eggs are laid at the base of the pubic hairs and hatch about a week later. Pubic lice puncture the skin to feed on blood, which causes the intense itching and irritation. Treatment is with insecticide lotion, available on prescription or from the pharmacist, applied to infected areas. Partners should also be treated to avoid re-infection, and clothes and bedding should be washed in very hot water.

Syphilis

Syphilis, a sexually transmitted disease caused by the bacterium *Treponema pallidum*, was introduced into Europe from North America during the late 15th century. It soon reached epidemic proportions, causing many deaths. Syphilis continued to spread in the following centuries, although its virulence abated. The discovery of penicillin in the 1940s brought it under control.

The bacterium enters the body via broken skin or the mucous membranes, in and around the mouth, genitals and anus. It is highly contagious and can be passed on by any intimate contact, including penetrative sex, oral sex, and even kissing. Unlike with most other STDs, condoms do not give total protection against syphilis.

The disease has four stages: primary, secondary, latent and tertiary. During the primary stage, the first symptoms of syphilis appear after an incubation period of just under a month. A small, painless ulcer will appear at the site of transmission, usually around the genitals or anus, but sometimes the lips, throat or fingers. This ulcer usually disappears after six weeks.

The secondary stage usually occurs up to three months after initial infection. It is marked by a variety of symptoms, the most common being a skin rash, but there may be fever, headaches, sore throat, swollen lymph nodes, aches and pains, loss of hair, and pink patches may appear on the skin. In some cases, there may be meningitis (inflammation of the membranes surrounding the brain), eye infection, or kidney problems.

If untreated, the sufferer enters the latent period, when symptoms may lie dormant for twenty years or more. Symptoms may recur in some sufferers. The tertiary phase is very serious and usually involves destruction of tissues and internal organs, such as damage to the heart, blood vessels, nervous system, and brain, resulting in heart disease, mental disorders, paralysis, and death.

Syphilis is usually identified with a blood test. The disease can be tackled effectively with penicillin or other antibiotics, although 50 per cent of infected people suffer a severe reaction to treatment as the body responds to the death of large numbers of bacteria.

Trichomoniasis

Trichomoniasis (TV) is an infection caused by a single-celled parasite, or protozoon, called *Trichomonas vaginalis*. This highly infectious microorganism is a common cause of vaginitis, or inflammation of the vagina, and is almost exclusively transmitted sexually.

Symptoms, if any, start between four days and three weeks after sexual contact and can show as a thin vaginal discharge that is yellow or green, and frothy, and usually has an offensive smell. In addition, some women may experience vaginal pain and itching, especially during sexual intercourse. These symptoms usually worsen during or after menstruation. Many women, however, suffer no symptoms at all.

Men don't usually show symptoms, although a few may notice a slight discharge and find urinating painful. The condition usually responds to treatment with the antiprotozoal drug metronidazole. The sexual partner should also be treated to avoid re-infection.

Index

adventurous positions 64-75
AIDS 124
anal intercourse 8-9, 10
arousal 22-3

barrier methods 11
bondage 97-9

clitoris 22, 25, 27-8, 48-50, 81
clothes 12-15, 90-3
coitus interruptus 120, 121
compatability 32-3
condoms 6-7, 9, 10-11, 118-19, 120
contraception 116-121
cross-dressing 92-3
cunnilingus 9, 26, 27-8, 33
diaphragm 118, 120
doggie position 69-70, 82
dominance 97-9
dressing up 90-3

ejaculation 59
  premature 112-13
erection 111-12
expressing sexuality 46-55

faking orgasm 60-1
fantasies 82-99, 114
fellatio 9, 26, 28-9
food fantasies 88-9
foreplay 16-25
French kissing 9-10

G-spot 53, 62
gonorrhoea 123

hepatitis 123-4
herpes 123
HIV 6, 7, 8-9, 124
hormones 22, 116-17, 120
hygiene 19, 31

impotence 111-12
IUDs 117, 119, 120
Kama Sutra 64-5
kissing 9-10, 16-18

latex barriers 11
lice 125
lust 102-5

man-on-top position 34, 36-45
master and slave 96
masturbation 10, 24, 76-81, 114
mirrors 83-4
"missionary position" 36
"morning-after" pill 119
multiple orgasms 61

natural family planning 120, 121
nipples 22, 23
NSU (non-specific urethritis) 124-5

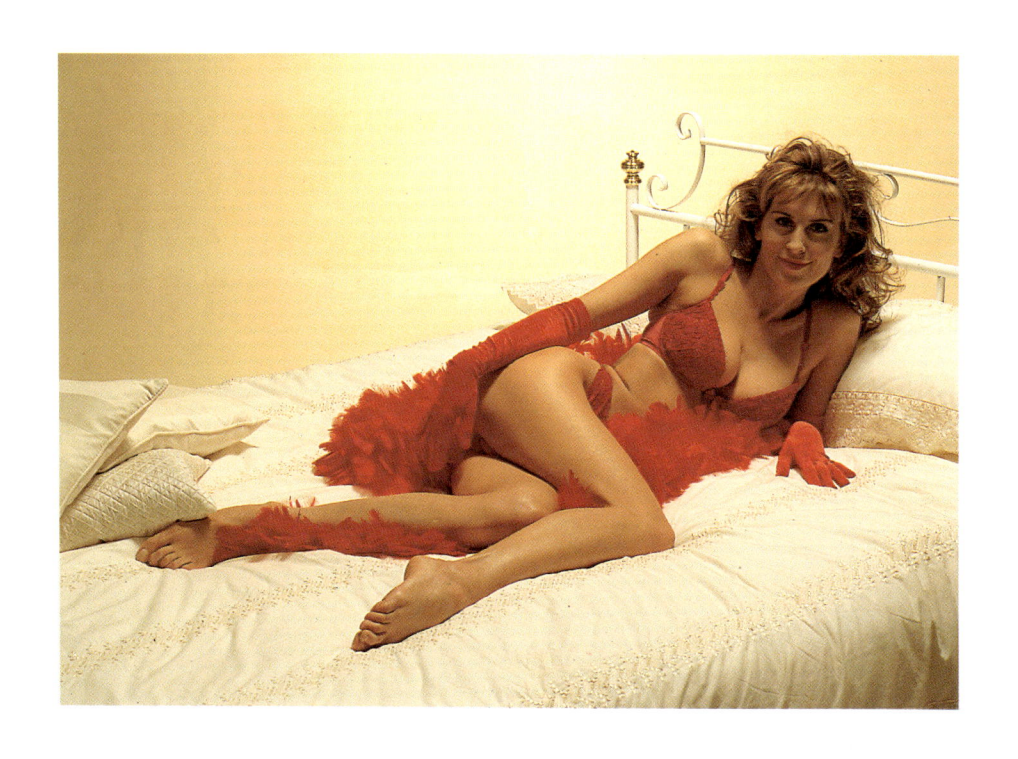

Index

oral contraceptive pill 116-17, 120
oral sex 9, 26-31
orgasm 56-7
  difficulties 114-5
  masturbation 76-7
  oral sex 28-9, 31

passion 102-5
penis
  condoms 10-11
  erection 111-12
  masturbation 78. 80-1
  squeeze technique 112-13
  touching 25
pregnancy 38, 116
premature ejaculation 112-13
problems 106-15
rear-entry sex 69-70, 82
resolution 63
restraint 68, 97-8, 99
rhythm method 121
"rimming" 11, 19

safer sex 6-11
semen 28, 30
sensate focus 106-15
sensual play 16-25
sex toys 9
sexually transmitted diseases (STDs) 6, 122-5
simultaneous orgasm 62-3
sitting positions 35, 54, 55, 70-4
sixty-nine 30-1
skin teasing 94-7
spermicides 117-18
sponges 119, 120
spontaneous sex 100-5
squatting positions 52-3
squeeze technique 112-13
standing positions 64-5, 101-2
sterilization 119-21
strip-tease fantasy 84-7
syphilis 125

teasing 94-7

therapy 83, 106-7
thrush 122
toes 22
tongue teasing 96
touch 106
trichomoniasis 125

underwear 85-7
undressing 12-15

vagina 22
vaginismus 115
vasectomy 119-21
vibrators 99
vulva 81

warts, genital 123
withdrawal method 121
woman-on-top position 34, 46-53

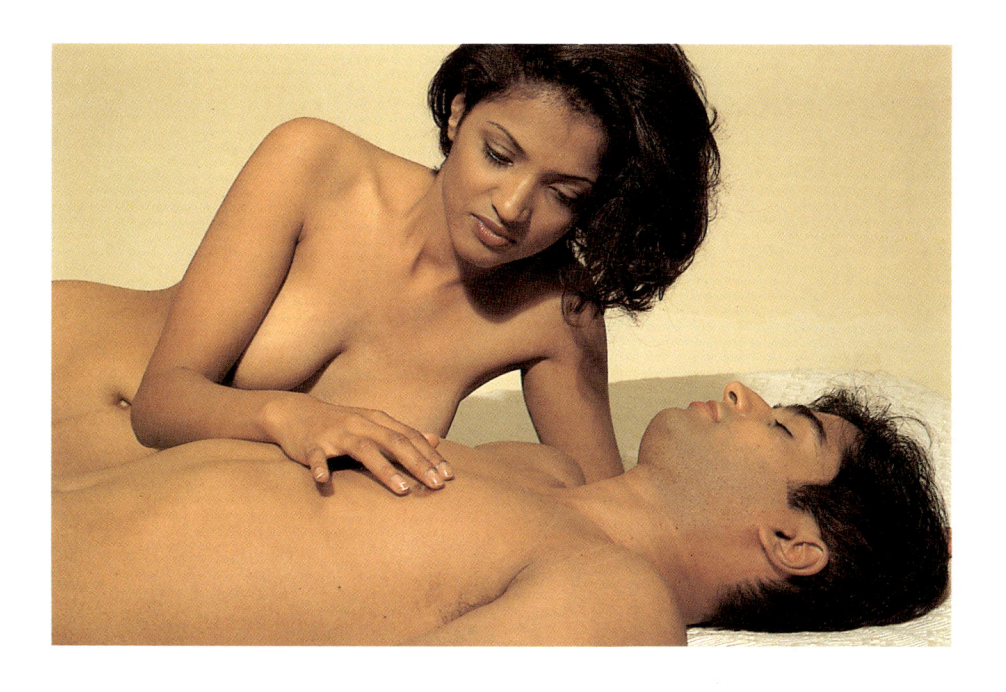

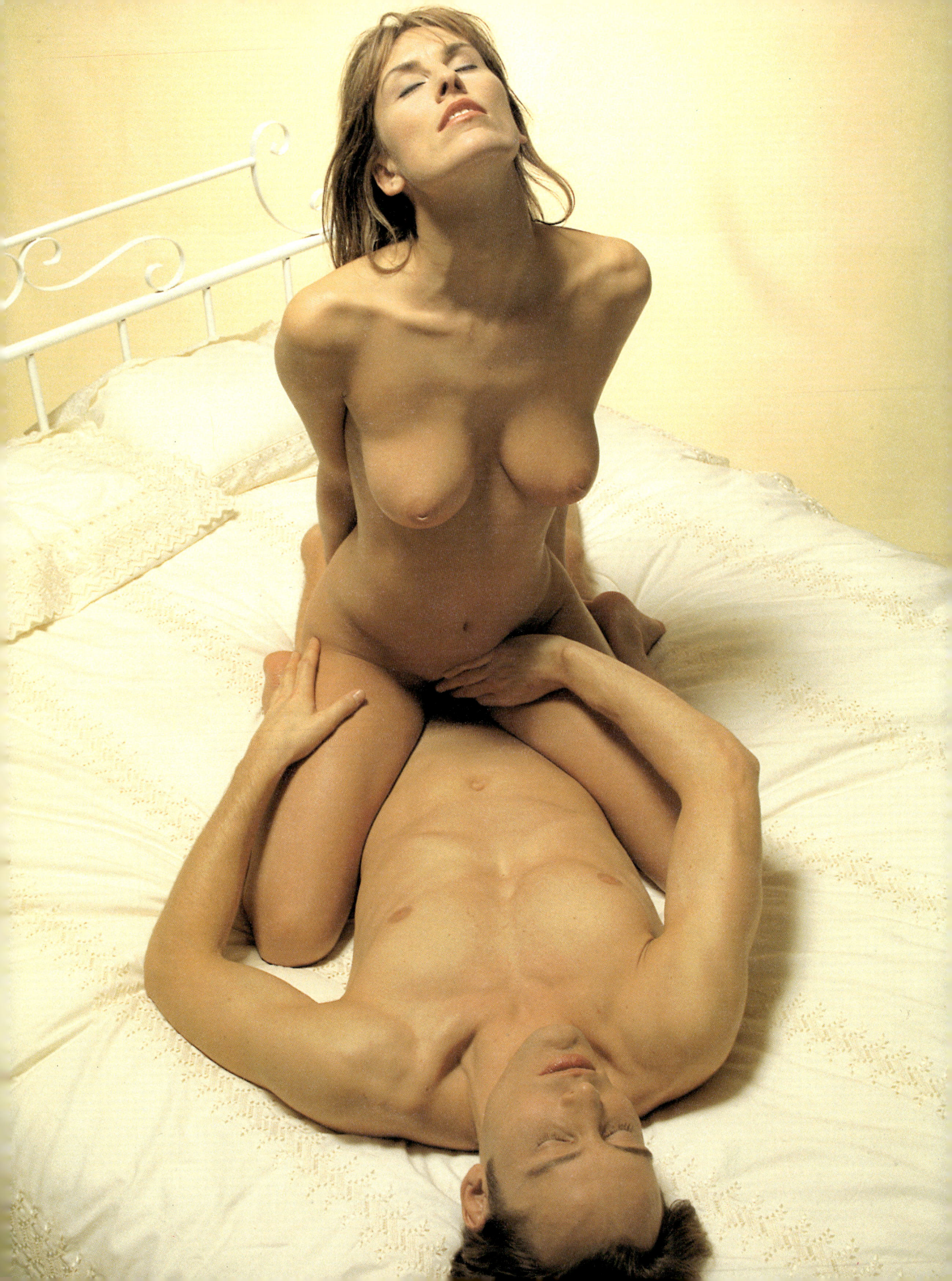